ALLERGIC RHINITIS

Edited by **Marek L. Kowalski**

Allergic Rhinitis
Edited by Marek L. Kowalski

Published by InTech
Janeza Trdine 9, 51000 Rijeka, Croatia

Publishing Process Manager Masa Vidovic

Technical Editor Teodora Smiljanic

Cover Designer InTech Design Team

Additional hard copies can be obtained from orders@intechopen.com

Allergic Rhinitis, Edited by Marek L. Kowalski
p. cm.
ISBN 978-953-51-0288-5

For EU product safety concerns:
IN TECH d.o.o., Prolaz Marije Krucifikse Kozulić 3, 51000 Rijeka, Croatia, info@intechopen.com or visit our website at intechopen.com.

Meet the editor

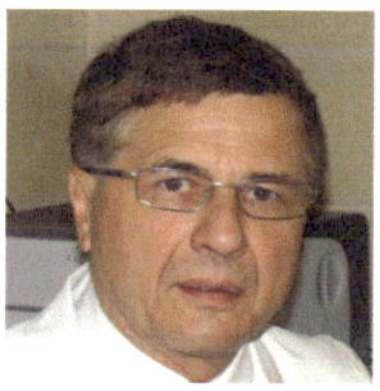

Marek L. Kowalski is an allergist trained in internal medicine and clinical immunology. He is a professor and the head of the Department of Immunology, Rheumatology and Allergy at the Medical University in Lodz, where he received medical and doctorate degrees. For three years he was a visiting fellow at the Allergic Diseases Section, National Institutes of Health, Bethesda, USA. He was the treasurer of the European Academy of Allergy and Clinical Immunology; and member of the WAO Board of Directors. Professor Kowalski is the sinusitis section editor of Current Allergy and Asthma Reports and and serves on the editorial boards of several other international journals. His major research interests include pathogenesis and management of rhinosinusitis, bronchial asthma and hypersensitivity to NSAID. He has authored or co-authored more than 300 publications.

Contents

Preface

During the last decades, an increasing prevalence of allergic diseases has been observed all over the world. According to recent estimates from the Global Allergy And Asthma European Network (GA2LEN), more than 50% of the European population will suffer from allergies by 2020. Allergic rhinitis is one of the most common allergic disorders affecting 20-40% of the population at all ages and the prevalence of the disease tends to increase all over the world. Allergic rhinitis adversely affects emotional well-being and social functions. It impairs cognitive functions and decreases the quality of life of patients . In children it is one of the most common causes of absence from school and, if untreated, may result in poorer learning ability.

Allergic rhinitis, while troublesome for a patient , may also be a challenge for the physician. Despite the progress in prevention, anti-inflammatory treatment and allergen- specific treatments (for example specific immunotherapy) a significant proportion of patients still suffer from serious symptoms of allergic rhinitis. That is why physicians must still learn more about the pathophysiology of the disease and why physicians and patients are looking forward for novel diagnostic and therapeutic approaches.

Allergic rhinitis may predispose to chronic sinusitis or otitis media and is associated with an increased risk of asthma. The fact that allergic rhinitis is not just a local disease, but is a manifestation of systemic allergy, has been appreciated by the doctor for a long time. In 1928 the Californian physician HP Merril concluded that allergic rhinitis "...is not a disease entity, but a local manifestation of a general hypersensitiveness to irritants, generally proteins, but probably to other substances as well. It is often accompanied by other types of allergic reaction, such as asthma, and like such must be considered as a symptom and not as a disease". Since that time the systemic nature of allergic rhinitis has been well documented and the concept of one-airway disease led to development of an ARIA document advocating a systemic approach to the management of allergic rhinits.

The chapters of this volume address a variety of important topics related to allergic rhinitis . They begin with a description of innovative translational approaches allowing for the unification of animal and human models. Contributing authors provide up-to-date reviews of clinical aspects of allergic rhinitis in children, its association with bronchial asthma and other co-morbid conditions. They also discuss the impact of allergic rhinitis on sleep and sports. Together with articles on diagnostic approaches as well as novel treatments, this book offers a comprehensive and stimulating review of the topic.

May this book find a wide readership among allergists and other physicians interested in allergic disease, and also among pediatricians, general practitioners and other specialists who increasingly have to deal with this seemingly benign, but sometimes extremely troublesome, disease.

Professor Marek L. Kowalski, M.D., Ph.D.
Medical University of Lodz, Lodz
Poland

1

From Mouse to Man: Translational Value of Animal Models of Allergic Rhinitis

James G. Wagner and Jack R. Harkema
Michigan State University
USA

1. Introduction

Allergic rhinitis (AR) is the most prevalent atopic disease in the world, affecting 10-20% of the population or up to 600 million people (Asher et al. 2006; Meltzer and Bukstein 2011). Data from multi-year international studies show that the incidence of upper airway allergy is greater than that for asthma, and since 1994 the prevalence of AR has increased more rapidly than allergic asthma (Asher et al. 2006; Weinmayr et al. 2008). The common clinical definition of AR is nasal obstruction, sneezing, rhinorrhea, and pruritus associated with known or suspected allergens. Comorbidity with asthma is common, with 50% to 100% of allergic asthma patients in the United States and Europe reporting AR symptoms (Gaugris et al. 2006). Furthermore, as much as 30% of individuals with AR have lower airway symptoms, such as bronchial hyperreactivity, and AR has emerged as a risk factor for eventually developing asthma (Ciprandi and Cirillo 2006; Ponikau et al. 2003). Because of the frequency of AR coexisting with allergic asthma, a role for common pathophysiologic linkages between asthma and AR has been a focus of discussion among clinical scientists. Comparison of the nasal and bronchial mucosa from allergic airways reveal similar inflammatory and epithelial cell alterations in both tissues, suggesting that common mechanisms of pathogenesis may contribute to each condition (Chanez et al. 1999). Given the clinical and pathologic commonalities of AR and asthma, recent efforts of physicians worldwide has led to Allergic Rhinitis and its Impact on Asthma (ARIA), a collaborative development of diagnostic and therapeutic strategies to treat AR as an asthma risk (Bousquet et al. 2001). A central tenet of ARIA is that AR and asthma represent a "united airway disease" and should be viewed as an interrelated disease with common etiology, features and treatments (Compalati et al. 2010; Marple 2010).

However the inherent differences in the anatomic, morphologic, and functional aspects of nasal versus pulmonary airways result in unique inflammatory and allergic responses in each site. For example, airway obstruction in upper and lower airways occurs by very different mechanisms. Smooth muscle contraction narrows conducting airways in lung, whereas acute vasodilation of vascular tissue limits airflow through nasal airways. Mucus overproduction and hypersecretion may also contribute to airway occlusion and obstruction in both nasal and bronchial airways. Excess mucus such as during rhinorrhea might be more easily cleared from the nose, but mucus plugging in pulmonary airways is a prominent feature associated with mortality in *status asthmaticus*. While the "one-airway" concept may be an attractive paradigm to describe relationships in allergic airways in support of the ARIA framework, differences in clinical opinions for treatment remain (Chipps et al. 2010).

Basic research directed at the study of each condition separately, as well as in tandem, is needed to fully understand the pathophysiology of allergic airways disease. AR is a unique pathophysiological entity that is part of a spectrum of atopic disease including eczema and asthma. The use of relevant animal models of allergic airways disease is necessary to provide the supportive data that defines the extent and nature of AR:asthma relationships. In the last decade, research efforts that focused on animal models of AR have begun to provide a scientific framework with which to understand the role of upper airways in allergic airways disease.

2. Insights from animal models of allergic asthma

Extensive work in susceptible rodent strains using ovalbumin as the test allergen, or environmentally-relevant allergens (e.g., house dust mite, cockroach), has helped describe both the acute and chronic immune and inflammatory responses in pulmonary airways.

The strengths and limitations of laboratory animal models has been debated (Shapiro 2006; Wenzel and Holgate 2006). Studies using mice, especially transgenics and knockout strains, have been important for understanding of the role of cytokines, adhesion molecules, and cell receptors in allergic inflammatory responses. Asthma is a chronic disease of inflammation that is marked by extensive airway remodeling. By comparison, most rodent models of asthma are relatively acute, with regular exposure to allergen challenges over a few days or weeks. As such, the reproduction of the human asthma pathophysiology is not perfect. While airway hyperreactivity, eosinophilic and lymphocytic infiltration, and mucus overproduction can be induced in experimental asthma, other features such as smooth muscle cell proliferation, myofibroblast activation, subepithelial fibrosis, and epithelial proliferation and shedding are often absent in allergic rodent models.

Given the limitations of acute rodent models, efforts to develop chronic asthma models that use frequent exposures to lower allergen concentrations can better portray exposure histories of allergic subjects to seasonal and episodic exacerbations. Specifically, airway remodeling in these mice include key features of human asthma, such as intraepithelial eosinophils, collagen deposition, epithelial hyperplasia and metaplasia, smooth muscle hyperplasia and hypertrophy, and increases in myofibroblasts (Lloyd and Robinson 2007; Nials and Uddin 2008; Yu et al. 2006).

Regardless of the rodent model (mouse, rat or guinea pig), the method to induce allergic responses in lower airways is similar across species and allergens. Primary sensitization to the allergen is accomplished by using either systemic (e.g., intraperitoneal, subcutaneous or dermal) or airway (aerosol inhalation, or instillation in the nose, pharynx, or trachea) routes of exposure, and given as a single or multiple administrations. An adjuvant, usually alum (potassium aluminium sulfate), may also be used. Sensitized animals are then challenged with a secondary exposure by either dermal, inhalation, or airway instillation, and with varying volumes and allergen concentrations or several days or weeks. Several groups have conducted comparisons of the different protocols and determined strengths and limitations of several approaches. (Farraj et al. 2006; Pauluhn and Mohr 2005; Samarasinghe et al. 2011; Southam et al. 2002; Ulrich et al. 2008).

3. Animal models of allergic rhinitis

Preclinical research on allergic airways disease has focused predominately on the lower airways and asthma. By comparison, animal models of AR are relatively underdeveloped and understudied. Until recently, AR models have relied on short-term protocols and therefore present the same weaknesses of focusing on acute inflammation and less attention on airway remodeling as acute asthma models discussed above. However more effort is being put into developing chronic models to address nasal obstruction, rhinorrhea, and remodeling that define human AR.

The standard laboratory guinea pig and, to a lesser extent, the Brown Norway rat and BALB/c mouse, have been the primary laboratory animals used to describe nasal responses to allergic stimuli. Occlusion of nasal passages, and the necessity for oral breathing, is the most common complaint from patients with AR. Nasal obstruction in response to an allergic stimulus is characterized by early and late phases of inflammation (Patou et al. 2006; Widdicombe 1990). An immediate and transient episode of itching and sneezing begins within seconds of exposure and lasts for 5 to 30 minutes. A secondary (late) phase is characterized by rhinorrhea and airway obstruction that can last for hours. The initial irritation and sneeze reflex is promoted by preformed mediators released from mast cells and basophils—specifically histamines, tryptase, cysteinyl leukotrienes (cysLTs), and platelet activating factor (PAF). Mucus hypersecretion with airway obstruction during the secondary phase is accompanied by a progression in mucosal swelling, tissue infiltration of eosinophils and neutrophils, and the synthesis and release of prostaglandins, interleukins, and reactive oxygen species (ROS).

In the allergic guinea pig, enumerating the frequency of nasal rubbing and sneezes is a subjective but useful measure, especially for testing the early phase mechanisms and therapies involving histamine- and leukotriene-dependent pathways (Al Suleimani et al. 2006; Szelenyi et al. 2000). For example observers will count between 3-6 sneezes and 6-10 rubbings per minute after acute exposure to allergen (Al Suleimani et al. 2008; Tsunematsu et al. 2007). However, the histopathology associated with nasal obstruction in both early and late phase responses in AR has not been extensively studied. This is in contrast to the detailed descriptions of airway remodeling and pathology that drive analogous responses in lower airways, i.e., early and late bronchoconstriction, which are well-studied in mice. Vasodilation-induced swelling of mucosa, remodeling of mucus-secreting apparatus, fibrosis and inflammatory cell infiltration are potential changes that can be detected in experimental AR. Nasal remodeling that occurs after chronic, multiple challenges to allergen may alter the early responses described above, and provide a more relevant approach to understand the complex pathophysiologic mechanisms in human AR.

3.1 Nasal obstruction in experimental AR

Approaches in humans to assess nasal airflow and acoustic rhinometry are not easily adapted to rodents (Kaise et al. 1999). However, direct and indirect methods have been developed and refined in recent years, which appear to provide a reproducible physiologic approach to determine nasal obstruction. Like direct measures of pulmonary function, invasive approaches are required to obtain direct measures of nasal flows and pressures in laboratory rodents. By retrograde cannulation of the trachea (directed toward the nasopharynx), ventilation patterns used to determine pulmonary function can be applied to the nasal cavity (Figure 1). For example, using the Flexivent system (Scireq, Montreal), direct nasal cavity pressure and flow measurements can be collected in mice during forced oscillation maneuvers using a small animal ventilator (Miyahara et al. 2005). More recently this approach was simplified to use a syringe pump to create flow through the nasal cavity while changes in nasal pressure were detected with a pressure transducer (Xie et al. 2009). Both studies found increased nasal resistance in allergic BALB/c mice without inducing changes in lower airways. However these are the only two examples of direct resistance measures in experimental AR, and pathological changes were not fully investigated.

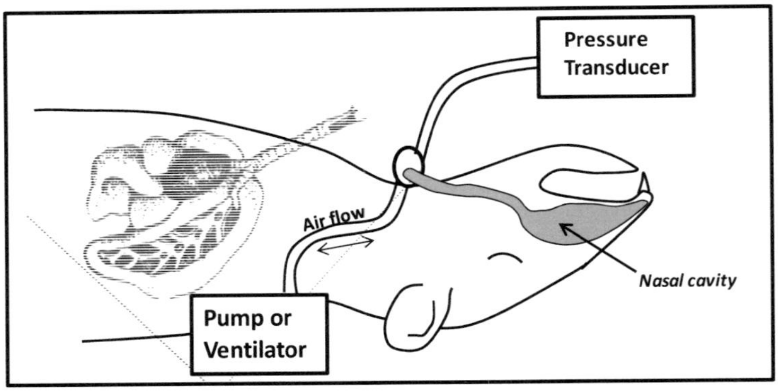

After retrograde cannulation of the trachea and ventilation of the nasal cavity, direct assessment of nasal resistance can be determined in anesthetized laboratory rodents. The lower airways can also be ventilated to determine pulmonary mechanics in the same animal.

Fig. 1. Direct measurement of nasal airway mechanics.

A second method employs a novel use of whole-body plethysmography (WBP) which, in nose-only breathing in rodents, would also detect contributions of flow and pressure changes from the upper airway (Figure 2). WBP has been used extensively to measure lower airway function in allergic rodents, and relies on a unit-less parameter called enhanced pause (Penh), the physiologic meaning has been debated over the last ten years (Bates et al. 2004; Frazer et al. 2011; Lomask 2006; Lundblad et al. 2007). Briefly, part of the derivation of the Penh parameter utilizes the change in the expiratory flow pattern, which some interpret as bronchoconstriction. It has been used to estimate lower airway reactivity in allergic rodents, and therefore a central criticism is that any upper airway obstruction (i.e., nasal) is ignored in the most data interpretations.

Some studies have taken advantage of WBP in rhinitis models where intranasal challenge protocols are designed for allergen delivery to be limited to the nose, and not to reach the deep lung. For example, Nakaya and coworkers measured increases in Penh after intranasal histamine or allergen challenge in allergic BALB/c mice (Nakaya et al. 2006). Although modest pulmonary inflammation was detected, there were no allergen-induced changes in lower airway resistance when analyzed by separate, invasive techniques that bypassed the nose. As such, it was concluded that changes in Penh were due solely to nasal obstruction.

It should be noted that this approach does not address another central criticism of Penh, that it simply represents ventilator timing, rather than airway obstruction. However a separate parameter that is reliably measured by WPB is respiratory frequency. In a series of studies by Miyahara and coworkers, decreased breathing rate in mice has been used as a reliable marker of increased nasal resistance (Miyahara et al. 2008; Miyahara et al. 2006; Miyahara et al. 2005). Respiratory frequency has also been used as an indicator of nasal obstruction in guinea pig models of AR, where it correlated well with histamine-induced airway reactivity (Zhao et al. 2005). Together these findings suggest that respiratory frequency, (i.e., ventilatory timing), is a reasonable indicator of nasal obstruction. An assumption of this model is that the contribution from lower airways or from neurogenic control of breathing is negligible in these rhinitis protocols that exploit WBP.

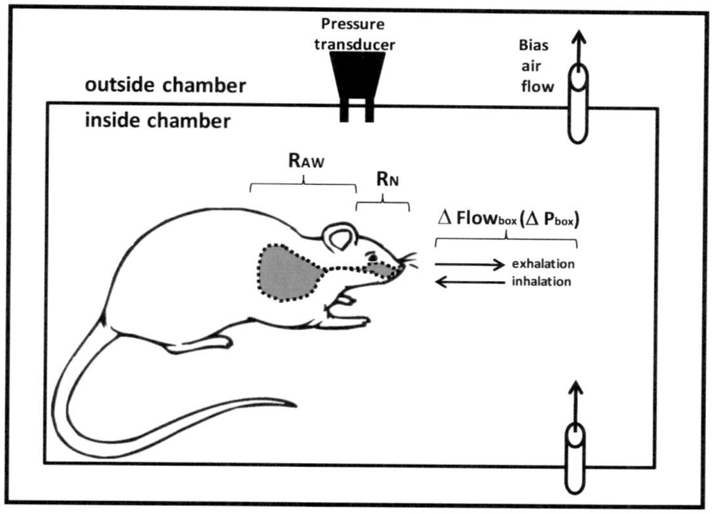

Total box pressure (P_{box}) fluctuates with the changes in box flow ($Flow_{box}$) caused by the animal's breathing. Changes in duration of inhalation and expiration are used to calculate enhanced pause (Penh), which has been used as a surrogate for airway resistance (R). Alternatively, respiration rate can be directly measured. Rodents are obligate nose breathers. AR models and their dosing regimens assume that nasal resistance (R_N) is greater than lower airway resistance (R_{AW}). If $R_N >> R_{AW}$, then changes in Penh or respiration rate are interpreted an indicator of R_N and of nasal obstruction.

Fig. 2. Whole body plethysmography to estimate nasal obstruction in rodents.

The relevance of AR models, especially using WBP to estimate nasal resistance, is to avoid the involvement of lower airways. Many AR models therefore target the upper airways by minimizing the instilled volume or by conducting intranasal challenges in conscious animals. Kinetic studies show that with instilled volumes of 10 µL or less, 70% of the instillate is retained in the nasal cavity of anesthetized mice, while 15% to 20% reaches the lung (Southam et al. 2002). In conscious mice, nasal retention of instillate can be achieved with volumes as large as 25 µL, where only 5% or less makes it to the lung. Although delivery to the nose is optimized with these approaches, subtle effects in the lung, either direct or indirect, cannot be completely discounted.

As discussed in the introduction to this chapter, the "united airway" hypothesis linking AR to asthma suggests that immunogenic responses in upper and lower airways are connected (Marple 2010; Pawankar 2006). While asthma:rhinitis relationships are clearly evident in clinical and epidemiological studies, reports from animals models are limited and without a consensus mechanism. For example allergen delivery to either upper or lower airways induced localized inflammation in either upper or lower airways, but not both (Li et al. 2005). However, serum eotaxin, interleukin (IL)-5, and eosinophils were equally elevated in all protocols, regardless of preferential inflammation in either nose or lung. In separate studies using mice, lower airway inflammation was dependent on circulating T-helper-2 lymphocytes and adhesion molecule expression (KleinJan et al. 2009). Thus, even with site-specific delivery of airway allergen, circulating cellular and inflammatory mediators associated with AR could affect pulmonary airway reactivity. Circulating cytokines and activated inflammatory cells during both AR and non-allergic are hypothesized to mediate lower airway pathologies, include hyperreactivity (Braunstahl 2009; Hellings and

Prokopakis 2010). As such, the only certain physiologic measure of nasal obstruction in allergic rodents, is to isolate the nasal cavity from the lower airway and perform modified pulmonary function techniques. Though presently in limited use, retrograde ventilation holds the most promise to understand mechanics of upper airway obstruction in rodents.

Other techniques that measure only the nasal pressure changes to estimate resistance (Δpressure/ Δflow), have also been correlated with allergen-induced AR indicators such as nasal rubbing, sneezes and secretions in guinea pigs (Al Suleimani et al. 2006; Fukuda et al. 2003). While these methods may provide a direct measure of nasal cavity physiology not available by WBP, one limitation is the need for euthanasia after measurements are taken.

In addition, some physiological responses in experimental AR may not be relevant for humans. For example, in guinea pigs, allergen-induced nasal resistance was reversed by antihistamines, but not by an adrenergic agonist (McLeod et al. 2002). These results disagree with the ameliorative effects of commonly used vasoconstrictors in humans. In separate studies using allergic mice, nasal resistance was dependent on immunoglobulin (Ig) E-mediated pathways but not on eosinophil accumulation (Miyahara et al. 2005). This result runs counter to the putative, causative role for eosinophils in the late response of airway obstruction (Ciprandi et al. 2004a). Taken together, the current approaches to measuring nasal obstruction show some limitations of acute AR models, and illustrate the need to develop chronic protocols that may better represent human AR.

3.2 Remodeling in experimental AR

In general, animal models of AR are less reported and lack the diversity of experimental animal models of asthma. Most experimental AR protocols range from hours to days of allergen challenge, with at most 12 exposures to allergen before measuring endpoints. These brief treatment regimens are most often designed to test the efficacy of pharmaceutical agents against acute exacerbations, leaving relatively few animal studies that model chronic AR of humans. Although these models have provided important insight into the early and late inflammatory and obstructive responses, accompanying histopathologic descriptions have been either vague or inaccurate.

Like asthma, AR is a chronic disease marked by episodic rounds of inflammation, yet few rodent AR models have been designed to examine long-term alterations and potential airway remodeling of the nasal mucosa. This limitation might easily have been filled, in part, by examining the nose from mice used in a number of well-designed, chronic experimental asthma models (Hirota et al. 2009; Ikeda et al. 2003; McMillan and Lloyd 2004; Yu et al. 2006). Repeated challenge with allergen for weeks or months produces many features of human asthma, including subepithelial fibrosis, smooth muscle and mucus cell hyperplasia, and epithelial exfoliation. In the few chronic experimental AR where histopathological changes are reported, some epithelial and inflammatory responses are consistent with human AR.

Multiple intranasal ovalbumin challenges in BALB/c mice over 3 months caused time- and challenge-dependent development of subepithelial fibrosis and goblet cell hyperplasia in the proximal aspects of nasoturbinates (Lim et al. 2007). Immunohistochemical detection of matrix metalloproteinase and tissue inhibitors of metalloproteinase was localized to the fibrotic lesions. Transient tissue infiltration of eosinophils occurred at early (1 week), but not later timepoints (1-3 months). Similar associations of decreasing inflammatory cell recruitment with repeated allergen provocation was found in C57BL/6 mice, where airway mucosal remodeling was evident only after 4-8 weeks of challenges, and eosinophil influx peaked after 2 weeks (Wang et al. 2008). In allergic BALB/c mice that were challenged 3 times a week, goblet cell hyperplasia in lateral walls occurred after 5, but not 2 weeks, and persists through 4 months; by 10 weeks of multiple challenges collagen deposition was evident (Nakaya et al. 2007). Despite the brevity in reports on experimental chronic AR, these studies nonetheless suggest that chronic remodeling of nasal mucosa after repeated exposures is preceded by a transient inflammatory response.

4. Translation to human AR

Translation of experimental results from animal studies to human AR is challenging. The distinct gross structural differences and distribution of epithelium of the rodent and human are important considerations. From a review of the literature, further examples of the limitations of histopathologic comparisons across and within human and experimental AR in animals include 1) inconsistencies in site-specific selection for evaluation, 2) misidentification of nasal anatomy in mice, and 3) the use of subjective quantitative and qualitative analyses (e.g., number of goblet cells versus amounts of stored mucosubstances). Interspecies variability in nasal gross anatomy has been emphasized in previous reviews (Harkema 1991; Harkema et al. 2006). Marked differences in airflow patterns among mammalian species are primarily due to variation in the shape of nasal turbinates. The human nose has three turbinates: the superior (st), middle (mt), and inferior (it) as depicted below in Figure 3.

These structures are relatively simple in shape compared to turbinates in most laboratory animals that have complex folding and branching patterns (Fig. 3). In mice, rats and guinea pigs, evolutionary pressures concerned chiefly with olfactory function and dentition have defined the shape of the turbinates and the type and distribution of the cells lining them. In the proximal nasal airway, the complex nasoturbinates (nt) and maxilloturbinates (mx) of small laboratory rodents probably provide better protection of the lower respiratory tract than the simple middle and inferior turbinates of the human nose. The posterior nasal cavity consists of ethmoturbinates (et) which are lined olfactory epithelium and comprised up to half of the rodent nasal cavity.

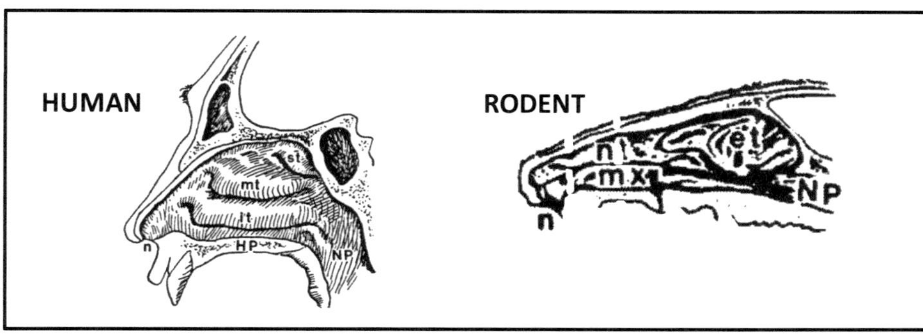

Diagrammatic representation of the exposed mucosal surface of the lateral wall and turbinates in the nasal airways of human and rat. The nasal septum has been removed to expose the nasal passage; illustration are not to scale. et – ethmoturbinates; HP – hard palate; it – inferior turbinate; mt – middle turbinate; mx – maxilloturbinate; n – naris; NP – nasopharynx; nt – nasoturbinate; st – superior turbinate.

Fig. 3. Comparative Nasal Anatomy.

Mucosal swelling in turbinates, especially where they are in close opposition to the septum and lateral wall, can impede both airflow and mucus drainage through the nasal cavity. Another major difference is the distribution of epithelial types in rodents and humans. Approximately 50% of the nasal cavity surface area in rats is lined by sensory neuroepithelium (Gross et al. 1982). By comparison, olfactory epithelium in humans is limited to an area of about 500 mm^2, which is only 3% of the total surface area of the nasal cavity. The majority of the nonolfactory nasal epithelium of laboratory animals and humans is ciliated respiratory epithelium. Although this pseudostratified nasal epithelium is similar to ciliated epithelium lining other proximal airways (i.e., trachea and bronchi), it also has unique features. Nasal respiratory epithelium in the rat is composed of six morphologically distinct cell types: mucous, ciliated, nonciliated columnar, cuboidal, brush, and basal. We have identified the nasal transitional epithelium, which consists of simple cuboidal cells and lines the proximal airways and maxilloturbinates of rodents, as a sensitive epithelium to undergo metaplastic responses to allergens (Wagner et al. 2002). It is unknown if similar metaplastic changes occur during human AR.

Most of the histopathologic analyses in both humans and rodents have been in regions populated with respiratory epithelium, where the character of the mucus-secreting apparatus and underlying mucosa are evaluated. The anterior portion of the middle and inferior turbinates are common sampling sites for biopsies in humans, partly because of their accessibility (Fig. 3). In rodents, by comparison, analyses are usually in the nasal septum and lateral wall (Figure 4; T1), as well as sites that unfortunately are not clearly identified in the methodological descriptions. The septal mucosa overlies cartilage, whereas the mucosa of turbinates overlies bone. Thus, when responses in respiratory epithelium of laboratory rodents and humans are compared, the surface epithelium may be similar, but the cellularity and vascularization of the underlying mucosa may be quite different and belie inaccurate conclusions with regard to structure/function relationships and its impact on the pathophysiology.

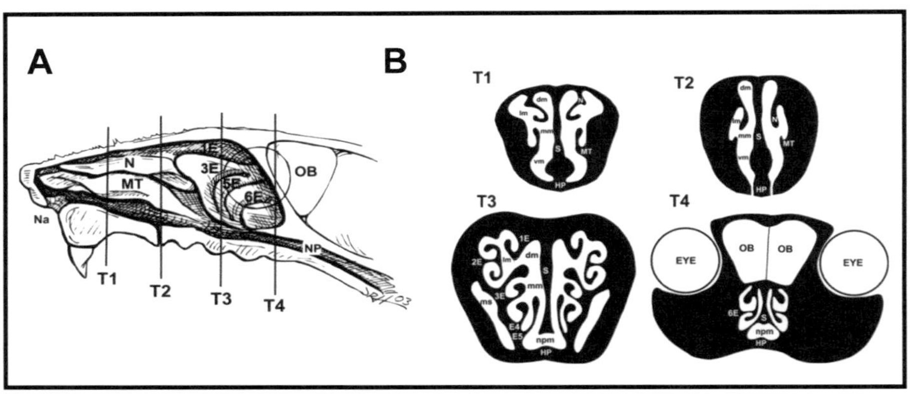

A) Diagrammatic representation of the right nasal passage of the laboratory mouse with the septum removed exposing the nasoturbinate (N), maxilloturbinate (MT), ethmoturbinates (1E-6E), and the nasal pharynx (NP). Lines T1-T4 represent the location of the transverse sections taken for light microscopic examination. B) Anterior face of tranverse sectionsT1-T4. Na, nares; N, nasoturbinate; MT, maxilloturbinate; 1E-6E, six ethmoid turbinates projecting from the lateral wall. HP, hard palate; OB, olfactory bulb of the brain; NP, nasopharynx; DM, dorsal medial meatus (airway); L, lateral meatus; MM, middle meatus; V, ventral meatus; S, septum; MS, maxillary sinus; NPM, nasopharyngeal meatus.

Fig. 4. Anatomic features the rodent nose.

There is no common approach for histologic evaluation by clinicians or by researchers in AR models, and thus comparisons are relatively limited. Veterinary pathologists have proposed a sampling regimen that captures the key anatomical features and epithelial populations in the rodent nose that respond to inhaled materials such as allergens (Young 1981). As depicted in Figure 4, four sampling sites (T1-4), from proximal to distal include respiratory epithelium (mucus-secreting cells) on the septum, nasoturbinates -and maxilloturbinates (T1 and T2 sections), olfactory epithelium in ethmoturbinates (T3), and respiratory epithelium of the nasopharynx (T3-4). Similar sampling strategies for humans have not been proposed, and biopsy are limited to disease and lesion status.

Early analyses of human responses focused on goblet cell enumeration, where modest increases during seasonal AR were not statistically significant (Berger et al. 1997b). Similar modest changes in the epithelial hyperplasia lining the nasal septum after acute allergen challenge has been reported in BALB/c mice (Miyahara et al. 2006) and Brown Norway rats (Wagner et al. 2002). However in the rat model there was a profound increase in the amount of intraepithelial mucosubstances (Wagner et al. 2002), suggesting that hypertrophy and hyperproduction of mucosubstances within individual cells, rather than an increase in mucous cells (hyperplasia), may underlie the hypersecretory mucosa associated with human AR. Supporting this notion are reports of secreted mucosubstances within the nasal lumen of allergic rats(Wagner et al. 2002; Wagner et al. 2008), which parallels the findings of Berger et al. (Berger et al. 1999) who found more actively secreting goblet cells in AR patients than in healthy controls. These features are likely overlooked with routine examination of hemotoxylin and eosin-stained tissue, and can be underestimated if mucus detection relies on only a single stain, rather than both periodic acid–Schiff (PAS) and alcian blue, which stain for neutral and acidic mucosubstances, respectively.

Mucosal and airway recruitment of eosinophils, neutrophils, and mast cells are commonly reported in both experimental and clinical AR (Miyahara et al. 2006; Nakaya et al. 2006; Wagner et al. 2002; Wagner et al. 2008). Furthermore, eosinophils in nasal biopsies or in nasal lavage fluid are highly correlated with most symptoms in AR patients (Ciprandi et al. 2004a; 2004b). Eosinophil products such as nitric oxide, cysteinyl leukotrienes, and interleukins are potential mediators of nasal obstruction (mucosal swelling) and goblet cell secretory responses during AR. However, at least two animal studies have found no causative role for eosinophils in AR responses. Blockade of IL-5 in guinea pigs inhibits eosinophil accumulation in nasal mucosa, but mucus secretion and nasal airway obstruction are unaffected after chronic allergen exposure (Yamasaki et al. 2002). Furthermore, in IgE-receptor–deficient mice, nasal obstruction is independent of eosinophil recruitment into nasal tissues (Miyahara et al. 2005). By comparison, eosinophils are strongly suggested, but not clinically proven to mediate late responses that lead to obstruction in human AR (Ciprandi et al. 2004a; 2004b). Furthermore eosinophil-independent pathways of airway hyperreactivity and mucus cell metaplasia have also been demonstrated in murine asthma models (Humbles et al. 2004; Singer et al. 2002). More studies with chronic models of AR are needed to clarify the role of eosinophils in both allergic asthma and AR.

Histamine-dependent pathophysiological responses initiated by activated mast cells are well defined in AR. Increases in degranulated mast cells are detected and identified in turbinate biopsies from patients with AR (Amin et al. 2001; Berger et al. 1997a). In kinetic studies of the response to allergen provocation in human AR, investigators have reported mast cell migration from the lamina propria into nasal epithelium where degranulation occurs (Fokkens et al. 1992). In allergic guinea pigs by comparison, mast cell migration, but not increased numbers or degranulation, was detected in the subepithelial mucosa (Kawaguchi et al. 1994). Beyond this example, comparative descriptions of nasal mast cell histopathology are rarely reported in experimental AR models. In a more recent report in a chronic mouse model of fungal AR, descriptions of mast cell kinetics into the epithelium and mucosa are very similar to that found in human AR (Lindsay et al. 2006). Despite the subjective evaluation and misidentification of nasal anatomy, this model reproduces many key features of human AR besides mast cell pathology. Specifically, the lesions include epithelial injury, shedding, invaginations, hyperplasia, and secretions, as well as thickening of lamina propria and progressive infiltration of eosinophils.

5. Paranasal airways

We have recently reported the involvement of paranasal airways in allergic Brown Norway rats that was enhanced by ozone inhalation (Wagner et al. 2009). Eosinophilic infiltrates and mucous cell metaplasia were detected in both the maxillary sinus and nasolacrimal duct, which is the first report of these responses in paranasal structures in experimental AR. Other reports of murine sinusitis models have appeared over the last decade. However most of these studies have been based on inappropriate application of mouse anatomy to human disease. Specifically, the airspaces between the ethmoid turbinates of mice (Figure 3B), have been misinterpreted to be analogous to human ethmoid sinuses (Bomer et al. 1998; Jacob and Chole 2006; Lindsay et al. 2006; Phillips et al. 2009). Ethmoid turbinates in mice do not enclose sinus airways, are lined predominantly by olfactory neuroepithelium, and receive significant airflow (Harkema et al. 2006; Kimbell et al. 1997). By comparison, the ethmoid sinuses of the human nasal cavity are true sinuses lined with respiratory epithelium and receive relatively less airflow. Inflammatory and immune processes in the mucosa underlying these distinct epithelial populations are likely to have different responses. As such caution is advised in the interpretation and design of rhinosinusitis studies, as the translational value of many existing reports from these mouse models is questionable. The rodent possesses a true maxillary sinus analogous to the sinus airways in human, consisting of respiratory epithelium and submucosal secretory glands, and as such is a more suitable structure to assess experimental sinusitis in mice.

6. Conclusions

Observations in human AR provide suggestive evidence that airway remodeling similar to allergic lower airways are also present in the nose, e.g., epithelial damage, basement membrane thickening, mesenchymal changes , eosinophilic infiltrates, mast cell migration, and alteration in the mucus-secreting apparatus (Ponikau et al. 2003; Salib and Howarth 2003). However these findings are inconsistent in rodent models of acute AR. Without a common methodological approach for the collection and analysis of both rodent and human tissues, relevant comparisons and meaningful conclusions will be difficult.

A critical knowledge gap concerns the histopathological changes in the rodent nose that occurs with chronic allergen challenge. Acute protocols have served well to describe inflammatory cell infiltration and reorganization of the mucus-secreting apparatus. It is not clear if the nasal structures in rodent AR exhibit notable tissue remodeling, such as neovascularization in mucosa, collagen deposition, or submucosal gland development. Subepithelial fibrosis can be induced in mouse nasal turbinates after 3 months (Lim et al.

2007), but additional reports in the literature are lacking. In order to provide a more clinically relevant model, more studies are needed that use repeated challenge regimens and extended low-dose exposures, similar to those used in mouse models of chronic asthma.

More systematic approaches need to be applied to the evaluation of nasal pathology in rodents. Strategies for histopathologic analyses should begin by consulting nasal diagrams generated by Mery et al. (Mery et al. 1994), or using the approach proposed by Young (Young 1981). We have recently identified sensitive sites to evaluate respiratory epithelial populations in nasal septum, lateral wall, turbinates, and nasopharynx (Farraj et al. 2003; Wagner et al. 2008). Analysis of the nasolacrimal duct as a sensitive site for allergic rhinoconjunctivitis is virtually absent in rodent models. Similarly, little attention is given to rodent sinus airways during experimental AR, though both structures are easily identified in rodent nasal maps. Many recent sinusitis models are limited by misidentification of nasal structures and irrelevance to human rhinosinusitis. A more thorough approach that combines descriptive and morphometric approaches would strengthen the translational value of animal models of AR. A integrated approach that unifies histopathologic and physiologic data from human and animal AR is needed to understand mechanisms of chronic responses in the allergic nose. Extension and incorporation of existing research on rodent asthma would greatly benefit the design and analysis of rodent models of AR.

7. References

Al Suleimani M, Ying D, Walker MJ. (2006). A comprehensive model of allergic rhinitis in guinea pigs. J Pharmacol Toxicol Methods 55(2):127-134.

Al Suleimani YM, Dong Y, Walker MJ. (2008). Differential responses to various classes of drugs in a model of allergic rhinitis in guinea pigs. Pulm Pharmacol Ther 21(2):340-348.

Amin K, Rinne J, Haahtela T, Simola M, Peterson CG, Roomans GM, Malmberg H, Venge P, Seveus L. (2001). Inflammatory cell and epithelial characteristics of perennial allergic and nonallergic rhinitis with a symptom history of 1 to 3 years' duration. J Allergy Clin Immunol 107(2):249-257.

Asher MI, Montefort S, Bjorksten B, Lai CK, Strachan DP, Weiland SK, Williams H. (2006). Worldwide time trends in the prevalence of symptoms of asthma, allergic rhinoconjunctivitis, and eczema in childhood: ISAAC Phases One and Three repeat multicountry cross-sectional surveys. Lancet 368(9537):733-743.

Bates J, Irvin C, Brusasco V, Drazen J, Fredberg J, Loring S, Eidelman D, Ludwig M, Macklem P, Martin J, Milic-Emili J, Hantos Z, Hyatt R, Lai-Fook S, Leff A, Solway J, Lutchen K, Suki B, Mitzner W, Pare P, Pride N, Sly P. (2004). The use and misuse of Penh in animal models of lung disease. Am J Respir Cell Mol Biol 31(3):373-374.

Berger G, Goldberg A, Ophir D. (1997a). The inferior turbinate mast cell population of patients with perennial allergic and nonallergic rhinitis. Am J Rhinol 11(1):63-66.

Berger G, Marom Z, Ophir D. (1997b). Goblet cell density of the inferior turbinates in patients with perennial allergic and nonallergic rhinitis. Am J Rhinol 11(3):233-236.

Berger G, Moroz A, Marom Z, Ophir D. (1999). Inferior turbinate goblet cell secretion in patients with perennial allergic and nonallergic rhinitis. Am J Rhinol 13(6):473-477.

Bomer K, Brichta A, Baroody F, Boonlayangoor S, Li X, Naclerio RM. (1998). A mouse model of acute bacterial rhinosinusitis. Arch Otolaryngol Head Neck Surg 124(11):1227-1232.

Bousquet J, Van Cauwenberge P, Khaltaev N. (2001). Allergic rhinitis and its impact on asthma. J Allergy Clin Immunol 108(5 Suppl):S147-334.

Braunstahl GJ. (2009). United airways concept: what does it teach us about systemic inflammation in airways disease? Proc Am Thorac Soc 6(8):652-654.

Chanez P, Vignola AM, Vic P, Guddo F, Bonsignore G, Godard P, Bousquet J. (1999). Comparison between nasal and bronchial inflammation in asthmatic and control subjects. Am J Respir Crit Care Med 159(2):588-595.

Chipps B, Spector S, Farrar J, Carr W, Meltzer E, Storms W, Kaliner M, Luskin A, Bukstein D, Oppenheimer J, Smart B, Derebery J, Harder J, Dykewicz M, Benninger M. (2010). Differences in recommendations between the Allergic Rhinitis and its Impact on Asthma Update 2010 and US Rhinitis Practice Parameters. Journal of Allergy and Clinical Immunology 127(6):1640-1641.

Ciprandi G, Cirillo I, Vizzaccaro A, Milanese M, Tosca MA. (2004a). Airway function and nasal inflammation in seasonal allergic rhinitis and asthma. Clin Exp Allergy 34(6):891-896.

Ciprandi G, Cirillo I, Vizzaccaro A, Milanese M, Tosca MA. (2004b). Correlation of nasal inflammation and nasal airflow with forced expiratory volume in 1 second in patients with perennial allergic rhinitis and asthma. Ann Allergy Asthma Immunol 93(6):575-580.

Ciprandi G, Cirillo I. (2006). The lower airway pathology of rhinitis. J Allergy Clin Immunol 118(5):1105-1109.

Compalati E, Ridolo E, Passalacqua G, Braido F, Villa E, Canonica GW. (2010). The link between allergic rhinitis and asthma: the united airways disease. Expert Rev Clin Immunol 6(3):413-423.

Farraj AK, Harkema JR, Jan TR, Kaminski NE. (2003). Immune responses in the lung and local lymph node of A/J mice to intranasal sensitization and challenge with adjuvant-free ovalbumin. Toxicol Pathol 31(4):432-447.

Farraj AK, Harkema JR, Kaminski NE. (2006). Topical application versus intranasal instillation: a qualitative comparison of the effect of the route of sensitization on trimellitic anhydride-induced allergic rhinitis in A/J mice. Toxicol Sci 92(1):321-328.

Fokkens WJ, Godthelp T, Holm AF, Blom H, Mulder PG, Vroom TM, Rijntjes E. (1992). Dynamics of mast cells in the nasal mucosa of patients with allergic rhinitis and non-allergic controls: a biopsy study. Clin Exp Allergy 22(7):701-710.

Frazer DG, Reynolds JS, Jackson MC. (2011). Determining when enhanced pause (Penh) is sensitive to changes in specific airway resistance. J Toxicol Environ Health A 74(5):287-295.

Fukuda S, Midoro K, Gyoten M, Kawano Y, Ashida Y, Nabe T, Kohno S, Nagaya H. (2003). Effects of TAK-427 on acute nasal symptoms and nasal obstruction in guinea pig model of experimental allergic rhinitis. Eur J Pharmacol 476(3):239-247.

Gaugris S, Sazonov-Kocevar V, Thomas M. (2006). Burden of concomitant allergic rhinitis in adults with asthma. J Asthma 43(1):1-7.

Gross EA, Swenberg JA, Fields S, Popp JA. (1982). Comparative morphometry of the nasal cavity in rats and mice. J Anat 135(Pt 1):83-88.

Harkema JR, Carey SA, Wagner JG. (2006). The nose revisited: a brief review of the comparative structure, function, and toxicologic pathology of the nasal epithelium. Toxicol Pathol 34(3):252-269.

Harkema JR. (1991). Comparative aspects of nasal airway anatomy: relevance to inhalation toxicology. Toxicol Pathol 19(4 Pt 1):321-336.

Hellings PW, Prokopakis EP. (2010). Global airway disease beyond allergy. Curr Allergy Asthma Rep 10(2):143-149.

Hirota JA, Ask K, Fritz D, Ellis R, Wattie J, Richards CD, Labiris R, Kolb M, Inman MD. (2009). Role of STAT6 and SMAD2 in a model of chronic allergen exposure: a mouse strain comparison study. Clin Exp Allergy 39(1):147-158.

Humbles AA, Lloyd CM, McMillan SJ, Friend DS, Xanthou G, McKenna EE, Ghiran S, Gerard NP, Yu C, Orkin SH, Gerard C. (2004). A critical role for eosinophils in allergic airways remodeling. Science 305(5691):1776-1779.

Ikeda RK, Miller M, Nayar J, Walker L, Cho JY, McElwain K, McElwain S, Raz E, Broide DH. (2003). Accumulation of peribronchial mast cells in a mouse model of ovalbumin allergen induced chronic airway inflammation: modulation by immunostimulatory DNA sequences. J Immunol 171(9):4860-4867.

Jacob A, Chole RA. (2006). Survey anatomy of the paranasal sinuses in the normal mouse. Laryngoscope 116(4):558-563.

Kaise T, Ukai K, Pedersen OF, Sakakura Y. (1999). Accuracy of measurement of acoustic rhinometry applied to small experimental animals. Am J Rhinol 13(2):125-129.

Kawaguchi S, Majima Y, Sakakura Y. (1994). Nasal mast cells in experimentally induced allergic rhinitis in guinea-pigs. Clin Exp Allergy 24(3):238-244.

Kimbell JS, Godo MN, Gross EA, Joyner DR, Richardson RB, Morgan KT. (1997). Computer simulation of inspiratory airflow in all regions of the F344 rat nasal passages. Toxicol Appl Pharmacol 145(2):388-398.

KleinJan A, Willart M, van Nimwegen M, Leman K, Hoogsteden HC, Hendriks RW, Lambrecht BN. (2009). United airways: circulating Th2 effector cells in an allergic rhinitis model are responsible for promoting lower airways inflammation. Clin Exp Allergy 40(3):494-504.

Li J, Saito H, Crawford L, Inman MD, Cyr MM, Denburg JA. (2005). Haemopoietic mechanisms in murine allergic upper and lower airway inflammation. Immunology 114(3):386-396.

Lim YS, Won TB, Shim WS, Kim YM, Kim JW, Lee CH, Min YG, Rhee CS. (2007). Induction of airway remodeling of nasal mucosa by repetitive allergen challenge in a murine model of allergic rhinitis. Ann Allergy Asthma Immunol 98(1):22-31.

Lindsay R, Slaughter T, Britton-Webb J, Mog SR, Conran R, Tadros M, Earl N, Fox D, Roberts J, Bolger WE. (2006). Development of a murine model of chronic rhinosinusitis. Otolaryngol Head Neck Surg 134(5):724-730; discussion 731-722.

Lloyd CM, Robinson DS. (2007). Allergen-induced airway remodelling. Eur Respir J 29(5):1020-1032.

Lomask M. (2006). Further exploration of the Penh parameter. Exp Toxicol Pathol 57 Suppl 2:13-20.

Lundblad LK, Irvin CG, Hantos Z, Sly P, Mitzner W, Bates JH. (2007). Penh is not a measure of airway resistance! Eur Respir J 30(4):805.

Marple BF. (2010). Allergic rhinitis and inflammatory airway disease: interactions within the unified airspace. Am J Rhinol Allergy 24(4):249-254.

McLeod RL, Young SS, Erickson CH, Parra LE, Hey JA. (2002). Characterization of nasal obstruction in the allergic guinea pig using the forced oscillation method. J Pharmacol Toxicol Methods 48(3):153-159.

McMillan SJ, Lloyd CM. (2004). Prolonged allergen challenge in mice leads to persistent airway remodelling. Clin Exp Allergy 34(3):497-507.

Meltzer EO, Bukstein DA. (2011). The economic impact of allergic rhinitis and current guidelines for treatment. Ann Allergy Asthma Immunol 106(2 Suppl):S12-16.

Mery S, Gross EA, Joyner DR, Godo M, Morgan KT. (1994). Nasal diagrams: a tool for recording the distribution of nasal lesions in rats and mice. Toxicol Pathol 22(4):353-372.

Miyahara S, Miyahara N, Lucas JJ, Joetham A, Matsubara S, Ohnishi H, Dakhama A, Gelfand EW. (2008). Contribution of allergen-specific and nonspecific nasal responses to early-phase and late-phase nasal responses. J Allergy Clin Immunol 121(3):718-724.

Miyahara S, Miyahara N, Matsubara S, Takeda K, Koya T, Gelfand EW. (2006). IL-13 is essential to the late-phase response in allergic rhinitis. J Allergy Clin Immunol 118(5):1110-1116.

Miyahara S, Miyahara N, Takeda K, Joetham A, Gelfand EW. (2005). Physiologic assessment of allergic rhinitis in mice: role of the high-affinity IgE receptor (FcepsilonRI). J Allergy Clin Immunol 116(5):1020-1027.

Nakaya M, Dohi M, Okunishi K, Nakagome K, Tanaka R, Imamura M, Baba S, Takeuchi N, Yamamoto K, Kaga K. (2006). Noninvasive system for evaluating allergen-induced nasal hypersensitivity in murine allergic rhinitis. Lab Invest 86(9):917-926.

Nakaya M, Dohi M, Okunishi K, Nakagome K, Tanaka R, Imamura M, Yamamoto K, Kaga K. (2007). Prolonged allergen challenge in murine nasal allergic rhinitis: nasal airway remodeling and adaptation of nasal airway responsiveness. Laryngoscope 117(5):881-885.

Nials AT, Uddin S. (2008). Mouse models of allergic asthma: acute and chronic allergen challenge. Dis Model Mech 1(4-5):213-220.

Patou J, De Smedt H, van Cauwenberge P, Bachert C. (2006). Pathophysiology of nasal obstruction and meta-analysis of early and late effects of levocetirizine. Clin Exp Allergy 36(8):972-981.

Pauluhn J, Mohr U. (2005). Experimental approaches to evaluate respiratory allergy in animal models. Exp Toxicol Pathol 56(4-5):203-234.

Pawankar R. (2006). Allergic rhinitis and asthma: are they manifestations of one syndrome? Clin Exp Allergy 36(1):1-4.

Phillips JE, Ji L, Rivelli MA, Chapman RW, Corboz MR. (2009). Three-dimensional analysis of rodent paranasal sinus cavities from X-ray computed tomography (CT) scans. Can J Vet Res 73(3):205-211.

Ponikau JU, Sherris DA, Kephart GM, Kern EB, Gaffey TA, Tarara JE, Kita H. (2003). Features of airway remodeling and eosinophilic inflammation in chronic rhinosinusitis: is the histopathology similar to asthma? J Allergy Clin Immunol 112(5):877-882.

Salib RJ, Howarth PH. (2003). Remodelling of the upper airways in allergic rhinitis: is it a feature of the disease? Clin Exp Allergy 33(12):1629-1633.

Samarasinghe AE, Hoselton SA, Schuh JM. (2011). A comparison between intratracheal and inhalation delivery of Aspergillus fumigatus conidia in the development of fungal allergic asthma in C57BL/6 mice. Fungal Biol 115(1):21-29.

Shapiro SD. (2006). Animal models of asthma: Pro: Allergic avoidance of animal (model[s]) is not an option. Am J Respir Crit Care Med 174(11):1171-1173.

Singer M, Lefort J, Vargaftig BB. (2002). Granulocyte depletion and dexamethasone differentially modulate airways hyperreactivity, inflammation, mucus accumulation, and secretion induced by rmIL-13 or antigen. Am J Respir Cell Mol Biol 26(1):74-84.

Southam DS, Dolovich M, O'Byrne PM, Inman MD. (2002). Distribution of intranasal instillations in mice: effects of volume, time, body position, and anesthesia. Am J Physiol Lung Cell Mol Physiol 282(4):L833-839.

Szelenyi I, Marx D, Jahn W. (2000). Animal models of allergic rhinitis. Arzneimittelforschung 50(11):1037-1042.

Tsunematsu M, Yamaji T, Kozutsumi D, Murakami R, Kimura S, Kino K. (2007). Establishment of an allergic rhinitis model in mice for the evaluation of nasal symptoms. Life Sci 80(15):1388-1394.

Ulrich K, Hincks JS, Walsh R, Wetterstrand EM, Fidock MD, Sreckovic S, Lamb DJ, Douglas GJ, Yeadon M, Perros-Huguet C, Evans SM. (2008). Anti-inflammatory modulation of chronic airway inflammation in the murine house dust mite model. Pulm Pharmacol Ther 21(4):637-647.

Wagner JG, Harkema JR, Jiang Q, Illek B, Ames BN, Peden DB. (2009). Gamma-tocopherol attenuates ozone-induced exacerbation of allergic rhinosinusitis in rats. Toxicol Pathol 37(4):481-491.

Wagner JG, Hotchkiss JA, Harkema JR. (2002). Enhancement of nasal inflammatory and epithelial responses after ozone and allergen coexposure in Brown Norway rats. Toxicol Sci 67(2):284-294.

Wagner JG, Jiang Q, Harkema JR, Ames BN, Illek B, Roubey RA, Peden DB. (2008). gamma-Tocopherol prevents airway eosinophilia and mucous cell hyperplasia in experimentally induced allergic rhinitis and asthma. Clin Exp Allergy 38(3):501-511.

Wang H, Lu X, Cao PP, Chu Y, Long XB, Zhang XH, You XJ, Cui YH, Liu Z. (2008). Histological and immunological observations of bacterial and allergic chronic rhinosinusitis in the mouse. Am J Rhinol 22(4):343-348.

Weinmayr G, Forastiere F, Weiland SK, Rzehak P, Abramidze T, Annesi-Maesano I, Bjorksten B, Brunekreef B, Buchele G, Cookson WO, von Mutius E, Pistelli R, Strachan DP. (2008). International variation in prevalence of rhinitis and its relationship with sensitisation to perennial and seasonal allergens. Eur Respir J 32(5):1250-1261.

Wenzel S, Holgate ST. (2006). The mouse trap: It still yields few answers in asthma. Am J Respir Crit Care Med 174(11):1173-1176; discussion 1176-1178.

Widdicombe JG. (1990). Nasal pathophysiology. Respir Med 84 Suppl A:3-9; discussion 9-10.

Xie J, Zhang Q, Lai K, Zhong N. (2009). Measurement of Nasal Airway Resistance and Response in Mice. Int Arch Allergy Immunol 151:262-264.

Yamasaki M, Mizutani N, Sasaki K, Nabe T, Kohno S. (2002). No involvement of interleukin-5 or eosinophils in experimental allergic rhinitis in guinea pigs. Eur J Pharmacol 439(1-3):159-169.

Young JT. (1981). Histopathologic examination of the rat nasal cavity. Fundam Appl Toxicol 1(4):309-312.

Yu M, Tsai M, Tam SY, Jones C, Zehnder J, Galli SJ. (2006). Mast cells can promote the development of multiple features of chronic asthma in mice. J Clin Invest 116(6):1633-1641.

Zhao Y, Woo JK, Leung PC, Chen GG, Wong YO, Liu SX, van Hasselt CA. (2005). Symptomatic and pathophysiological observations in a modified animal model of allergic rhinitis. Rhinology 43(1):47-54.

2

Clinical Implications and Facts About Allergic Rhinitis (AR) in Children

Zorica Zivkovic[1,2], Sofija Cerovic[2],
Ivana Djuric-Filipovic[1], Zoran Vukasinovic[3,4],
Jasmina Jocic-Stojanovic[2] and Aleksandra Bajec-Opancina[5]

[1]US Medical School, European University, Belgrade
[2]Children's Hospital for Lung Diseases and Tuberculosis, Medical Center "Dr Dragisa Misovic", Belgrade
[3]Faculty of Medicine, University of Belgrade, Belgrade
[4]Institute of Orthopaedic Surgery „Banjica", Belgrade
[5]Mother and Child Health Care Institute, Belgrade
Serbia

1. Introduction

The upper airways symptoms in childhood are the most frequent reasons that make children and their parents to seek the doctor's help. The truth is that the symptoms occur as viral infections of the upper airways specially in preschool age children. Up to 30% of preschool age children with acute upper airway problems will suffer at least one wheezing episode, which brings them to the pediatrician for treatment. (Asher et al., 2006) It means that for the first 6 years of life every 3rd child will be treated by bronchodilators, antibiotics or even anti-inflammatory therapy such as corticosteroids.

However, data from hundreds of papers and from our experience as well, shows that it is "normal and expected for a healthy child". What is not expected is more than 3 wheezing episodes in early life that coexists with numerous upper airways diseases. (Lemanske et al., 2005) Children with such a history should be observed more carefully and if the symptoms gradually get worse, should be referred to a specialist for further investigations. (Sigurs et al. 2000; Sigurs et al., 2005) Frequently, these children are atopic with the family history of atopy or some comorbid condition that may confirm the allergic background, even if the skin prick tests on aeroallergens remains negative. (Ng Man Kwong et al., 2001) Usually, child with recurrent wheezing episodes will be suspected of having childhood asthma and successfully treated by antiasthma drugs (inhaled corticosteroids and/or leukotriens antagonists) not taking into account her/his recurrent or chronic upper airways problems. Despite the lack of severe asthma symptoms in these patients, they still suffer from blocked, congested upper airways, runny, itchy nose and eyes, reactive cough and mild wheezy episodes particularly during the physical activities. This is the scenario that we are facing in our everyday practice and this is the reason for involving the investigation and subsequent treatment of the upper airways problem in our work. We cannot expect to solve the childhood asthma problem completely if the allergic rhinitis persists.

2. Quality of life and allergic rhinitis (AR) in childhood

Although it is frequently seen as a mild and intermittent AR is capable of changing and disturbing the quality of life of the children, as well as their well-being, learning and physical activity. Apparently, the severity, and not necessarily the duration of the AR, has a more relevant effect on the quality of life of the patients with AR, with main consequences on sleep quality and learning ability. (Juniper et al., 1999) The impact that AR severity had on quality of life-sleep, activities of daily living and school performance was more significant than was the duration of the disease. (Craig et al., 2004) More than 80% of the patients with more severe forms reported impairment in their activities due to the disease, compared with only 40% of those with mild forms. Disease-specific questionnaires are the instruments most widely used in order to "measure the quality of life". In the case of allergic rhinoconjunctivitis, the disease-specific questionnaire most commonly used is the Rhinoconjunctivitis Quality of Life Questionnaire (RQLQ). (Nascimento Silva et al., 2001; Santos et al., 2006) It is fundamental to highlight that AR-related physical, psychological and social impairments are experienced not only by adults but also by children and adolescents. Although adolescents experience problems similar to those of the adults, they present greater difficulty in concentrating, particularly on their school work. Younger children, however, present a slightly different profile: they feel unhappy and unsatisfied, however, they tend to experience less limitation in their activities of daily living and do not exhibit the emotional disturbance experienced by adults and adolescents. Our experience in assessment of quality of life of children with AR alone or associated with asthma, basically shows disturbances in physical domen specially during the pollen season in children suffering from hay fever. (Cerovic et al., 2009) It was shown by other authors that quality of life (QOL) in individuals with perennial chronic rhinitis was worse in relation to persons with mild to moderate asthma. (Bousquet 2008a, 1994b, 1994c) Our results on quality of life in children with asthma revealed bad score only for physical activities in children while very bad score for parents and very high level of anxiety related to their children's asthma. (Cerovic et al., 2009) Our survey didn't divide patients with asthma and allergic rhinitis from patients with only one condition, and definitely children are less susceptible to QOL disturbances independently of their real condition. However, untreated and undertreated symptoms of allergic rhinitis in children, definitely impair overall quality of life mainly due to persistent nasal congestion and subsequent feeling of fatigue, headache, cognitive impairment and school problems. (Walker et al., 2007) Nasal congestion has been defined as the most troublesome condition since it may affect negatively sleep time, resulting in reduced daytime activities and particularly sports involvement that is the most important and popular among children and adolescents. (Sundberg et al., 2007; Broide 2007) Occasionally, recurrent upper airways diseases and clearly allergic rhinitis are the conditions that precede or progress to asthma, while in the other cases these are the causes of worsening of already existing asthma symptoms. Both conditions lead to continuous usage of drugs, from symptomatic once (decongestive medications, antitussive drugs) to evidence-based antiallergic, antiasthmatic drugs. Even more, in children with or without obvious signs of complications (otitis media, bronchitis, pneumonia) antibiotics are frequently advised in every respiratory episode. Overtreatment of these children exists in all cases of children hospitalized due to an acute severe bronchiolitis in the first 12 months of age or hospitalized due to repeated acute asthmatic attacks. (Rodić et al., 2006; Radić et al., 2009) So far, not only usual predictive or risk factors for developing asthma should be taken into consideration. We suggest the hypothesis that individuals with the early life upper airways problem similar to so called "common cold symptoms", should attract our attention for earlier and better investigations in terms of proper diagnosis and treatment as early as possible. Basically, the possibility of developing asthma after 6 years of age after having allergic rhinitis from 3rd to 6th year of life, has been estimated at about 30% in children (not administered allergen specific hyposensitization). (Meltzer 2005; Martinez et al., 1995) In real life, detailed investigations (that have to be performed before the decision on immunotherapy) in children of preschool ages are difficult due to weak cooperation of a child and parents as well. Secondly, the lack of information and standardized protocols on allergen specific immunotherapy (ASIT) among pediatricians, allergologists and all relevant subspecialties make this situation even more complicated.

Our aim is to present some numbers on prevalence of allergic rhinitis in childhood and some considerations about ASIT in children. Long-term benefits have also been seen with the use of immunotherapy, although some patients, especially children, resist the injections used in subcutaneous immunotherapy. Recent studies with sublingual immunotherapy have indicated that it might be an effective and well-tolerated alternative to immunotherapy injections.

3. Epidemiology of allergic rhinitis in children

Reference list of the articles dealing with the prevalence and epidemiology of childhood atopic diseases, mainly asthma, dermatitis and rhinitis, is extremely long and extended. The numbers from thousands of surveys varied from too low to too high, rarely can rely on approved methodological and statistical background and cannot deserve enough attention for valid conclusions. However, the International Study of Asthma and Allergies (ISAAC) Phase Three has valuable power involving 98 countries worldwide and 236 Phase Three Centers, in other words around 1 059 053 children of 2 age groups from 236 centres in 98 countries.(Ait-Khaled et al., 2009) (Obviously, this multicentric, multiethnic, multicultural study present "a new and greatly enlarged world map of symptom prevalence". The average prevalence of current symptoms of allergic rhinoconjunctivitis across all centres was 14.6% for the 13- to 14-year old children. However, extensive variation in the prevalence of diagnosis of allergic rhinitis within regions, countries and centres was observed (values range from 1% in India to 45.1% in Paraguay). The highest regional prevalence rates of current rhinoconjunctivitis were observed in Africa (18.0%) and Latin America (17.3%) and the lowest in Northern and Eastern Europe (9.2%). In each region, there were major differences in prevalence between countries. Variation in the prevalence of severe rhinoconjunctivitis symptoms was also observed between regions (range 0.4% in Western Europe to 2.1% in Africa), and between countries within regions. The prevalence of severe rhinoconjunctivitis symptoms was generally the highest (more than 1%) in centres from middle and low income countries. These are important and valuable observations that socio-economic impact of the country and regions have been related to the severity of the AR. In the 13- to 14-year age group, the prevalence of current AR was substantially lower in centres in low income countries compared with those in high income countries. From the other hand, centres in low income countries had an increased prevalence of severe AR related to the centres in high income countries. (Ait-Khaled et al., 2009)

These results are sufficient for conclusion that economic burden of allergic rhinitis worldwide is enormous and directly related to high morbidity in countries with poor health resources.

The prevalence rate of allergic rhinitis, asthma and eczema in Serbia has been investigated as a part of the ISAAC phase 3. The survey was conducted in five regional centers with different geographical and urban characteristics. Around 14000 children were enrolled, aged 6- to 7-year and 13- to 14- years. Prevalence rate of asthma has been 6,59% in 6- to 7- year group and 5,36% in 13- to 14- year group respectively. Prevalence of allergic rhinitis has been 7,17% in 6- to 7- year age group while 14,89% in the 13- to 14- year age group. We found statistically significant difference between groups. Prevalence of eczema has been 14,04% in younger and 14,45% in older children. When counted prevalence rate in total we found asthma in 5,91%, rhinitis in 11,46% and eczema in 14,27%. From the whole number of children around 40% presented repeatedly for upper airway problems, 26% presented at least once with symptoms of upper and lower airways simultaneously and 11% more than 4 times for the both conditions for the last 12 months. It means that expenses only for their acute episodes highly cross over the expected annual budget for outpatients clinics. In addition, AR is commonly associated with other respiratory diseases, and the cost resulting from these comorbidities increases even more the socioeconomic impact of the disease. (Zivkovic et al., 2010) Not less important conclusion that we made has been that prevalence rate has been higher in urban than rural areas except in certain villages near by large air-pollutants (power stations and chemical industry). This is the conclusion that leads us to multifactorial origin of the rhinitis in childhood and particularly for the youngest ages seems to be difficult to distinguish allergic from nonallergic rhinitis.

Our special clinical interest was association of allergic rhinitis in children and wheezing episodes or asthma. The majority of children suffer from both conditions from the early childhood. From the infancy they experience waterish nasal discharge or congestion all over the year, frequently unrelated to day care respiratory infections. Later in childhood they present with wheezing episodes, cough or asthma that deserve more attention and investigations. (Brand et al., 2008; Zivkovic et al., 2009) Usually, the allergic background of the nasal symptoms has been revealed many years after their occurrence. From our study it is evident that delay in diagnosis of asthma is around 4,5 years and of allergic rhinitis more than 5,7 years. (Zivkovic Z et al., 2009) Analysing the course of allergic symptoms of upper and lower airways we found allergic rhinitis frequently associated with pollen allergy, long-term usage of medication, unsatisfaction of patient and parents and deterioration of quality of life. The important effort in the literature was made in assessment of allergic inflammation in children with comorbid conditions in regard of treatment of clinically silent forms or inappropriate response on therapy. (Pijnenburg et al., 2005; Arnal et al., 1997) We measured exhaled NO in children with asthma and allergic rhinitis, 6 to 16 years of life, in September - December 2009. (Zivkovic et al., 2009) Clearly, the higher was fraction of exhaled NO, the more symptoms allergic rhinitis we detected in children as well as higher levels of nasal eosinophils. In conclusion, we stated importance of follow up of a child with asthma and AR through the seasons are mostly valuable since atopic conditions are developing in terms of season or years. (Zivkovic et al., 2008) What is the main result of our studies and clinical surveys? The AR in children is an early life presenting problem, recurrent or persistent during the early childhood, frequently associated with the lower airway diseases, over treated or maltreated, and finally completely confusing and disturbing in terms of quality of life of children and their families. So far, the various aspects of treatments might be successful but over time they become bothersome and hardly acceptable for young persons and adolescents. Obviously, we are looking for efficient, easy to use and inexpensive treatment, but it is probably not possible. (Mçsges et al., 2007) Therefore, we were searching through the literature and clinical practice for the benefits of the allergen specific immunotherapy, particularly sublingual immunotherapy (SLIT) as the causative way of treatment and would like to present in the other part some of our findings and comments.

SLIT is widely known as an effective treatment for children requiring immunotherapy who normally prefer oral administration compared to subcutaneous therapy. (Mahr et al., 2007; Canonica et al., 2003) Concerns and dilemmas still remain in relation to the optimal dose and treatment protocol . In addition, there are no standardized code for administration of SLIT therapy. Studies are underway to evaluate an FDA-approved product for SLIT. Hopefully these studies will assist clinicians in clarifying the role of SLIT therapy in the management of AR. (Cox et al., 2006; Hankin et al., 2010)

There are many studies on clinical effectiveness of sublingual immunotherapy and we would like to point out one of the meta-analyses. Meta-analysis of SLIT for AR in children 4–18 years of age involved 10 trials and 484 subjects. The results of this meta-analyses showed that SLIT was significantly more effective than placebo, by improving AR symptom scores and usage of rescue medication. Related to the possible, mainly local side effects it seems that SLIT is better tolerated than subcutaneous route of administration of allergen specific immunotherapy. Despite many clinical studies confirming the clinical efficacy there are still unmet needs for SLIT in children : the optimal dose and dosing frequency of allergen administration, time of administration of SLIT in patients unresponsive to pharmacotherapy, duration of SLIT, long-term efficacy, preventive capacity, other allergic processes beyond respiratory allergy, usage of SLIT in children in preschool ages etc. (Moingeon et al., 2006; Penagos et al., 2008)

4. More about immunotherapy and sublingual immunotherapy in children

The first data concerning immunotherapy dated from the beginning of 19th century. The main aim of the immunotherapy was to redirect inappropriate immunological response in atopic patients. It has proven to be efficacious to treat type I allergies to a variety of allergens. (Pichler et al., 2001; Moller et al., 2002) Since Food Drug Agency (FDA) reported more seriously adverse reaction post subcutaneous immunotherapy new routes of administration (sublingual and intranasal) have been widely considered. (Canonica et al., 2003) After more than 500 million doses of SLIT administered to humans SLIT is proven to be much safer than subcutaneous immunotherapy (SCIT), with no evidence of anaphylactic shock recorded. (Wilson et al., 2003; Frew et al., 2001; Agostinis et al., 2005; et al., 2002) SLIT was firstly accepted as a viable alternative to SCIT in the World Health Organization (WHO) position paper, published in 1998, and then included in the ARIA guidelines. (Sub-Lingual Immunotherapy World Allergy Organization Position Paper 2009) The main targets for using SLIT are patients of all ages with good correlation between clinical symptoms of allergy and positive allergen specific IgE. Monosenzitized patients are the best candidates for SLIT. Recent studies have investigated using SLIT for the patients with food allergy, latex allergy, atopic dermatitis and allergy on insect venoms. (Sub-Lingual Immunotherapy World Allergy Organization Position Paper 2009) SLIT is also a good choice for patients uncontrolled with optimal pharmacotherapy (SCUAD), patients in whom pharmacotherapy induces undesirable side effects, patients refusing injections, patients who do not want to be on constant or long-term pharmacotherapy. (Sub-Lingual Immunotherapy World Allergy Organization Position Paper, 2009).

Allergens using in SLIT persist in tablets and drops forms. (Casale , 2004) The most frequent schedule for using SLIT considers induction (build up) and retention phases. The best time for starting SLIT is 4/5 months before pollen season. (Allergy and Immunology Society of Serbia and Montenegro, Position Paper, 2005).

Optimal allergen extracts dose is a dose which is sufficient for improving clinical symptoms in a great number of patients without adverse reaction. (Moingeon et al., 2006). Despite excellent clinical experience in using SLIT the exact immunological mechanism is still undefined. The central paradigm for successful immunotherapy has been to reorient the pattern of allergen-specific T-cell responses in atopic patients from a Th2 to Th1 profile.

There is currently a growing interest in eliciting regulatory T cells, capable of down regulating both Th1 and Th2 responses through the production of interleukin (IL)-10 and/or transforming growth factor (TGF)-β. SLIT induces three categories of immunological changes: modulation of allergen-specific antibody responses; reduction in recruitment and activation of proinflammatory cells and changes in the pattern of allergen specific T-cell responses.

5. Modulation of allergen-specific antibody responses

SLIT was shown to increase allergen-specific IgG4 levels compared with placebo, with a more limited impact on specific IgE responses. A decrease in the IgE/IgG4 ratio has been observed in a number of SLIT studies (Bahceciler et al., 2005), with some exceptions. (Rolinck-Werninghaus et al., 2005).

A meta analysis of six SLIT studies with detailed analysis of antibody responses concluded on a consistent increase in allergen-specific IgG4 levels. (Torres Lima et al., 2002) Such changes in the IgE/IgG4 ratio were found to correlate with a decrease in the late-phase skin reaction to the allergen and with the overall clinical efficacy of the vaccine in some studies (Torres Lima et al., 2002). In a recent phase I/II trial with grass pollen tablets, SLIT was shown to elicit allergen-specific seric IgAs in a dose-dependent fashion (Malling et al., 2005) and a small up regulation of IgA responses was also observed when SLIT was used in house dust mite allergic patients. Altogether, allergen-specific IgG (and IgA) antibodies induced by immunotherapy are thought to contribute to the positive clinical response through distinct and nonexclusive mechanisms: these antibodies can compete with IgEs for binding to the allergen, thereby preventing both basophil or mastocyte deregulation (Mothes et al., 2003; Niederberger et al., 2004), as well as allergen capture and presentation to T lymphocytes by FcεRI+ and CD23+ antigen-presenting cells (APCs). and such antibodies may act as blocking antibodies by engaging low-affinity Fc receptors for immunoglobulins (e.g. FcγRII) expressed by B lymphocytes, basophils, or mast cells. FcγRII receptors contain immunoreceptor tyrosine-based inhibitory motifs (ITIM), they transduce, as a consequence, negative signals preventing cellular activation and release of soluble pro-inflammatory mediators following co-aggregation with FcεRI receptors. (Wachholz et al., 2003; Flicker et al., 2003) SLIT prevented the recruitment of eosinophils in the eyes or in the nose after allergen challenge. (Marcucci et al., 2001; Marcucci et al., 2003; Silvestri et al., 2002) SLIT with grass pollen extracts was shown to decrease local or systemic levels of eosinophil cationic protein (ECP), without any increase in tryptase. (Marcucci et al., 2001).

Changes in the pattern of allergen specific T-cell responses. Recent studies focused on the impact of SLIT on CD4+ T cells responses. It is well known that allergic patients usually mount strong allergen-specific Th2 cells immune response, characterized by the secretion of high amounts of interleukin IL-4, IL-5 and IL-13 cytokines.
(El Biaze et al., 2003). Concerning that a central goal for immunotherapy has been to reorient allergen specific T-cell responses in atopic patients from a Th2 to Th1 profile [the latter being rather associated with the production of interferon (IFN)-γ and IL-12cytokines]. (Laaksonen et al., 2003; et al., Gabrielsson et al., 2001; et al., 2001; Faith et al., 2003; Oldfield et al., 2002;) Comparing with SCIT there is a less evidence on the impact of SLIT on T-cell responses. In several studies conducted in children or adults with seasonal allergic rhinoconjunctivitis to grass pollen, no significant effect of SLIT on T-cell functions (i.e. cytokine production, proliferation) was observed. (Rolinck-Werninghaus et al., 2005; Torres Lima et al., 2002) SLIT does not induce any detectable changes in the numbers of dendritic cells (DCs) nor T lymphocytes in the epithelium or lamina propria of the oral mucosa. Immunization through the sublingual route was nevertheless shown in other studies to decrease the production of the Th2 cytokine IL-13 and the proliferation of peripheral blood mononuclear cells (PBMCs) from patients allergic to house dust mite. (Ippoliti et al., 2003; Fenoglio et al., 2005) As of today, there is still no firm evidence that SLIT can induce regulatory T cells. A preliminary study suggests that SLIT increases IL-10 production in PBMCs from house dust mite (HDM) allergic patients following in vitro stimulation with Dermatophagoides farinae antigens, but also with recall antigens (e.g. Candida albicans) or PHA, when compared with untreated allergic patients. (Ciprandi et al. 2005) The fact that some IL-10-secreting T cells are not allergen-specific raises the possibility of a bystander immunosuppressive effect of SLIT. Of note, high-dose SLIT regimens with ovalbumin in mice induce specific T cells producing TGF-β in the spleen of sensitized animals.

6. Regulatory T cells and allergy vaccines

Although both anergy and T-cell depletion are known to contribute to the establishment of peripheral tolerance against environmental antigens, it is now broadly admitted that antigen-specific T-cell populations with suppressive/regulatory function play a key role in controlling immune responses to both self- and nonself-antigens. (Blaser et al., 2004; Umetsu et al., 2003; Jonuleit et al., 2003; Hawrylowicz et al.,2005) These cells, termed regulatory T cells, are heterogeneous, and include both: (i) naturally occurring CD4+CD25+ T cells and (ii) cells induced in the periphery following antigen exposure (e.g. Tr1 cells, Th3 cells, and CD8+ regulatory T cells). There is a growing evidence supporting the role of regulatory T cells in controlling the development of asthma and allergic disease in a variety of models , although it is not clear yet which of the various regulatory T cell subsets are the most important in this regard. (Taylor et al., 2004) A revised version of the hygiene hypothesis proposes that a limited exposure to infectious pathogens during infancy, most particularly telluric mycobacteria and parasites, may prevent the establishment of not only a Th1, but also a T reg repertoire, thereby explaining in part the observed increase in prevalence of allergies in developed countries. (Yazdanbakhsh et al., 2002)
Several studies documented an association between atopy and a defect in T reg functions. For example, children born with a dysfunctional Fox p3 gene presented with a deficit in CD4+CD25+ regulatory T cells, develop severe autoimmune diseases often associated with eczema, elevated IgE levels, eosinophilia and food allergy [the polyendocrinopathy,

enteropathy, and X-linked inheritance (IPEX) syndrome]. (Gambineri et al., 2003) Moreover, for at least some atopic subjects with active disease, the suppressive activity of CD4+CD25+ regulatory T cells is significantly decreased in vitro when compared with nonatopic individuals, potentially explaining the loss of tolerance against allergens. (Ling et al., 2004)
Studies showed that DCs from children with allergic rhinitis can be impaired in their capacity to produce IL-10. (Grindebacke et al., 2004) Interestingly, allergen-specific IL-10-secreting Tr1 cells are highly represented in healthy individuals in comparison with allergen-specific IL-4-secreting Th2 cells, suggesting that regulatory T cells are predominant during natural immune responses to environmental allergens in nonatopic donors. (Gentile et al., 2004; Akdis et al., 2004) Regulatory T lymphocytes can control an established allergic response via distinct mechanisms: IL-10 and TGF-β decrease IgE production and enhance IgG4 and IgA production, respectively. Both cytokines lower the release of proinflammatory mediators by downregulating IgE-dependent activation of basophils and mast cells and by decreasing survival and activation of eosinophils. IL-10 and TGF-β also inhibit the production of Th2 cytokines such as IL-4 and IL-5. (Akdis et al., 2004;, Blaser et al., 2004; Akdis et al., 2001) In addition, regulatory T cells exhibit a direct inhibitory effect on Th1 and Th2 T cells, through cell–cell contact, or by decreasing the antigen presenting function of DCs.
Regulatory T cells producing IL-10 and/or TGF-b are induced not only in atopic patients by successful immunotherapy, but also during natural allergen exposure in healthy people. As per the hygiene hypothesis, limited exposure to bacteria and parasites in developed countries may result in a poor establishment of a T reg repertoire during childhood, thereby contributing to an increase in the frequency of allergies. Regulatory T cells can control and regulate all effectors mechanisms activated during allergy and Th2 responses through the production of IL-10/TGF- β and/or cell–cell contact. IL-10 is a potent suppressor of total and allergen-specific IgEs, whereas it induces an antibody isotype switch towards IgG4. TGF-β also decreases IgE production and induces immunoglobulin isotype switch towards IgA. IL-10 and TGF- β act directly or indirectly on human airways to decrease both mucus production and airway hyper-reactivity.

7. Oral mucosa and immune responses

7.1 SLIT and induction of peripheral tolerance

Sublingual immunotherapy takes advantage of an important physiological mechanism (i.e. oral tolerance), which has been evolutionarily conserved to ensure immune tolerance to various antigenic stimuli from the environment, especially from food and commensal bacteria. During SLIT, as for immunization at any mucosal surface, the allergen is captured locally (i.e. within the oral mucosa) by Langerhans-like DCs following either phagocytosis, macropinocytosis or receptor-mediated endocytosis. Subsequent to allergen capture, DCs mature and migrate to proximal draining lymph nodes (e.g. submaxillary, superficial cervical and internal jugular), as a consequence of changes in expression of surface receptors (e.g. the CCR7 chemokine receptor) involved in adhesion and trafficking. Those lymph nodes represent specialized microenvironments favoring the induction of mucosal tolerance through the production of blocking IgG antibodies (IgG2b in mice) and the induction of T lymphocytes with suppressive function. (Van Helvoort et al., 2004) Importantly, the magnitude of CD4+ T-cell responses elicited within lymph nodes is directly proportional to the number of allergen carrying DCs that migrate to lymph nodes, which clearly represents a limiting step. (Martin-Fotecha et al., 2003) Eventually, as a consequence of the circulation of allergen-specific activated effector T cells throughout the body and the persistence of memory cells, a local (i.e. sublingual) administration of the allergen during desensitization results in both systemic and mucosal protective immune responses. Dendritic cells in the sublingual mucosa exhibit morphological characteristics of Langerhans cells, including the presence of intracytoplasmic Birbeck granules. (Allam et al., 2003) Interestingly, Langerhans-like cells from the oral mucosa constitutively express both low- (CD23) and high- (FCeRI) affinity receptors for IgEs, which may facilitate IgE-mediated allergen capture in atopic individuals. (Allam et al., 2003) Perhaps, more importantly, upon engagement of such IgE receptors, oral Langerhans-like cells produce IL-10, TGFb and up regulate indoleamine 2-dioxygenase (IDO), a rate-limiting enzyme-metabolizing tryptophan, thereby resulting in a decrease in T-cell proliferation. (Allam et al., 2003; Von Bubnoff et al., 2004) As discussed above, there is still no formal evidence of Treg induction via the sublingual route. Nevertheless, on the basis of its aforementioned characteristics, the immune system in the oral mucosa appears prone to induce active tolerance mechanisms against allergens and antigens from the environment. Consistent with this, there is preliminary evidence that SLIT elicits IL-10-producing T cells in humans (Ciprandi et al., 2005) and antigen-specific TGF-b+ T cells in murine. (Moingeon, et al., 2004).

8. Clinical efficacy

Usually clinical efficacy of SLIT is measured by the Rhinoconjunctivitis Total Symptom Score (RTSS), which included the 6 most common symptoms of pollinosis (sneezing, rhinorrhea, nasal pruritus, nasal congestion, ocular pruritus, and watery eyes). A score ranging from 0 to 3, according to the Center for Drug Evaluation and Research guidance (April 2000), was used for each individual symptom: 0/5 no symptoms, 1/5 mild symptoms (symptoms clearly present, but minimal awareness; easily tolerated), 2/5 moderate symptoms (definite awareness of bothersome but tolerable symptoms), and 3/5 severe symptoms (symptoms hard to tolerate and/or cause interference with activities of daily living and/or sleeping).

From approximately a month before and during the pollen season, patients completed a daily diary card to score nasal and ocular symptoms using the RTSS. The average RTSS was calculated during the entire pollen season. In addition, the effect of immunotherapy on the 6 individual symptom scores (sneezing, runny nose, itchy nose, nasal congestion,watery eyes, and itchy eyes) was analyzed as secondary outcomes. The proportion of symptom-free days (%) during the pollen season was also assessed. A symptom-free day was a day on which"0/ 5 absent" was recorded for each of the 6 individual rhinoconjunctivitis symptoms.

Allergen specific immunotherapy (ASIT) is very important in pediatric population. It has been shown to have possibility to change natural course of allergic diseases and to prevent new sensibilisation. ASIT is the only therapeutic method with causal effects in children population. Sublingual route of allergen administration is very comfortable, simple and non-traumatic especially for children.

The first evidence of the effect of SLIT in children came from an 18-month study of 2 different doses of SLIT for tree-pollen allergy in 88 children suffering seasonal allergic rhinitis, confirmed by skin prick test, specific serum IgE, and conjunctival allergen challenge. Eighteen months of SLIT with tree pollen extract provided dose-dependent benefits in terms of significantly reduced symptoms and medication use.(Valovirta E et al., 2006) Two adequately powered, well-designed double blind placebo controlled (DBPC)

randomized controlled trial (RCTs) have now been published, both showing a clear effect of allergen tablets in childhood. A statistically significant reduction in rhinitis symptoms (28%) and medication (64%) score was shown during the pollen season in 114 children receiving active grass allergen tablets (with 15g Phl p 5) compared with 120 children in the placebo group.(Wahn U et al., 2009). The other DBPC/RCT evaluated the efficacy of 5-grass tablets (with 25g group 5 major allergen) administered pre- and coseasonally to 227 children with seasonal allergic rhino-conjunctivitis. In those receiving the 5-grass tablets a significant improvement was found in symptom and medication scores.(Roder E et al., 2007) All these studies, clearly show the efficacy of SLIT in reducing the symptom score during pollen season in children with rhinitis; furthermore, there were also a significant reduction in medication use. The allergens that have been used with success in SLIT in the pediatric age group for rhinitis are pollen from *Phleum pratense,* 5-grass mix, *Parietaria* and *Betulaceae* pollens and HDM. SLIT with olive pollen showed only improvement in symptoms and one grass study was negative.(Bufe A et al. 2004)
23 DBPC studies in the period of 1990-2002. documented clinical efficacy of SLIT. Pediatric population was involved in 16 of those studies. SLIT has been shown to reduce bronchial hyperreactivity, symptoms and medication scores in adolescents population treated with SLIT containing extracts of grass pollen. (Robinson et al., 2004)

9. Safety in children

The sublingual route was introduced with the aim of reducing side effects and increasing the safety of immunotherapy. Recent studies showed that there is no difference in the incidence of adverse events (AE) between children and adults (Passalacqua G, et al., 2007) and SLIT has been shown to be safe. The most frequently reported AEs (mostly self-limiting) are local in the oral mucosa (itching and swelling) and of the digestive system. Just a few cases were considered moderate/severe requiring medical intervention. Experience must be gained in the use of single versus multiple-allergens. SLIT with a single allergen is the most common practice in Europe whereas multiple allergens are used mainly in USA, Latin America and some other parts of the world. In adults, in one study, use of SLIT with multiple allergens was reported to be as safe as SLIT with a single allergen.(Agostinis F et al., 2008)
It is also very important to mention that there are three studies, 2 observational and one postmarketing survey, specifically designed to assess the safety of SLIT in young children. A total of 231 children younger than 5-years-old, who were treated with various pollen and mite allergens (33 patients received allergoid) were included.(Agostini et al, 2005; Fiocchi A,et al. , 2005; Rienzo VD et al. , 2005) AEs were reported in 5 to 15% of patients in a total of 68,975 doses with rates of 0.268, 0.766, and 1.767 AEs per 1,000 doses in the 3 studies. Most reactions appeared to be mild or moderate and resolved without treatment. Dose reduction by changing from a sublingual-swallow to a sublingual-spit method controlled gastrointestinal reactions in one study. One further RCT with HDM SLIT in 138 children aged 2–5 years with asthma or rhinitis showed only mild to moderate local AEs. (Rodriguez-Santos O. Et al., 2008)

10. Our clinical experience

In our practice, we have started using the allergen specific immunotherapy in children more than 10 years ago, however, more frequently for the last 4 to 5 years. Number of children on SLIT is 37, but 31 successfully followed the protocol. The data about the patients, their outcomes and clinical results are about to be analyzed in another article. The youngest child on SLIT is 7 years old, and the upper age limit doesn't exist. The adolescent patients started at 17 years of age continue the treatment after their pediatric ages. Patients sensitized with Dermatophagoides pteronyssinus are the most frequent cases for SLIT, slightly less frequent is the group of patients sensitized with ragweed pollen (Ambrosia elatior or Artemisia). Predominantly, current symptoms are allergic rhinitis, allergic rhinoconjuncitivitis (hay fever), and 70% of all patients claimed asthma symptoms in the early childhood. At the moment of inclusion to a group for SLIT, asthmatic symptoms were mild or absent. Couple of patients stopped the SLIT from their own reasons, and 2 of the patients had to follow protocol with reduced maintenance doses due to the adverse reactions (sneezing, coughing, tickling of the throat). The final results and outcomes will be announced and published elsewhere, but we have sufficient data to state: good clinical efficacy, lack of hay fever symptoms or diminishing the symptoms after 3 years of therapeutic regime, satisfaction with collaboration and treatment adherence, valuable improvement of patients and their families' quality of life. (Z. Zivkovic: personal communication)

11. Acknowledgment

This work was supported by Ministry of Education and Science, Republic of Serbia (Grant No. 41004).

12. References

Agostinis F, Tellarini L, Canonica GW, Falagiani P, Passalacqua G. Safety of sublingual immunotherapy with a monomeric allergoid in very young children. Allergy 2005;60: 133-138.

Agostinis F, Foglia C, Landi M, Cottini M, Lombardi C, et al. The safety of sublingual immunotherapy with one or multiple pollen allergens in children. Allergy. 2008;63:1637–1639.

Ait-Khaled N, Pearce N, Anderson HR, Ellwood P, Montefort S, Shah J, and the ISAAC Phase Three Study Group (...Zivkovic Z ...). Global map of the prevalence of symptoms of rhinoconjunctivitis in children: The International Study of Asthma and Allergies in Childhood (ISAAC) Phase Three. Allergy 2009; 64: 123-148.

Akdis M, Verhagen J, Taylor A, Karamloo F, Karagiannidis C, Crameri R et al. Immune responses in healthy and allergic individuals are characterized by a fine balance between allergenspecific T regulatory 1 and T helper 2 cells. J Exp Med 2004; 199:1567–1575.

Akdis C, Blaser K, Akdis M. Genes of tolerance. Allergy 2004; 59:897–913.

Akdis C, Joss A, Akdis M, Blaser K. Mechanisms of IL10 induced T cell inactivation in allergic inflammation and normal response to allergens. Int Arch Allergy Immunol 2001;124:180–182.

Allergen Specific Immunotherapy: National Consensus/Working Group for National Consensus. Editor Rajica M. Stosovic: Association of Allergologist and Clinical Immunologist of Serbia and Montenegro 2005; Loznica, Mladost group.

Allam JP, Novak N, Fuchs C, Asen S, Berge S, Appel T et al. Characterization of dendritic cells from human oral mucosa: a new Langerhans cell type with high constitutive FC epsilon RI expression. J Allergy Clin Immunol 2003;112:141–148.

Asher MI, Montefort S, Bjorksten B et al. Worldwide time trends in the prevalence of symptoms of asthma, allergic rhinoconjunctivitis, and eczema in childhood: ISAAC Phases One and Three repeat multicountry cross-sectional surveys. Lancet 2006;368:733–743.

Bahceciler N, Arikan C, Taylor A, Akdis M, Blaser K, Barlan I et al. Impact of sublingual immunotherapy on specific antibody levels in asthmatic children allergic to house dust mite. Intern Arch Immunol Allergy 2005;136:287–294.

Bousquet J, Khaltaev N, Cruz A et al. Allergic Rhinitis and its Impact on Asthma (ARIA) 2008. Allergy 2008: 63 (Suppl. 86): 8–160.

Bousquet J, Knani J, Dhivert H, et al. Quality of life in asthma. Internal consistency and validity of the SF-36 questionnaire. Am J Respir Crit Care Med 1994; 149:371-375.

Brand P, Baraldi E, Bisgaard H, Boner AL, Castro-Rodriguez A, Custovic A, de Blic J, de Jongste JC, Eber E, Everard M, Frez U, Gappa M, Garcia-Marcos L, Grigg J, Lenney W, le Souef P, Mc Kenzie S, Merkus PJ, Midulla F, Paton JZ, Piacentini G, Pohunek P, Rossi GA, Seddon P, Silverman M, Sly PD, Stick S, Valiulis A, van Aalderen WMC, Wildhaber JH, Wennergren G, Wilson N, Živković Z, Bush A. ERS Task Force. Definition, assessment and treatment of wheezing disorders in preschool children: an evidence-based approach. Eur Respir J 2008; 32: 1096-1110.

Broide D. The pathophysiology of allergic rhinoconjunctivitis. Allergy Asthma Proc 28:398 - 403, 2007; doi: 10.2500/aap.2007.28.3011)

Bufe A, Eberle P, Franke-Beckmann E, Funck J, Kimmig M, et al. Safety and efficacy in children of an SQ-standardized grass allergen tablet for sublingual immunotherapy. J Allergy Clin Immunol. 2009;123:167–173.

Bufe A, Ziegler-Kirbach E, Stoeckmann E, Heidemann P, Gehlhar K, et al. Efficacy of sublingual swallow immunotherapy in children with severe grass pollen allergic symptoms: a double-blind placebo-controlled study. Allergy. 2004;59:498 –504.

Canonica GW, and Passalacqua G. Noninjection routes for immunotherapy. J Allergy Clin Immunol 2003: 111:437- 448.

Ciprandi G, Fenoglio D, Cirillo I, Vizzaccaro A, Ferrero A, Tosca MA et al. Sublingual HDM-specific immunotherapy induces IL10 production: Preliminary report. Ann Allergy Asthma Immunol 2005;95:38–44.

Cerovic S, Zivkovic Z, Milenkovic B, Jocic-Stojanovic J, Opancina-Bajec A, Vukasinovic Z The Serbian Version of the Pediatric Asthma Quality of Life Questionnaire in Daily Practice. J Asthma 2009; 46:936-939.

Cox LS, Linnemann DL, Nolte H, et al. Sublingual immunotherapy: A comprehensive review. J Allergy Clin Immunol 2006; 117: 1021–1035..

Craig TJ, McCann JL, Gurevich F, Davies MJ. The correlation between allergic rhinitis and sleep disturbance. J Allergy Clin Immunol 2004;114(Suppl. 5):S139–S145.

El Biaze M, Boniface S, Koscher V, Mamessier E, Dupuy P, et al. T activation, from atopy to asthma: more a paradox than a paradigm. Allergy 2003; 58:844–853.

Faith A, Richards DF, Verhoef A, Lamb JR, Lee TH, Hawrylowicz CM. Impaired secretion of interleukin-4 and interleukin-13 by allergen-specific T cells correlates with defective nuclear expression of NF-AT2 and jun B: relevance to immunotherapy. Clin Exp Allergy 2003;33:1209–1215.

Fenoglio D, Puppo F, Cirillo I, Vizzaccaro A, Ferrera A, Tosca MA et al. Sublingual specific immunotherapy reduces PBMC proliferations. Eur Ann Allergy Clin Immunol 2005;37:147–151.

Fiocchi A, Pajno G, La Grutta S, Pezzuto F, Incorvaia C, et al. Safety of sublingual-swallow immunotherapy in children aged 3 to 7 years. Ann Allergy Asthma immunology. 2005;95:254 -258.

Flicker S, Valenta R. Renaissance of the blocking antibody concept in type I allergy. Int Arch Allergy Immunol 2003;132:13–24.

Frew AJ, Smith HE. Sublingual immunotherapy. J Allergy Clin Immunol 2001;107:441–444.

Gabrielsson S, Soderlund A, Paulie S, van der Pouw Kraan TC, Troye- Blomberg M, Rak S. Specific immunotherapy prevents increased levels of allergen-specific IL-4 and IL-13-producing cells during pollen season. Allergy 2001; 56:293–300.

Gambineri E, Torgerson T, Ochs H. Immune dysregulation, polyendocrinopathy, enteropathy, and X-linked inheritance (IPEX), a syndrome of systemic autoimmunity caused by mutations of Foxp3, a critical regulator of T cell homeostasis. Curr Opin Rhumatol 2003; 15:430–435.

Gentile D, Schreiber R, Howe-Adams J, Trecki J, Patel A, Angelini B et al. Diminished dendritic cell interleukin 10 production in atopic children. Ann Allergy Asthma Immunol 2004; 92:538- 544.

Grindebacke H, Wing K, Andersson AC, Suri-Payer E, Rak S, Rudin A. Defective suppression of Th2 cytokines by CD4+CD25+ regulatory T cells in birch allergics during birch pollen season. Clin Exp Allergy 2004; 34:1364- 1372.

Grosclaude M, Bouillot P, Alt R, Leynadier F, Scheinmann P, Rufin P et al. Safety of various dosage regimens during induction of sublingual immunotherapy. Int Arch Allergy Immunol 2002;129:248–253.

Guerra F, Carracedo J, Solana-Lara R, Sanchez-Guijo P, Ramirez R. Th2 lymphocytes from atopic patients treated with immunotherapy undergo rapid apoptosis after culture with specific allergens. J Allergy Clin Immunol 2001; 107:647–653.

Hankin C, Cox L,Lang D. Allergen immunotherapy and health care cost benefits for children with allergic rhinitis: a large-scale, retrospective, matched cohort study Ann Allergy Asthma Immunol. 2010;104:79–85.

Hawrylowicz CM, O'Garra A. Potential role of interleukin-10 secreting regulatory T cells in allergy and asthma. Nature Rev Immunol 2005; 5:271–283.

Ippoliti F, De Santis W, Volterrani A, Lenti L, Canitano N, Lucarelli S et al. Immunomodulation during sublingual therapy in allergic children. Pediatr Allergy Immunol 2003;14:216–221.

Juniper EF, Thompson AK, Ferrie PJ, Roberts JN. Validation of the standardized version of the Rhinoconjunctivitis Quality of Life Questionnaire. J Allergy Clin Immunol 1999;104:364–369.

Laaksonen K, Junikka M, Lahesmaa R, Terho EO, Savolainen J. In vitro allergen-induced mRNA expression of signaling lymphocytic activation molecule by PBMC of patients with allergic rhinitis is increased during specific pollen immunotherapy. J Allergy Clin Immunol 2003; 112:1171–1177.

Ling EM. Relation of CD4+CD25+ regulatory T-cell suppression of allergen-driven T-cell activation to atopic status and expression of allergic disease.Lancet 2004; 363:608–615.

Lemanske R, Jackson DJ, Gangnon RE, et al. Rhinovirus illnesses during infancy predict subsequent childhood wheezing. J Allergy Clin Immunol 2005; 116: 571-7

Ling EM, Smith T, Nguyen XD, Pridgeon C, Dallman M, et al. Relation of CD4+CD25+ regulatory T-cell suppression of allergen-driven T-cell activation to atopic status and expression of allergic disease. Lancet 2004; 363:608–615.

Mahr T. Therapy in allergic rhinoconjunctivitis: New horizons. Allergy Asthma Proc 28:404 –409, 2007; doi: 10.2500/aap.2007.28.3012).

Malling HJ, Lund L, Ipsen H, Poulsen LK. Safety and immunological changes during tablet based specific immunotherapy. J Allergy Clin Immunol 2005;115:S161.

Marcucci F, Sensi L, Frati F, Senna GE, Canonica GW, Parmiani S et al. Sublingual tryptase and ECP in children treated with grass pollen sublingual immunotherapy (SLIT): safety and immunologic implications. Allergy 2001; 56:1091–1095.

Marcucci F, Frati F, Bernardini R, Novembre E, Barbato A, Pecora S. Effects on inflammation parameters of a double blind, placebo controlled one year course of SLIT in children monosensitized to mites. Allergy 2003; 58:657–662.

Martin-Fotecha A, Sebastiani S, Hopken U, Uguccioni M, Lipp M, et al. Regulation of dendritic cell migration to the draining lymph node: impact on T lymphocyte traffic and priming. J Exp Med 2003; 198:615–621.

Mçsges R, Klimek L. Todays allergic rhinitis patients are different: new factors that may play a role. Allergy 2007: 62: 969–975.

Meltzer E. The Relationships of Rhinitis and Asthma. Allergy and Asthma Proc 2005; 26:336 –340.

Moingeon P, Batard T, Fadel R, Frati F, Sieber L. Immune mechanisms of allergen-specific sublingual immunotherapy Allergy 2006; 61: 151–165.

Moller C, Dreborg S, Ferdousi HA, Halken S, Host A, Jacobsen L et al. Pollen immunotherapy reduces the development of asthma in children with seasonal rhinoconjunctivitis (the PATStudy). J Allergy Clin Immunol 2002;109:251–256.

Mothes N, Heinzkill M, Drachenberg KJ, Sperr WR, Krauth MT, Majlesi Y et al. Allergen-specific immunotherapy with a monophosphoryl lipid A-adjuvanced vaccine: reduced seasonnaly boosted immunoglobulin E production and inhibition of basophil histamine release by therapy-induced blocking antibodies. Clin Exp Allergy 2003;33:1198–1208.

Nascimento Silva M, Naspitz C, Sole D. Evaluation of quality of life in children and teenagers with allergic rhinitis: adaptation and validation of the Rhinoconjunctivitis Quality of Life Questionnaire (RQLQ). Allergol Immunopathol 2001;29: 111-118.

Ng Man Kwong G, Proctor A, Billings C, et al. Increasing prevalence of asthma diagnosis and symptoms in children is confined to mild symptoms. Thorax 2001; 56: 312-314.

Niederberger V, Horak F, Vrtala S, Spitzauer S, Krauth MT, Valent P et al. Vaccination with genetically engineered allergens prevents progression of allergic disease. Proc Natl Acad Sci USA 2004;101(Suppl. 2):14677–14682.

Oldfield WL, Larche´ M, Kay AB. Effect of T-cell peptides derived from Fel d 1 on allergic reactions and cytokine production in patients sensitive to cats: a randomised controlled trial. Lancet 2002; 360:47–53.

Passalacqua G, Guerra L, Compalati E, Canonica GW. The safety of allergen specific sublingual immunotherapy. Curr Drug Saf. 2007;2: 117–123.

Pichler CE, Helbling A, Pichler WJ. Three years of specific immunotherapy with house-dust-mite extracts in patients with rhinitis and asthma: significant improvement of allergen-specific parameters and of non-specific bronchial hyperreactivity. Allergy 2001;56:301–306.

Pijnenburg MW, Hofhuis W, Hop WC, de Jonste JC. Exhaled nitric oxide predicts asthma relapse in children with clinical asthma remission. Thorax. 2005;60:215-218.

Penagos M, Passalacqua G, Compalati E et al. Metaanalysis of the efficacy of sublingual immunotherapy in the treatment of allergic asthma in pediatric patients, 3 to 18 years of age. Chest. 2008;133:599–609.

Radic S, Zivkovic Z, Cerovic S, Calovic O, Rodic V, Drobnjak M, Jocic-Stojanovic J, Maksimovic T. Relationship between time of the first exacerbation of childhood asthma and asthma prognosis at the age of 30. ERS Annual Congress, Vienna, Austria 2009; P1245, 217s

Rienzo VD, Minelli M, Musarra A, Sambugaro R, Pecora S, et al. Post-marketing survey on the safety of sublingual immunotherapy in children below the age of 5 years. Clin Exp Allergy. 2005;35:560 -564.

Robinson DS, Larch´e M, Durham SR, Tregs and allergic disease. J Clin Invest 2004;114:1389–1397.

Rodic V, Cerovic S, Zivkovic Z, Radic S, Milanovic V, Lakovic G, Veljkovic P Uticaj pušenja na udruženu pojavu alergijskog rinitisa, atopijskog dermatitisa i astme. IV Kongress pedijatara Srbije i Crne Gore , Novi Sad, 2006; 406-407.

Rodriguez-Santos O. Sublingual immunotherapy for Allergic rhinitis and asthma in children from two to five years of age with mite allergy. Revista Allergia Mexico. 2008;55:71–75.

Rolinck-Werninghaus C, Kopp M, Liebke C, Lange J, Wahn U, Niggemann B. Lack of detectable alterations in immune responses during sublingual immunotherapy in children with seasonal allergic rhinoconjunctivitis to grass pollen. Int Arch Allergy Immunol 2005;136:134–141

Santos CB, Pratt EL, Hanks C, McCann J, Craig TJ. Allergic rhinitis and its effect on sleep, fatigue, and daytime somnolence. Ann Allergy Asthma Immunol. 2006;97:579–586;

Sigurs N, Gustafsson PM, Bjarnason R, Lundberg F, Schmidt S, Sigurbergsson F, Kjellman B. Severe respiratory syncytial virus bronchiolitis in infancy and asthma and allergy at age 13. Am J Respir Crit Care Med. 2005; 171: 137-41.

Silvestri M, Spallarossa D, Battistini E et al. Changes in inflammatory and clinical parameters and in bronchial hyperreactivity in asthmatic children sensitized to house dust mites following sublingual immunotherapy. J Invest Allergol Clin Immunol 2002;12:52–59. Sub-Lingual Immunotherapy World Allergy Organization:Position Paper.*2009*

Sundberg R, Toren K, Hoglund D et al. Nasal symptoms are associated with school performance in adolescents. J Adolesc Health. 2007; 40:581–583.

Taylor A, Verhagen J, Akdis CA, Akdis M. T regulatory cells in allergy and health: a question of allergen specificity and balance. Int Arch Allergy Immunol 2004;135:73–82.

Torres Lima M, Wilson D, Pitkin L, Roberts A, Nouri-Aria K, Jacobson M et al. Grass pollen sublingual immunotherapy for seasonal rhinoconjunctivitis: a randomized controlled trial. Clin Exp Allergy 2002; 32:507–514.

Valovirta E, Jacobsen L, Ljorring C, Koivikko A, Savolainen J. Clinical efficacy and safety of sublingual immunotherapy with tree pollen extract in children. Allergy. 2006;61:1177–1183.

Van Helvoort JM, Samsom J, Chantry D, Jansen W, Schadee-Eestermans I,Thepen T et al. Preferential expression of IgG2b in nose draining cervical lymph nodes and its putative role in mucosal tolerance induction. Allergy 2004; 59:1211–1218.

von Bubnoff D, Fimmers R, Bogdanov M, Matz H, Koch S, et al. Asymptomatic atopy is associated with increased indoleamine 2,3-dioxygenase activity and interleukin 10 production during seasonal allergen exposure. Clin Exp Allergy 2004; 34:1056–1063.

Wachholz PA, Durham SR. Induction of blocking IgG antibodies during immunotherapy. Clin Exp Allergy 2003; 33:1171–1174.

Walker S, Khan-Wasti S, Fletcher M et al.Seasonal allergic rhinitis is associated with a detrimental effect on examination performance in United Kingdom teenagers: case-control study. J Allergy Clin Immunol. 2007; 120:381–387.

Wahn U, Tabar A, Kuna P, Halken S, Montagut A, et al. Efficacy and safety of 5-grass-pollen sublingual immunotherapy tablets in pediatric allergic rhinoconjunctivitis. J Allergy Clin Immunology 2009;123:160–166.

Weiner HL. Induction and mechanism of action of transforming growth factorbeta-secreting Th3 regulatory cells. Immunol Rev 2001; 182:207–214.

Wilson D, Torres Lima M, Durham S. Sublingual immunotherapy for allergic rhinitis. Cochrane Database Syst Rev 2003;2:CD002893.

Yazdanbakhsh M, Kremsner PG, Van Ree R. Allergy, parasites and the hygiene hypothesis. Science 2002; 296:490– 494.

Zivkovic Z, Vukasinovic Z, Cerovic S, Radulovic S, Zivanovic S, Panic E, Hadnadjev M, Adzovic Prevalence of childhood asthma and allergies in Serbia and Montenegro. World J Pediatr 2010; 6 (4): 331-336.

Zivkovic Z, Cerovic S, Vukasinovic Z, Jocic-Stojanovic J. News in treatment of childhood asthma. Srp Arh Celok Lek 2009; 137 (9-10):558-561.

Zivkovic Z, Cerovic S, Jocic-Stojanovic J, Sedlarevic I, Radic S, Smiljanic S, Micic-Stanojevic M, Andric A. Predicting exacerbations: asthma, allergy and exhaled NO. ERS Annual Congress, Vienna, Austria 2009; P2154, 371s.

Zivkovic Z, Cerovic S, Jocic-Stojanovic J, Sedlarevic I, Radic S, Smiljanic S, Micic-Stanojevic M, Andric A.The effects of gender and age on exhaled nitric oxide in children with asthma. ERS Annual Congress, Vienna, Austria 2009; P4093, 734s

Zivkovic Z, Radic S, Cerovic S, Vukasinovic Z. Asthma School Program in children and their parents. World J Pediatr 2008; 4:267-273.

3

The Impact of Allergic Rhinitis on Asthma: Current View

Betül Ayşe Sin
Ankara University, School of Medicine, Department of Pulmonary Diseases, Division of Immunology and Allergy, Ankara Turkey

1. Introduction

Although allergic rhinitis and asthma have been assessed and treated as separate diseases, they often occur together. The connection between asthma and rhinitis is not a new discovery. This association has been recognized since earlier times. In the second century, Galen hypothesized that sinonasal disease caused lung disease through a direct anatomic connection. But, the nature of the link between the nose and the lung has been poorly understood until recent years (McFadden, 1986). Because the prevalence rates of rhinitis and asthma, as with all allergic diseases, are increasing worldwide, there is a growing interest in the interaction between upper and lower airways (Bousquet et al.,ARIA Workshop Group. World Health Organization, 2001).

Allergic rhinitis (AR) is the most common atopic disease all over the world affecting almost 10% to 30% of population (Berger, 2003; Settipane, 2003). Although it generally is not considered a severe disorder, the socioeconomic costs of AR are substantial . It adversely affects quality of life of the patients, work productivity and school performance as well as increasing health care costs (Bachert et al., 2002; Meltzer et al., 2004). Patients who have asthma and rhinitis tend to have more severe disease with higher treatment costs. Treatment of rhinitis may improve asthma control, and early treatment of allergies may prevent the development of asthma (Marple, 2010).

The connection between upper and lower airways has become a topic of great interest over the past few decades. It is now well established that rhinitis and asthma frequently co-exist, with approximately 20-50% of AR patients have concomitant asthma and over the 80% of asthmatics have nasal symptoms (Bousquet et al., 2003; Braunstahl & Fokkens, 2003).

During this time of period, a body of evidence concerning the relationship between allergic rhinitis and asthma lead to the concept of unified airways or "one airway one disease". Recent advances in the understanding and knowledge of the underlying mechanisms has been integrated into the "Allergic rhinitis and its impact on asthma" international report (Bousquet et al., ARIA Workshop, 2001). This document have been provided an comprehensive overview of current knowledge on allergic rhinitis and asthma, and evidence-based guidelines for the treatment. Neverthless not all patients with rhinitis present with asthma, the reason why are unknown. The "united airway disease" hypothesis proposes that upper and lower airway disease are both manifestations of a single inflammatory process of entire respiratory tract (Togias, 2003).

2. Epidemiologic evidences

Several cross-sectional studies have demonstrated that allergic rhinitis, rhinosinusitis and asthma frequently coexist in the same patients, despite some methodologic limitations (Leynaert et al., 2000). In fact, allergic rhinitis is a ubiquitous disorder in patients with asthma. Because the prevalence of allergic rhinitis among patients with asthma is as high as 90% when the diagnosis of rhinitis was made by using strict diagnostic criteria. (Kapsali et al.,1997). The prevalence of allergic rhinitis among patients with asthma is as much as 80% which is significantly higher than the 20% prevalence rate in the general population. However, up to 40% of patients with allergic rhinitis suffer from asthma symptoms but only 5% to 10% of the general population (Danielsson & Jessen, 1997).

The Copenhagen Allergy Study investigated the frequency of asthma and rhinitis related to exposure to pollen, animal dander or mites. For people with pollen allergy, 41% of those with pollen-related rhinitis also had pollen-related asthma. Pollen-related asthma was almost not present (0.1%) in those without pollen-related rhinitis (Linneberg et al., 2001). Most patients with asthma have complaints of seasonal or perennial allergic rhinitis. It has been shown however, that perennial rhinitis is a risk factor for asthma, independent of allergy. By investigating cross-sectional data from the European Community Respiratory Health Survey. Leynaert et al found the adjusted odds ratios for the association between perennial rhinitis and asthma to be 8.1 among atopic and 11.6 among nonatopic subjects 20 to 44 years old. (Leynaert et al.,1999). Similarly, Guerra et al reported that the presence of rhinitis had a strong predictive value for the adult-onset asthma in both atopic and nonatopic patients regarding to skin test responses . In their study, there was a tendency of more stronger in the group of subjects with high total IgE levels (Guerra et al., 2002).

3. Etiopathogenesis

Allergic disorders such as allergic rhinitis and asthma, have a multifactorial origin. Both diseases are characterized by chronic airway inflammation based on common genetic and environmental factors. Rhinitis and asthma are often co-exist, and they share common causative risk factors including genetic such as atopy, and environmental exposure. Same triggers that provoke the diseases of the nose and the lungs contribute to the development of the allergic airway syndrome, and comprise inhalant allergens, viral infection, cold-dry air, tobacco smoke and air pollution (Bachert et al., 2004; Braunstahl, 2005; Slavin, 2008).

The inflammation is a central component of both conditions, in which eosinophils, mast cells and T-lymphocytes are predominant effector cells. As antigen-presenting cells, dendritic cells form a network that is localized within the epithelium and submucosa of the entire respiratory mucosa, capture allergens, break them into allergenic peptides, and migrate to lymph nodes, where they present them to naive CD4+ T lymphocytes. After sensitization process and production of allergen specific IgE antibodies by B cells, their binding to high-affinity IgE receptors (FcεRI) on the surface of mast cells and basophils, rendering them "sensitized". Within minutes of contact of sensitized individuals with allergens, the IgE-allergen interaction takes place, leading to mast cell and basophil degranulation and the release of preformed mediators such as histamine and tryptase, and the *de novo* generation of other mediators, including cysteinyl leukotrienes (CysLTs) and prostaglandins, some of which induce the early-phase symptoms. The late-phase response is characterized by the recruitment and activation of inflammatory cells like eosinophils, basophils and T cells into the mucosa of end-organ. This infiltration of inflammatory cells can also be orchestrated by

T-helper type 2 (Th2) cells within the local microenvironment. It is likely that cell migration is due to the chemokines and cytokines released by the primary effector cells acutely and over several hours after allergen exposure leading to chronic on-going inflammation and the development of hyperresponsiveness (Rimmer & Ruhno, 2006; Sin & Togias, 2011).

The natural course of atopic disorders is called the "atopic march". It has been suggested that atopic dermatitis is a starting point for subsequent allergic disease according to this theory (Spergel, 2005). The German Multicenter Atopy study evaluated the atopic march in 1314 children during a 7-year study period. The authors found that 46% of children with severe atopic dermatitis had an increased risk of early wheezing compared to patients with mild atopic dermatitis (32%) (Lau et al.,2002). However, another study of Illi S et al was found to be not completely consistent with the hypothesis in which atopic dermatitis preceded wheezing in 56% whereas wheezing preceded atopic dermatitis in 33% (Illi et al.,2004). Furthermore, the presence of BHR and rhinitis or both for the development of clinical asthma has traditionally been interpreted as the progression of a common airway diseases because they are associated with atopic background.

Yet, the question remains as to why some individuals only manifest symptoms of rhinitis and not asthma. The hypothesis would be that those patients may still be part of the continuum, but have a milder form of the disease. If so, not only are their lower airways less affected (no asthma), but their upper airways should be less severe as well (Pawankar, 2006). In supporting this hypothesis, Hanes et al, have reported that patients with AR and concomitant asthma showed more severe nasal symptoms when they were exposed to cold-dry air than if they had AR alone (Hanes et al., 2006).

4. Clinical aspects

Asthma and rhinitis also represent the two ends of the clinical spectrum in the respiratory tract in which have wide range of changing severity. Allergic rhinitis alone without bronchial hyperresponsiveness is a mildest form of the spectrum (Togias, 2003). However, from previous studies also known that patients with rhinitis and no clinical evidence of asthma may have BHR to inhaled allergens and chemical or physical stimulants (Ramsdale, et al.,1985). Some individuals with allergic rhinitis exhibit only seasonal lung symptoms. This patients have been shown increased bronchial reactivity during the natural exposure or experimental setting to allergen and also nonspecific stimuli as well which may be thought as subclinical asthma (Boulet et al., 1989). Therefore, presence of BHR accompanying allergic or non-allergic rhinitis is considered as high risk factor for onset of asthma on follow-up. But, the factors that determine the progression of rhinitis to asthma are not yet clear.

The effect of rhinitis on the onset of asthma has been investigated in longitudinal studies. The one study of the Settipane et al, which had a 23-year follow-up, demonstrated that allergic rhinitis at inclusion resulted in a 3-fold risk of asthma development compared to the group without rhinitis (Settipane et al., 1994). Similarly, patients aged 18 to 45 years with hay fever have been shown to be at increased risk for asthma in a prospective cohort study in Finland (Huovinen et al., 1999).

Patients with rhinitis have been reported three times more likely to develop asthma than healthy control subjects. Therefore, it is suggested that rhinitis is an important risk factor for the development of asthma, especially when bronchial hyperresponsiveness (BHR) is present.

One of the main clinical features of asthma is an increase in non-specific airway hyperresponsiveness to methacholine or histamine. However, BHR can be present in some patients with allergic rhinitis without clinical evidence of asthma when exposed to an allergen to which they were sensitized (Boulay & Boulet, 2003). However, which factors determine BHR in these subjects are clearly unknown. The development of BHR can depend on duration of an inflammatory process, such as the one that has been described in the lower airways of adult subjects with allergic rhinitis, or on other factors. BHR seems to reflect not only the airway inflammation but also the remodelling process. (Foresi et al., 1997; Polosa et al., 2000).

BHR among patients with hay fever has been shown to increase during the pollen season and to be predictive of the onset of lower airway symptoms (Braman et al., 1987; Madonini et al., 1987). In a study of Prieto et al, airway responsiveness to either methacholine or adenosine monophosphate was found significantly increased in patients with allergic rhinitis alone during the season compared with out of the pollen season. In addition, BHR in the asthmatic range was detected during the season in these subjects (Prieto et al., 2002). A recent paper by Sin et al. showed that in contrast to the population with both allergic rhinitis and asthma, patients with seasonal allergic rhinitis alone did not show a higher degree of airway hyperresponsiveness to exercise challenge test when compared to the methacholine challenge test during the pollen season (Sin et al., 2009).

Furthermore, Ciprandi et al, evaluated patients with perennial allergic rhinitis symptoms alone. The authors observed that 54 patients out of 100 showed positive methacholine challenge test and impairment of spirometric parameters especially reduced forced expiratory flow at 25 and 75% of pulmonary volume (FEF_{25-75}) values as a sensitive measure of lower airways (Ciprandi et al., 2004). A study of patients with allergic rhinitis showed impaired lung function. A lack of bronchodilator response to deep inhalation is a characteristic physiological abnormality of asthmatic patients. People with rhinitis had blunted response to a deep inhalation suggesting altered airway smooth muscle function (Skloot & Togias, 2003).

It has also been shown that BHR was associated with longer duration of AR and more severe nasal inflammation in the absence of asthma symptoms. Based on these data, the current concept is that AR precedes asthma in most patients, and worsening of one disease negatively affects the course of asthma. It has been postulated that patients with asthma and broad extent symptoms of rhinitis may have more severe asthma than those asthmatic patients who have minimal or no rhinitis (DREAMS study). From this point of view, it has been suggested that the severity of rhinitis and asthma follows a parallel track in correlation with the overall severity of the chronic allergic respiratory syndrome that allows for cross-talk between the upper and lower airways (Togias, 2003).

Allergic rhinitis may also be contributing factor in 25% to 30% of patients with acute maxillary sinusitis and in as many as 60% to 80% of patients with chronic sinusitis (Spector, 1997). At least, allergic rhinitis is associated with, and probably a predisposing factor in the development of rhinosinusitis (Meltzer et al., 2004). Despite the pathophysiologic link between allergic rhinitis and asthma have been well-studied, understanding of paranasal sinus diseases and its possible relationship with asthma still remain largely unclear. Chronic upper airway diseases include allergic rhinitis, non-allergic rhinitis (NAR), chronic rhinosinusitis (CRS) with and without nasal polyposis, and occupational rhinitis. They are commonly associated with asthma, and increase the complexity of management and costs Bousquet et al., 2009). The overall prevalence of CRS have been reported 10.9% in Europe and it was found to be more common in smokers.

In children, nasal sinus disease may lead to less asthma control. Peroni et al. studied the CT findings in children with severe asthma. They concluded that severe asthma patients appear to have the most relevant abnormalities on CT scanning of the paranasal sinuses (Peroni et al., 2007).

Co-morbidity of other upper airway diseases including chronic rhinosinusitis with or without nasal polyps have also been linked to asthma severity. Many studies have reported that the severity of nasal and sinus disease parallel that of the lower airway disease (Pearlman et al., 2009; Ponte et al., 2008). On the other hand, the presence of nasal polyposis accompanying chronic rhinosinusitis and the duration of diseases were found to be correlated with extensive paranasal sinus computed tomography findings, and were related to the severity of asthma in adults (Dursun et al., 2006).

Sinus disease and lower airway comorbidity often present as severe clinical symptoms of the diseases such as nasal polyps, aspirin-exacerbated respiratory disease (AERD), and late-onset severe intrinsic asthma. However, many patients with aspirin hypersensitivity appear with SCUAD (extensive nasal polyposis and anosmia) and accompanying severe asthma (Bousquet et al., 2009).

AERD is a clinical syndrome combining from nasal polyps, chronic hypertrophic eosinophilic sinusitis, asthma and sensitivity to aspirin and other non-steroidal anti-inflammatory drugs that inhibits cyclooxygenase-1 (COX-1) enzymes. Its prevalence rises to 10-20% of asthmatics and up to 30-40% in those asthmatics with nasal polyposis despite occurring in 0.3-0.9% of the general population. Asthma may precede the sinonasal disease or develop later. Patients with AERD suffer from frequent attacks of upper and lower airway reactions such as nasal congestion with anosmi, rhinorrhea, progression to pansinusitis and nasal polyps, and also bronchospasm (Lee et al., 2011). Nasal polyps are consistently associated with severe asthma. It has been reported that patients with nasal polyposis and asthma have the highest rates of exacerbation and hospital admissions (Ceylan et al., 2007).

In fact, most severe forms of both upper and lower airway disease may occur in nonatopic patients. AERD develops according to a pattern, characterized by a sequence of symptoms. First, persistent rhinitis, appearing at a mean age of 29 years, then asthma, aspirin intolerance, and finally nasal polyposis. In half of the patients, asthma is severe, and steroid dependent (Szczeklik et al., 2000).

5. Proposed mechanisms for the interaction between upper and lower airways

The mechanisms by which allergic rhinitis may be a risk factor for asthma are not entirely understood, although a few studies have addressed this question. It seems that allergic rhinitis and asthma result from similar inflammatory processes induced by allergens in the upper as well as in the lower airways of sensitized subjects. The nose and lung should thus be seen as a continuum, with "information" travelling in both directions, rather than as two distinct compartments. In this regard, the concept of "united airways" has been proposed, and increasing numbers of studies have agreed with this model (Boulay & Boulet, 2003; Rimmer & Ruhno, 2006). The main difference between the upper and lower airways is that upper airway patency is largely influenced by vascular tone, whereas, in the lower airway, airflow is influenced predominantly by smooth muscle function. Despite some anatomical differences between asthma and rhinitis, they share common airway mucosa and epithelium with similar immunopathological features (Rowe-Jones, 1997). Both diseases are characterized by chronic inflammation of the entire respiratory mucosa and involve similar inflammatory process. Many cells and cellular elements play a role in particular, mast cells, eosinophils, T lymphocytes (Th2, Tregulatory), macrophages and epithelial cells (Bourdin et al., 2009; KleinJan, et al, 2010; Sin & Togias, 2011). Several potential mechanisms have been proposed to explain the interaction between the nose and the lung. Among them, some strong evidences suggest that not only local or neural-vascular, but also systemic induction of inflammatory cells is involved in this relationship. Indeed, cells (Th2 effector cells), cytokines, chemokines and mediators from the upper airways are drained by the systemic circulation and can subequently affect tissues at a distance. In this regard, bidirectional relationship also exists between upper and lower airways. Although the precise mechanisms have not yet been elucidated in naso-bronchial cross-talk, there appear to be important links (Fasano, 2010; Togias, 2000, 2003).

One of them is that of a shift from nasal to mouth breathing due to the nasal congestion. In AR, loss of nasal warming, humidifying and filtering functions may result in an increased exposure of the lower airways to allergens and irritants. This condition may lead to inflammatory changes and an increase in BHR in susceptible subjects. As another possible explanations are the aspiration of nasal contents or secretions and the nasobronchial reflex (Alvarez et al., 2000; Togias, 1999). Today, most data suggest a systemic link between mucosal sites, involving bloodstream, bone marrow and the lymphoid tissues. Several studies using nasal allergen challenge models have demonstrated that patients with allergic rhinitis alone may have inflammatory changes within the lower airways such as increased sputum eosinophils which is suggestive as predictor of asthma (Braunstahl et al., 2001; Inal et al., 2008; Sin et al., 2002). In keeping with the united airways concept, it has been shown that provocation with relevant allergens of the nose induces lower airway inflammation. Indeed, Braunstahl et al., demonstrated that nasal allergen challenge results in an increase of eosinophils as well as increased expression of intercellular adhesion molecule-1 in both nasal and bronchial biopsies of allergic rhinitis patients without asthma. (Braunstahl et al., 2001a). In another study of these authors, a decrease in the mast cell numbers in the nose has been detected 24 h after segmental bronchoprovocation with allergen in nonasthmatic patients with allergic rhinitis, interpreted as a result of enhanced degranulation. At the same time, there was evidence for an influx of basophils from the blood into the nasal and bronchial mucosa. (Braunstahl et al.,2001b). Similarly, in patients with asthma, nasal biopsies showed eosinophilic inflammation, even in those who do not have symptoms of rhinitis. (Gaga et al., 2000).

As a similar phenomenon, segmental bronchial allergen challenge in nonasthmatic patients with allergic rhinitis induces increased numbers of nasal eosinophils, IL-5 expression in nasal epithelium and eotaxin-positive cells in nasal lamina propria (Braunstahl et al., 2000). Therofore, investigators concluded that the inflammatory response following allergen challenge is not restricted to a local effect. Systemic propogation of allergic inflammation from the nasal to the lower airway mucosa has been proposed to explain the rhinitis and asthma link (Togias, 1999, 2003). Local absorption of inflammatory mediators at the site of initial inflammation presumably leads to a more generalized systemic response involving mucosa-associated lymphoid-tissue and bone-marrow as well. (Braunstahl & Hellings, 2006).

Two parts of the systemic aspect are the systemic circulation and the nervous system. They probably include classical mediators of the acute allergic reaction, production of several cytokines and chemokines, the vascular endothelium and adhesion molecules, antigen-presenting dendritic cells and their interaction with T-lymphocytes, as well as a strong bone marrow component. (Togias, 2004). Furthermore, local tissue factors, such as microbial stimuli and systemic inflammatory mechanisms appear to have a role in the clinical expression of the allergic airway diseases. Increasing evidence indicates a major involvement of airway epithelial cells in the pathogenesis of both rhinitis and asthma (Compalati et al., 2010).

Chronic airway inflammation has been considered an important hallmark in both asthma and rhinitis. However, collagen deposition to upper airways is not typically observed in the allergic rhinitis in contrast to the bronchi. Very few studies have investigated upper and lower airways simultaneously. Even increased basement membrane thickness together with eosinophilic inflammation was also shown in the bronchial mucosa of atopic nonasthmatics and allergic rhinitis alone (Chakir et al., 1996). In a publication by Ediger et al., authors reported that infiltration of inflammatory cells particularly eosinophils both in the nasal and the bronchial tissues obtained from same subjects do not remarkably differ between patients with nasal polyp alone without BHR and asthmatic patients with nasal polyp (Ediger et al., 2005).

Recent studies suggest that the *Staphylococcus aureus* enterotoxins (SAEs) may act as superantigens by amplifying eosinophilic inflammation and possibly inducing local IgE formation in severe persistent airway disease in AERD (Kowalski et al., 2011). Bachert et al also reported that within the group for chronic rhinosinusitis with nasal polyp, patients with Th_2-biased eosinophilic inflammation have increased risk of severe asthma development (Bachert et al., 2010). However, nasal tissue and bronchial biopsies reveal extensive eosinophilic infiltration and degranulated mast cells in patients with AERD. Furthermore, once the disease established, production of proinflammatory cytokines and Th_2 type cytokines (IL-2, IL-3, IL-4, IL-5, IL-13, GM-CSF) have been found to be increased. Most patients with AERD synthesize excessive amounts of leukotrienes even before the exposure the disease. Recent evidences showed high expression of transforming growth factor beta (TGF-β) and the deposition of collagen in CRS with or without nasal polyp (Stevenson et al., 2006). Furthermore, increased epithelial desquamation has also been detected in the lower airways of atopic subjects, even before the onset of clinical symptoms whereas no structural changes was found in the nasal mucosa of allergic patients despite the presence of inflammatory cells (Braunstahl et al., 2003). The reasons why remodeling appears to be less extensive in the nasal mucosa than in the bronchial mucosa are still unclear (Bousquet et al., 2004).

6. Therapeutic implications

AR, even though not a serious disease, is a clinically relevant while it may responsible for some complications and affects quality of life. In a number of retrospective database analyses, the severity of allergic rhinitis was demonstrated to be directly correlated with asthma severity. Those patients whose allergic rhinitis was mild or well controlled, had better asthma control. Therefore, this data suggest that effective treatment of one disease may improve the other (Henriksen & Wenzel, 1984; Ponte et al, 2008).

The study by Crystal-Peters et al. was a retrospective cohort design to evaluate the treatment effects of AR on asthma-related health care resource utilization. In their analysis, the risk of emergency room visit or hospitalization due to the acute asthma attacks was almost 50% lower for patients treated with nasal steroids or oral antihistamines compared to those who did not receive these drugs (Crystal-Peters et al., 2002). Moreover, another studies have demonstrated that among patients with asthma and concomitant AR, those receiving therapy for AR have a significantly lower risk of subsequent asthma-related events than those not treated. (Bousquet et al., 2005; Corren et al., 2004).

In a study conducted by Shaaban et al, it has been shown that subjects with rhinitis sensitized to indoor allergens such as mites or cat, were probably at increased onset of BHR. The authors also reported that BHR remission was more frequent in patients with rhinitis treated by nasal steroids than in those not treated. (Shaaban et al., 2007).

Although rhinosinusitis plays an important role in initiating or exacerbating asthma, there is no concensus whether its treatment is effective on asthma control. Some authors considered rhinosinusitis as a trigger factor, whereas others support the idea of comorbidity. (Smart, 2006). In either case, rhinosinusitis has been shown to worsen the symptoms of asthma. Therefore, controlling upper airway infection, inflammation, and symptoms may also improve the asthma outcomes (Pawankar & Zernotti, 2009). Both medical therapy and sinus surgery has been found to have a positive impact on improvement of asthma. (Ragab et al., 2006).

In some cases, the presence of upper airway inflammation like sinus disease or nasal polyposis renders the clinical course of asthma more severe and treatment more cumbersome. Several studies demonstrated that appropriate treatment of sinonasal disease reduces lower airway symptomatology, and improves asthma control (Dixon, 2009). Management options for AERD are the standard medical and surgical interventions with complete avoidance of COX-1 inhibiting drugs or aspirin desensitization and continuously receiving aspirin drug (Lee et al., 2011). Patients mostly require long-term therapy with oral corticosteroids. Furthermore, leukotriene modifiers improve the control of asthma in patients using high dose inhaled corticosteroids (Bousquet et al., 2009).

Nasal therapy has a beneficial effect on bronchial hyperresponsiveness and airway inflammation. (Corren et al., 1992). In a recent study, the combination of intranasal and intrabronchial administration of corticosteroid preparation has been resulted in the highest reduction of blood eosinophil count and serum ECP, and better quality of life as well. (Nair et al.,2010). Scichilone et al., reported that in patients with allergic rhinitis and mild asthma, intranasal corticosteroids caused important fall in nasal eosinophils and effective asthma control associated with improvement in health- related quality of life. (Scichilone et al., 2011). However, although optimal medical treatment of allergic rhinitis is known to be a prerequisite for a good therapeutic result in asthma, it remains to be clarify whether early and timely introduction of drugs may prevent the progression to asthma. (Koh & Kim, 2003). Allergen specific immunotherapy has demonstrated benefit in allergic rhinitis and allergic asthma in appropriately selected patients. It may also prevent the subsequent development of asthma and new sensitizations in children. (Fiocchi & Fox, 2010; Pipet et al., 2009). Furthermore, patients with moderate to severe persistant allergic asthma has been observed to achieve significant additional clinical benefit for their symptoms of concomitant allergic rhinitis and improvement in quality of life after receiving Omalizumab, a recombinant, humanized, monoclonal anti-IgE antibody. (Humbert et al., 2009; Vignola et al., 2004).

Better understanding of mechanisms related to inflammation in the nose and the lung has lead to combined therapeutic approaches targeting both diseases. (Greenberger, 2008; Nathan, 2009). Current ARIA guidelines strongly encourage dual evaluation of these patients and given therapies. Therefore, the effectively treatment of upper airway disease can significantly improve established asthma outcomes as well as may prevent the future development of asthma (Brozek et al., 2010). Consequently, a therapy that addresses the systemic aspects of AR is more beneficial than a therapy with only local effects because it improves both AR and concomitant inflammatory disorders that might be present. (Borish, 2003).

It should be emphasized that because upper and lower airway diseases commonly comorbid conditions, it is important to consider the respiratory system as an integrated unit. By increasing the awareness of sinonasal and lung involvement in any patient, appropriate diagnostic and therapeutic options will significantly improve the level of care among those different specialties or primary care physicians. (Krouse et al., 2007; Rimmer & Ruhno, 2006).

In conclusion, elegant studies confirm that sinonasal disorders are very crucial co-morbidities in people with asthma, and they should be treated with an integrated approach. Further investigations are needed to determine if early intervention of rhinitis and/or sinusitis could prevent or delay the onset of asthma.

7. References

Alvarez MJ., Olaguibel JM., & Garcia BE., et al. (2000). Comparison of allergen-induced changes in bronchial hyperresponsiveness and airway inflammation between mildly allergic asthma patients and allergic rhinitis patients. *Allergy*, Vol. 55, pp. 531-539.

Bachert C., Claeys SEM., Tomassen P., van Zele T.,& Zhang N.(2010). Rhinosinusitis and asthma: A link for asthma severity. *Curr Allergy Asthma Rep*, Vol. 10, pp. 194-201.

Bachert C., van Cauwenberge P., & Khaltaev N. (2002). World Health Organization. Allergic rhinitis and its impact on asthma. In collaboration with the World Health Organization. Executive summary of the workshop report. *Allergy*, Vol. 5, pp. 841-855.

Bachert C., Vignola AM., & Gevaert P., et al. (2004). Allergic rhinitis, rhinosinusitis, and asthma: one airway disease. *Immunol Allergy Clin N Am*, Vol. 24, pp: 19-43.

Berger WE. (2003). Overview of allergic rhinitis. *Ann Allergy Asthma Immunol*, Vol. 90 (suppl. 3), pp. 7-12.

Borish L. (2003). Allergic rhinitis: Systemic inflammation and implications for management. *J Allergy Clin Immunol*, Vol. 112, pp. 1021-1031.

Boulay M-E., & Boulet L-P. (2003). The relationship between atopy, rhinitis and asthma: pathophysiological considerations. *Curr Opin Allergy Clin Immunol*, Vol. 3, No. 1, pp.51-55

Boulet L-P., Morin D., & Milot J., et al. (1989). Bronchial responsiveness increases after seasonal antigen exposure in non-asthmatic subjects with pollen-induced rhinitis. *Ann Allergy*, Vol. 63, pp. 114-119.

Bourdin A., Gras D., & Vachier I., et al. (2009). Upper airway-1: Allergic rhinitis and asthma: United disease through epithelial cells. *Thorax*, Vol. 64, pp. 999-1004.

Bousquet J., Bachert C., & Canonica GW., et al. (2009). Unmet needs in severe chronic upper airway disease (SCUAD). *J Allergy Clin Immunol*, Vol.124, pp. 428-433.

Bousquet J., Gaugris S., & Sazonov Kocevar V., et al. (2005). Increased risk of asthma attacks and emergency visits among asthma patients with allergic rhinitis: a subgroup analysis of the improving asthma control trial. *Clin Exp Allergy*, Vol. 35, pp. 723-727.

Bousquet J., Jacquot W., & Vignola M., et al. (2004). Allergic rhinitis: A disease remodeling the upper airways? *J Allergy Clin Immunol*, Vol. 113, pp. 43-49.

Bousquet J., Van Cauwenberge P., & Khaltaev N. (2001). ARIA Workshop Group. World Health Organization. Allergic rhinitis and its impact on asthma. *J Allergy Clin Immunol*, Vol. 108 (suppl 5), pp. S147-S334.

Bousquet J., Vignola AM., & Demoly P. (2003). Links between rhinitis and asthma. *Allergy*, Vol. 58, pp. 691-706.

Braman SS., Barrows AA., & DeCotiis BA., et al. (1987). Airway hyperresponsiveness in allergic rhinitis. A risk factor for asthma. *Chest* , Vol. 91, pp. 671-674.

Braunstahl G-.J, & Hellings PW. (2006). Nasobronchial interaction mechanisms in allergic airways. *Curr Opin Otolaryngol Head Neck Surg*, Vol. 14, pp. 176-182.

Braunstahl G-J. (2005). The unified immune system: Respiratory tract-nasobronchial interaction mechanisms in allergic airway disease. *J Allergy Clin Immunol*, Vol. 115, pp. 142-148.

Braunstahl G-J., & Fokkens W. (2003). Nasal involvement in allergic asthma. *Allergy*, Vol. 58, pp. 1235-1243.

Braunstahl GJ., Fokkens WJ., & Overbeek SE., et al. (2003). Mucosal and systemic inflammatory changes in allergic rhinitis and asthma: a comparison between upper and lower airways. *Clin Exp Allergy*, Vol. 33, pp. 579-587.

Braunstahl GJ., Kleinjan A., & Overbeek SE., et al. (2000). Segmental bronchial provocation induces nasal inflammation in allergic rhinitis patients. *Am J Respir Crit Care Med*, Vol. 161, pp. 2051-2057.

Braunstahl GJ., Overbeek SE., & Fokkens WJ., et al. (2001b). Segmental bronchoprovocation in allergic rhinitis patients affects mast cell and basophil numbers in nasal and bronchial mucosa. *Am J Respir Crit Care Med*, Vol. 164, pp. 858-865.

Braunstahl GJ., Overbeek SE., & Kleinjan A., et al. (2001a). Nasal allergen provocation induces adhesion molecule expression and tissue eosinophilia in upper and lower airways. *J Allergy Clin Immunol*, Vol. 107, pp. 469-476.

Brozek JL., Bousquet J., & Baena-Cagnani CE., et al. (2010). Allergic rhinitis and its impact on asthma (ARIA) guidelines: 2010 revision. *J Allergy Clin Immunol*, Vol.126, pp. 466-476.

Ceylan E., Gencer M., & San I. (2007). Nasal polyps and the severity of asthma. *Respirology*, Vol.12, pp. 272-276.

Chakir J., Laviolette M., & Boutet M., et al. (1996). Lower airways remodeling in nonasthmatic subjects with allergic rhinitis. *Lab Invest*, Vol. 75, pp. 735-744.

Ciprandi G., & Passalacqua G. (2008). Allergy and the nose. *Clin Exp Immunol*, Vol. 153 (suppl. 1), pp. 22-26.

Ciprandi G., Cirillo I., & Tosca MA., et al. (2004). Bronchial hyperreactivity and spirometric impairment in patients with perennial allergic rhinitis. *Int Arc Allergy Immunol*, Vol. 133, pp. 14-18.

Cirillo I., Pistorio A., & Tosca M., et al. (2009). Impact of allergic rhinitis on asthma: effects on bronchial hyperreactivity. *Allergy*, Vol. 64, pp. 439-444.

Compalati E., Ridolo E., & Passalacqua G., et al. (2010). The link between allergic rhinitis and asthma: the united airways disease. *Expert Rev Clin Immunol*, Vol. 6, pp. 413-423.

Corren J. (1997). Allergic rhinitis and asthma: How important is the link? *J Allergy Clin Immunol*, Vol. 99, pp. S781-786.

Corren J., Adinoff AD., & Buchmeier AD., et al. (1992). Nasal beclomethasone prevents the seasonal increase in bronchial responsiveness in patients with allergic rhinitis and asthma. *J Allergy Clin Immunol*, Vol. 90, pp. 250-256.

Corren J., Manning BE., & Thompson SF., et al. (2004). Rhinitis therapy and the prevention of hospital care for asthma: a case-control study. *J Allergy Clin Immunol*, Vol. 113, pp. 415-419.

Crystal-Peters J., Neslusan C., & Crown WH., et al. (2002). Treating allergic rhinitis in patients with comorbid asthma: the risk of asthma-related hospitalizations and emergency department visits. *J Allergy Clin Immunol*, Vol. 109, pp. 57-62.

Danielsson J., & Jessen M. (1997). The natural course of allergic rhinitis during 12 years of follow-up. *Allergy*, Vol. 52, pp. 331-334.

Dixon AE. (2009). Rhinosinusitis and asthma: the missing link. *Curr Opin Pulm Med*, Vol. 15, pp. 19-24.

Dursun AB., Sin BA., & Dursun E., et al. (2006). Clinical aspects of the link between chronic sinonasal diseases and asthma. *Allergy Asthma Proc*, Vol. 27, pp. 510-515.

Ediger D., Sin BA., & Heper A., et al. (2005). Airway inflammation in nasal polyposis: immunopathological aspects of relation to asthma. *Clin Exp Allergy*, Vol. 35, pp. 319-326.

Fasano MB. (2010). Combined airways: impact of upper airway on lower airway. *Curr Opin Otolaryngol Head Neck Surg*, Vol. 18, pp.15-20.

Fiocchi A., & Fox AT. (2010). Preventing progression of allergic rhinitis: the role of specific immunotherapy. *Arch Dis Child Educ Pract Ed*. Published online November 3,2010. doi: 10.1136/adc.2010.183095.

Foresi A., Leone C., & Pelucchi A., et al. (1997). Eosinophils, mast cells, and basophils in induced sputum from patients with seasonal allergic rhinitis and perennial asthma: relationship to methacholine responsiveness. *J Allergy Clin Immunol*, Vol. 100, pp. 58-64.

Gaga M., Lambrou P., & Papageorgiou N., et al. (2000). Eosinophils are a feature of upper and lower airway pathology in non-atopic asthma, irrespective of the presence of rhinitis. *Clin Exp Allergy*, Vol. 30, pp. 663-669.

Greenberger PA. (2008). Allergic rhinitis and asthma connection: Treatment implications. *Allergy Asthma Proc*, Vol. 29, pp. 557-64.

Guerra S., Sherrill D.,& Martinez FD., et al. (2002). Rhinitis as an independent risk factor for adult-onset asthma. *J Allergy Clin Immunol*, Vol. 109, pp. 419-425.

Hanes LS., Issa E., & Proud D., et al. (2006). Stronger nasal responsiveness to cold air in individuals with rhinitis and asthma, compared to rhinitis alone. *Clin Exp Allergy*, Vol. 36, pp. 26-31.

Henriksen JM., & Wenzel A. (1984). Effect of an intranasally administered corticosteroid (budesonide) on nasal obstruction, mouth breathing, and asthma. *Am Rev Respir Dis*, Vol. 130, pp. 1014-1018.

Humbert M., Boulet LP., & Niven RM., et al. (2009). Omalizumab therapy: patients who achieve greatest benefit for their asthma experience greatest benefit for rhinitis. *Allergy*, Vol. 64, pp. 81-84.

Huovinen E., Kaprio J., & Laitinen LA., et al. (1999). Incidence and prevalence of asthma among adults Finnish men and women of the Finnish Twin Cohort from 1975 to 1990, and theirrelation to hay fever and chronic bronchitis. *Chest*, Vol. 115, pp. 928-936.

Illi S., Von Mutius E., & Lau S., et al. (2004). The natural course of atopic dermatitis from birth to age 7 years and the association with asthma. *J Allergy Clin Immunol*, Vol. 113, pp. 925-31.

Inal A., Kendirli SG., & Yilmaz M., et al. (2008). Indices of lower airway inflammation in children monosensitized to house dust mite after nasal allergen challenge. *Allergy*, Vol. 63, pp. 1345-1351.

Kapsali T., Horowitz E., & Togias A. (1997). Rhinitis is ubiquitous in allergic asthmatics. *J Allergy Clin Immunol*, Vol. 99, pp. S138.

KleinJan A., Willart M., & van Nimwegen M., et al. (2010). United airways: circulating Th2 effector cells in an allergic rhinitis model are responsible for promoting lower airways inflammation. *Clin Exp Allergy*, Vol. 40, pp. 494-504.

Koh YY., & Kim CK. (2003). The development of asthma in patients with allergic rhinitis. *Curr Opin Allergy Clin Immunol*, Vol. 3, pp. 159-164.

Kowalski ML., Cieslak M., Perez-Novo CA., Makowska JS., & Bachert C. (2011). Clinical and immunological determinants of severe/refractory asthma (SRA): association with staphylococcal superantigen-specific IgE antibodies. *Allergy*, Vol. 66 (1), pp. 32-38.

Krouse JH., Veling MC., & Ryan MW., et al. (2007). Executive summary: Asthma and the unified airway. *Otolaryngology-Head Neck Surgery*, Vol. 136, pp. 699-706.

Lau S., Nickel R., & Niggemann B., et al. (2002). The development of childhood asthma: lessons from the German Multicentre Allergy Study (MAS). *Paed Resp Rev*, Vol. 3, pp. 265-272.

Lee RU.,& Stevenson DD. (2011). Aspirin-exacerbated respiratory disease: Evaluation and management. *Allergy Asthma Immunol Res*, Vol. 3 (1), pp. 3-10.

Leynaert B., Bousquet J., & Neukirch C., et al. (1999). Perennial rhinitis: an independent risk factor for asthma in nonatopic subjects: results from the European Community Respiratory Health Survey. *J Allergy Clin Immunol*, Vol. 104, pp. 301-304.

Leynaert B., Neukirch F., & Demoly P., et al. (2000). Epidemiologic evidence for asthma and rhinitis comorbidity. *J Allergy Clin Immunol*, Vol. 106, pp. S201-205.

Linneberg A., Nielsen NH., & Madsen F., et al. (2001). Secular trends of allergic asthma in Danish adults. The Copenhagen Allergy Study. *Respir Med*, Vol. 95, pp. 258-264.

Madonini E., Briatico-Vangosa G., & Pappacoda A., et al. (1987). Seasonal increase of bronchial reactivity in allergic rhinitis. *J Allergy Clin Immunol*, Vol. 79, pp. 358-363.

Marple BF. (2010). Allergic rhinitis and inflammatory airway disease: interactions within the unified airspace. *Am J Rhinol*, Vol. 24, pp. 249-54.

McFadden ERJr. (1986). Nasal-sinus-pulmonary reflexes and bronchial asthma. *J Allergy Clin Immunol*, Vol. 78 pp. 1-3.

Meltzer EO., Svwarcberg J., & Pill MW. (2004). Allergic rhinitis, asthma, and rhinosinusitis: Diseases of the integrated airway. *J Manag Care Pharm*, Vol. 10, pp. 310-317.

Nair A., Vaidyanathan S., & Clearie K., et al. (2010). Steroid sparing effects of intranasal corticosteroids in asthma and allergic rhinitis. *Allergy*, Vol. 65, pp. 359-67.

Nathan RA. (2009). Management of patients with allergic rhinitis and asthma: literature review. *South Med J*, Vol. 102, pp. 935-941.

Pawankar R. (2006). Allergic rhinitis and asthma: are they manifestations of one syndrome? *Clin Exp Allergy*, Vol. 36, pp. 1-6.

Pawankar R., & Zernotti ME. (2009). Rhinosinusitis in children and asthma severity. *Curr Opin Allergy Clin Immunol*, Vol. 9, pp. 151-153.

Pearlman AN., Chandra RK., & Chang D., et al. (2009). Relationship between severity of chronic rhinosinusitis and nasal polyposis, asthma, and atopy. *Am J Rhinol Allergy*, Vol. 23, pp. 145-148.

Peroni DG., Piacentini GL., & Ceravolo R., et al. (2007). Difficult asthma: possible association with rhinosinusitis. *Pediatr Allergy Immunol*, Vol. 18 (suppl.18), pp. 25-27.

Pipet A., Botturi K., & Pinot D., et al. (2009). Allergen-specific immunotherapy in allergic rhinitis and asthma. Mechanisms and proof of efficacy. *Respir Med*, Vol. 103, pp. 800-12.

Polosa R., Ciamarra I., & Mangano G., et al. (2000). Bronchial hyperresponsiveness and airway inflammation markers in nonasthmatics with allergic rhinitis. *Eur Respir J*, Vol. 15, pp. 30-35.

Ponte EV., Franco R., & Nascimento HF., et al. (2008). Lack of control of severe asthma is associated with co-existence of moderate-to-severe rhinitis. *Allergy*, Vol. 63, pp. 564-569.

Prieto L., Uixera S., & Gutierrez V., et al. (2002). Modifications of airway responsivenss to adenosine 5´-monophosphate and exhaled nitric oxide concentrations after the pollen season in subjects with pollen-induced rhinitis. *Chest*, Vol. 122, pp. 940-947.

Ragab S., Scadding GK., & Lund VJ., et al. (2006). Treatment of chronic rhinosinusitis and its effects on asthma. *Eur Respir J*, Vol. 28, pp. 68-74.

Ramsdale EH., Morris MM., & Robers RS., et al. (1985). Asymptomatic bronchial hyperresponsiveness in rhinitis. *J Allergy Clin Immunol*, Vol. 75, pp. 573-577.

Rimmer J., & Ruhno JW. (2006). Rhinitis and asthma: united airway disease. *MJA Practice Essentials-Allergy*, Vol. 185, No.10, pp. 565-571.

Rowe-Jones JM. (1997). The link between the nose and lung,perennial rhinitis and asthma- is it the same disease? *Allergy*, Vol. 52 (suppl. 36), pp. 20-28.

Scichilone N., Arrigo R., & Paterno A., et al. (2011). The effect of intranasal corticosteroids on asthma control and quality of life in allergic rhinitis with mild asthma. *J Asthma*, Vol. 48, pp. 41-47.

Settipane RA. (2003). Rhinitis: A dose of epidemiologic reality. *Allergy Asthma Proc*, Vol. 24, pp. 147-154.

Settipane RJ., Hagy GW., & Settipane GA. (1994). Long-term risk factors for developing asthma and allergic rhinitis: a 23-year follow-up study of college students. *Allergy Proc*, Vol. 15, pp. 21-25.

Shaaban R., Zureik M., & Soussan D., et al. (2007). Allergic rhinitis and onset of bronchial hyperresponsiveness: a population-based study. *Am J Respir Crit Care Med*, Vol. 176, pp. 659-66.

Shaaban R., Zureik M., & Soussan D., et al. (2008). Rhinitis and onset of asthma: a longitudinal population-based study. *Lancet*, Vol. 372, pp. 1049-1057.

Sin B., & Togias A. (2011). Pathophysiology of allergic and nonallergic rhinitis. *Proc Am Thorac Soc*, Vol. 8, pp.106-114.

Sin B., Wu X., & Hoenig T., et al. (2002). Nasal allergen challenge induces inflammatory cell influx in sputum and peripheral eosinophilia. *J Allergy Clin Immunol*, Vol. 109, pp. S100-S101.

Sin BA., Yıldız OA., & Dursun AB., et al. (2009). Airway hyperresponsiveness: a comparative study of methacholine and exercise challenges in seasonal allergic rhinitis with or without asthma. *J Asthma*, Vol. 46, pp. 486-491.

Skloot G., & Togias A. (2003). Bronchodilation and bronchoprotection by deep inspiration and their relationship to bronchial hyperresponsiveness. *Clin Rev Allergy Immunol*, Vol. 24, pp. 55-72.

Slavin RG. (2008). The upper and lower airways: the epidemiological and pathophysiological connection. *Allergy Asthma Proc*, Vol. 29, pp. 553-56.

Smart BA. (2006). Is rhinosinusitis a cause of asthma? *Clin Rev Allergy Immunol*, Vol. 30, pp. 153-164.

Spector SL. (1997). Overview of comorbid associations of allergic rhinitis. *J Allergy Clin Immunol*, Vol. 99, pp. S773-S780.

Spergel JM. (2005). Atopic march: link to upper airways. *Curr Opin Allergy Clin Immunol*, Vol. 5, pp. 17-21.

Stevenson DD., & Szczeklik A. (2006). Clinical and pathologic perspectives on aspirin sensitivity and asthma. *J Allergy Clin Immunol*, Vol. 118, pp. 773-786.

Szczeklik A., Nizankowska M., & Duplaga M., on behalf of the AIANE Investigators. (2000). Natural history of aspirin-induced asthma. *Eur Respir J*, Vol. 16, pp.432-436.

Togias A. (1999). Mechanisms of nose-lung interaction. *Allergy*, Vol. 54 (suppl. 57), pp. 94-105.

Togias A. (2003). Rhinitis and asthma: evidence for respiratory system integration. *J Allergy Clin Immunol*, Vol. 111, pp. 1171-1183.

Togias A. (2004). Systemic effects of local allergic disease. *J Allergy Clin Immunol*, Vol. 113, pp. S8-S14.

Togias AG. (2000). Systemic immunologic and inflammatory aspects of allergic rhinitis. *J Allergy Clin Immunol*, Vol. 106 (suppl. 5), pp. S247-S250.

Vignola AM., Humbert M., & Bousquet J., et al. (2004). Efficacy and tolerability of anti-immunoglobulin E therapy with omalizumab in patients with concomitant allergic asthma and persistent allergic rhinitis: SOLAR. *Allergy*, Vol. 59, pp. 709-717.

4

Allergic Rhinitis and Its Impact on Bronchial Asthma

Katerina D. Samara[1], Stylianos G. Velegrakis[2] and Alexander D. Karatzanis[2]
[1]*Department of Thoracic Medicine, University of Crete Medical School*
[2]*Department of Otolaryngology, University of Crete Medical School*
Crete,
Greece

1. Introduction

Allergic rhinitis and bronchial asthma are two entities often coexisting. In fact, during recent years the concept "one airway, one disease" has been proposed. Many asthmatic patients, particularly those with allergic asthma, also have allergic rhinitis (AR). The mucosa of the upper and lower airways is continuous, and the type of inflammation in AR and asthma is very similar, involving T-helper type 2 lymphocytes, mast cells, and eosinophils. It is now well understood that the epidemiological association between bronchial asthma and AR is very strong. In addition, the two entities seem to share common genetic and environmental risk factors, while the immunopathology of rhinitis and asthma are virtually the same. Current evidence indicates that co-morbid AR may have clinically relevant effects on asthma. Consequently, new knowledge about the pathophysiologic mechanisms of allergic inflammation of the human airways has resulted in better therapeutic strategies. In this chapter, a detailed presentation of the similarities between AR and bronchial asthma is performed giving emphasis on the interactions between the upper and lower airways and any associated clinical implications. Moreover, a few important differences between the two entities are discussed based on original research previously published by the authors.

2. Epidemiologic relationship between asthma and rhinitis

Epidemiologic studies have consistently shown that asthma and rhinitis often coexist [Dixon, 2006; Leynaert, 2000; Greisner, 1998]. The Allergic Rhinitis and its Impact on Asthma (ARIA) guidelines first developed in 1999 by the World Health Organization and an international panel of experts and updated in 2008, recognizes the importance of this relationship [Bousquet J, 2008]. Prevalence rates of allergic rhinitis range from 15% to 40%. Similarly, asthma is a prevalent disorder that affects approximately 7% of the United States population [Meltzer, 2005]. Asthma and AR, however, occur together at rates that greatly exceed what would be expected from the baseline prevalence of each disorder alone (Fig. 1). AR is associated with asthma in 40% of patients, whereas 80% to 95% of patients with allergic asthma also have rhinitis. In a classical, 23-year follow-up study in more than 1800 college students initially evaluated for the presence of asthma, AR, and positive allergen skin tests, those presenting with AR and positive skin tests were three times more likely to eventually develop asthma [Settipane, 1994]. This study was confirmed by two other studies in Sweden [Plaschke, 2000] and the United States [Guerra, 2002]. In the Copenhagen Allergy Study, which relied on direct questioning and examination of study subjects, 100% of subjects who had allergic asthma induced by pollen had AR from pollen. Eighty-nine percent of subjects who had allergic asthma caused by animals had AR from animals, and 95% of subjects who had allergic asthma caused by mites had AR from mites. When re-evaluated eight years after initial screening, all patients who developed allergic asthma also had AR to the same allergens, leading the investigators to the conclusion that AR and allergic asthma are manifestations of the same disease entity [Linneberg, 2002]. However, epidemiologic differences may exist when comparing the developing world to western countries. One study showed that AR is far less common among asthmatic subjects in rural China (6%) than in asthmatic subjects in industrialized countries with a western lifestyle [Celedon, 2001].

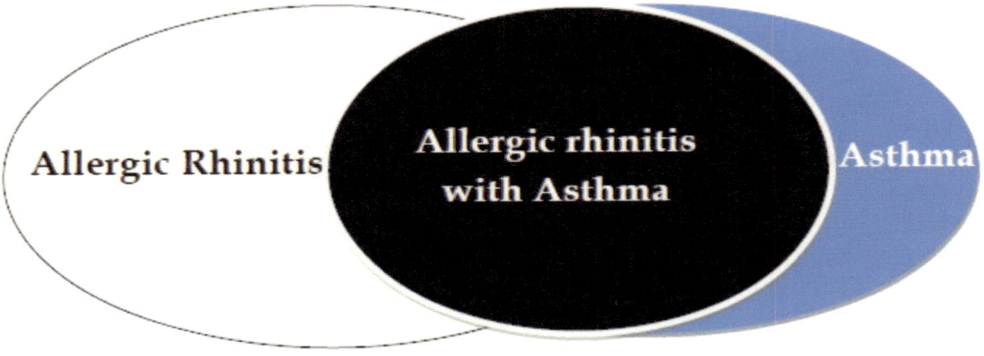

Fig. 1. Relative populations with asthma, allergic rhinitis, or a combination of both.

When assessing AR cases for asthma, a unique subset of rhinitis patients may be identified with a physiologic behaviour that separates them from patients with asthma and normal subjects. They exhibit increased bronchial sensitivity to methacholine or histamine, especially during and slightly after the pollen season. Bronchial hyper-responsiveness is common in people with AR, even if they have no asthma symptoms, and asymptomatic airway hyper-responsiveness is associated with increased risk for developing asthma [Boulet, 2003; Porsbjerg, 2006]. In one study, up to 40% of patients with AR showed hyper-responsiveness to methacholine challenge; those showing hyper-responsiveness were more likely to develop asthma over the following 4-5 years [Braman, 1987]. There are large differences in the magnitude of airway reactivity between asthmatics and people with rhinitis that are not explained by the allergen type or degree of reactivity. The finding that patients who have rhinitis without asthma diagnosis or asthma symptoms have bronchial hyperreactivity lends further support to the notion that asthma and rhinitis are different manifestations of a single respiratory system disease.

3. Rhinitis as a risk factor for asthma

AR is considered a risk factor for the development of asthma; an association which has been supported by multiple studies [Greisner, 1998; Settipane, 1994; Wright, 1994; Guerra, 2002].

The Children's Respiratory Study in 1994 showed that the presence of AR in infancy was independently associated with doubling of the risk for asthma by age 11 years [Wright, 1994]. The age of onset of atopy seems to be an important factor for the development of asthma and rhinitis or rhinitis alone. In an Australian study, atopy diagnosed at an early age (<6 years) was a significant predictive factor for the persistence of asthma into late childhood, whereas atopy presenting later in life was associated only with seasonal allergic rhinitis [Peat, 1990]. Burgess et al also reported that childhood AR was significantly associated with overall presence of asthma: 42% of participants with AR had asthma, compared to only 12.9 % of asthmatics without AR [Burgess, 2007]. In accord with these findings the term "allergic march" was introduced to describe the progression of allergic disease from the nose and sinuses down to the airways of the lung [Almqvist, 2007]. Patients with persistent and severe rhinitis have the highest risk for asthma. It is not clear whether AR represents an earlier clinical manifestation of allergic disease in atopic subjects who eventually develop asthma or if the nasal disease itself is causative for asthma. However, the presence of rhinitis appears to be associated with more severe asthma. In a study of hospital admissions in 2961 children from Norway, even when correcting for severity of asthma, children with AR had a higher risk of hospital readmission and more hospital days per year when compared to asthmatic patients without rhinitis [Kocevar, 2004]. Similar findings have been noted in the United Kingdom. Using a general practice database, the investigators estimated that asthmatic children who had a recorded diagnosis of AR had more general practitioner visits and were more likely to be hospitalized during the 12-month follow- up period of the study compared with children who had asthma alone [Thomas, 2005]. Moreover, when asthma and rhinitis coexist, in addition to increased severity of disease, healthcare costs are also increased. In a study of 1245 asthmatics in the USA, yearly medical care charges were 46% higher in those patients who had concomitant asthma and rhinitis [Yawn, 1999]. Halpern and colleagues [Halpern, 2004] performed an analysis of a medical claims database, and found that the presence of AR was associated with more asthma medication prescriptions and higher asthma prescription costs. These studies suggest that the diagnosis of AR may be more common in individuals who have severe asthma and that those individuals who exhibit both rhinitis and asthma symptoms suffer a more severe disease complex than those who have only upper or lower airway symptoms. Environmental factors may also affect the progression of disease to the lower airways in patients with AR. One environmental factor that should be addressed in allergic patients is tobacco smoke. In a study of patients with allergic rhinitis smoking increased the risk of developing asthma by approximately threefold [Polosa, 2008]. Another common factor that is now recognized as a risk factor for asthma, obesity, does not appear to affect the presence or progression of the allergic march. A population based study showed that obesity was associated with an increased prevalence of asthma, but not AR, suggesting that the pathogenesis of asthma in the obese may be through a different pathway than that linking AR and asthma [Loerbroks, 2008]. Family history has also been shown to play an important predictive role in the development of asthma and AR. A Swedish study concluded that adults with a family history of asthma or rhinitis had a 3- to 4-fold higher risk for developing asthma and a 2- to 6-fold higher risk for developing AR compared with adults without family history [Lundback, 1998]. Another report by the Multi-centre Allergy Study (MAS) group found that history of maternal asthma and/or maternal smoking were strong predictive factors of childhood asthma, even more than early atopic sensitization and AR. The MAS authors suggest that this predisposition to asthma precedes the pattern of allergic sensitization, contrary to the view that asthma results from a sequential progression of atopic sensitization beginning in childhood with early food allergy and AR [Illi, 2001]. Most patients with asthma present seasonal or perennial AR symptoms. Rhinitis, however, may be a risk factor even in non-atopic subjects, as shown in the Tucson Epidemiologic Study of Obstructive Lung Diseases. After adjustment for atopic status, age, sex, smoking status, and presence of chronic obstructive pulmonary disease, rhinitis still significantly increased the risk for asthma, in both atopic and non-atopic patients [Guerra, 2002]. In the European Community Respiratory Health Survey, an association between asthma and rhinitis was also observed in non-atopic individuals [Leynaert, 2004]. These results cannot be fully explained by shared risk factors and support the hypothesis that upper airway disorders may directly affect the lower airways.

4. Inflammation in allergic rhinitis and asthma

AR and asthma exhibit important similarities in their pathophysiology and involve common inflammatory mechanisms. The nasal and bronchial mucosas are histologically similar; both have ciliated pseudostratified columnar epithelium and an underlying basement membrane. The inflammation in rhinitis is similar to that seen in the bronchial mucosa of asthmatics, consisting mainly of mononuclear cells, lymphocytes, and eosinophils. Additionally, the cytokines, adhesion molecules, and other inflammatory mediators are the same in both diseases [Bachert, 2004]. The same inhaled allergens and irritants stimulate both upper and lower respiratory tracts resulting in a Th2 pattern of proinflammatory cytokine activity [Casale, 2004]. Both AR and asthma symptoms are triggered by atopic sensitization and the allergic cascade, resulting in the generation of allergen-specific IgEs. Circulating levels of allergen-specific IgEs, and the presence of increased total serum IgE is a risk factor for asthma even in non-allergic individuals [Sherrill, 1999; Beeh, 2000]. After sensitization occurs, antigenic fragments of the allergens are presented to T-helper cells, which release cytokines that induce allergen-specific IgE antibody production by B lymphocytes and plasma cells. These antibodies then bind to the surface receptors of mast cells and basophils present in the mucosa of both the upper and lower airways. Re-exposure to the airborne allergen, triggers antigenic binding to the cell-surface specific IgE and activates the mast cells and basophils, resulting in degranulation and release of inflammatory mediators, including histamine, leukotrienes (LTC4, LTD4, LTE4), various proteases and cytokines. These mediators, in turn, trigger vasomotor and glandular responses in the upper airway, and smooth muscle contraction and mucosal edema in the lower airway, leading to airway obstruction [Casale, 2004; Marshall, 2000]. A late-phase reaction occurs approximately 4 to 8 hours after the initial IgE-mediated reaction to allergen exposure. In both the upper and lower airways, this late reaction is characterized by obstruction (nasal congestion, bronchoconstriction), and chronic inflammatory changes involving T cells, mast cells and eosinophils. There is also evidence to suggest that basophils may also play an important role in the late phase of AR [Arshad, 2001]. Recent studies have suggested that additional pathways may contribute to the pathophysiology of AR including local synthesis of IgE in the nasal mucosa, the epithelial expression of cytokines that regulate Th2 cytokine responses (i.e., thymic stromal lymphopoietin, IL-25, and IL-33), and the activation of histamine receptors other than H1 and H2, such as H4-histamine receptors [Broide, 2010].

Systemic inflammation affecting first the upper and then the lower airways plays a major role in the relationship between AR and asthma. AR and asthma exhibit many elements of a systemic disease in that effector cells are recruited from the circulation, white cell progenitors are stimulated in the bone marrow, and systemic effector cells are primed. Exposing the lower airways of animals to allergens causes the white cell progenitors in the bone marrow to proliferate and differentiate, and leads to high number of eosinophils in the lung, suggesting there is communication between the lung and bone marrow after allergen exposure. Eosinophilic inflammation is a common finding of AR and allergic asthma. The pathways involved include interleukin (IL)-5, supporting the hypothesis of a common pathway in allergic disease [Inman, 2000]. IL-5 is one of several cytokines with a central role in Th2-driven allergic responses in the airways and novel anti-IL-5 strategies have emerged for the treatment of severe persistent eosinophilic asthma [Castro, 2011; Walsh, 2009]. Evidence of inflammation in the lower airway has been documented after local nasal allergen provocation. In a study by Braunstahl et al, nasal allergen provocation was performed in subjects with seasonal allergic rhinitis with bronchial and nasal biopsy specimens obtained before and 24 hours after the provocation. Eosinophils and expression of intercellular adhesion molecule (ICAM)-1, vascular cell adhesion molecule (VCAM)-1, and E–selectin were increased in bronchial epithelium 24 hours after nasal provocation, suggesting that the airway inflammation occurs through upregulation of adhesion molecules [Braunstahl, 2001]. In another study, exhaled nitric oxide (eNO) was measured in children with allergic rhinitis and asthma after allergen-specific nasal challenge and found to be significantly higher than in control groups [Marcucci, 2007].

Differences between the upper and lower airways do exist however. The nose filters irritants and allergens from the inhaled air, thus, reducing the exposure of the airways to environmental allergens and pollutants and constituting a critical barrier. The nose has a complex microcirculation that serves multiple functions, including the heating and humidifying of inspired air and the regulation of airflow, via vasodilation and vasoconstriction. The exudation of plasma into the submucosa provides the necessary fluid for copious secretions. Inflammation and excessive mucosal secretions lead to nasal congestion and rhinorrhea and are the hallmarks of AR. The lower airway has a much larger surface area than that of the upper airway. Its patency is mainly controlled by smooth muscle. In allergic asthma, the characteristic response is bronchial smooth muscle contraction or bronchoconstiction. The latter is mediated by various inflammatory and neurogenic factors, including muscarinic pathways specific to the lower airway, resulting in reduced airflow. Other hallmarks of chronic asthma are structural changes or remodelling of the lower airway, which takes the form of epithelial shedding, sub-basement membrane thickening, and smooth muscle hypertrophy and hyperplasia. The pathologic extent of nasal remodelling in patients with rhinitis seems to be far less extensive than that in the bronchi of asthmatic patients. In AR, the epithelium of the nasal mucosa tends to remain intact and the reticular basement membrane does not appear to be largely thickened; moreover, epithelial apoptosis is far greater in the bronchial mucosa of asthmatic patients than in the nasal mucosa of patients with AR [Bousquet, 2004]. The degree and clinical importance of upper airway remodelling are less pronounced than in allergic asthma [Chanez, 1999]. The reasons why remodelling appears to be less extensive in the nasal mucosa than in the bronchial mucosa are still under investigation, but two hypotheses have been proposed: on one hand, the cytokine production of smooth muscle cells might partly explain differences in remodeling of the two sites of the airways. On the other hand, the genes of the embryologic differentiation might persist in the nose and bronchi or might be re-expressed in asthma and rhinitis. Because the nose is of ectodermal origin and the bronchi of endodermal origin, these genes might also govern remodelling patterns. A better understanding of nasal and bronchial remodelling might help to identify new pathways and new therapeutic strategies to reduce bronchial remodelling in asthma [Bousquet, 2004].

5. Therapeutic links between rhinitis and asthma

Treatment of rhinitis has been shown by many studies to reduce asthma severity. In one study, subjects with allergic rhinitis and asthma were treated with intranasal corticosteroid (beclomethasone) or placebo for the entire allergy season. Intranasal beclomethasone therapy prevented the increase in bronchial hyper-responsiveness that was seen in the placebo group [Corren, 1992]. This beneficial effect of intranasal corticosteroids on bronchial hyperresponsiveness was confirmed by another study in asthmatic patients with allergic rhinitis. The subjects who used intranasal fluticasone propionate during the allergy season exhibited less nasal symptoms and the expected increase in bronchial hyper-responsiveness was attenuated [Foresi, 1996]. Treatment of AR in asthmatic patients has also been shown to decrease asthma-related emergency room visits and hospitalizations. A large, retrospective cohort study involving approximately 5000 subjects with allergic asthma showed that asthma related events requiring emergency room visits or hospitalizations occurred more often in those not receiving treatment for AR compared with those receiving regular treatment (6.6% vs. 1.3%) [Crystal-Peters, 2002]. Another retrospective cohort study performed in 13,844 asthmatics over the age of 5 concluded that patients who received intranasal corticosteroids had a reduced risk for emergency department visit compared to those who did not receive this treatment [Adams, 2002]. An important therapeutic issue under debate is allergen immunotherapy, as several studies have shown that apart from treating AR symptoms, immunotherapy may also decrease the development of asthma in children and adults. Immunotherapy can alter the atopic phenotype by restoring the normal equilibrium between Th1 and Th2 lymphocytes [Moller, 2002]. In one study, patients with seasonal AR but no asthma were randomized to receive either immunotherapy or placebo and followed for 3 years. Although sputum eosinophils and bronchial hyperresponsiveness to methacholine did not change, immunotherapy appeared to prevent progression to asthma (14% in immunotherapy group vs. 47% in placebo group) [Polosa, 2004]. The Preventive Allergy Treatment (PAT) study in children who received specific immunotherapy for grass and/or birch pollen or no immunotherapy for 3 years, showed significantly less asthma in the immunotherapy group two years after the end of treatment [Niggemann, 2006]. Patients with AR should be evaluated for asthma periodically by good history taking, physical examination, and pulmonary function testing so that early intervention can be started when asthma is detected. However, all patients with asthma should always be examined and aggressively treated for concomitant AR. A systemic approach using medications that treat both rhinitis and asthma, including corticosteroids (intranasal and inhaled), leukotriene receptor antagonists, immunotherapy, and immunomodulation, is advocated by many physicians. In detail, the intranasal treatment of rhinitis using corticosteroids was found to improve asthma and there is strong evidence to support this as first-line treatment. Drugs administered by the oral route may have an effect on nasal and bronchial symptoms. Oral H1 antihistamines are routine treatment for AR. Although studies have found some effect on asthma symptoms at the recommended dose in the treatment of seasonal asthma, these drugs are not recommended for the treatment of asthma [Baena-Cagnani, 2003; Van-Ganse, 1997]. Oral administration of leukotriene receptor antagonists (montelukast) has been shown to be effective in the maintenance treatment of asthma and to relieve symptoms of seasonal allergies [Meltzer, 2000]. While other allergy treatments (such as antihistamines or corticosteroids) treat only the symptoms of allergic disease, immunotherapy is the only available treatment that can modify the natural course of allergic disease, by reducing sensitivity to allergens. A three-to-five-year individually tailored regimen of injections may result in long-term benefits [Durham, 1999]. Allergen-specific immunotherapy based on the allergen sensitization rather than on the disease itself, is particularly likely to be successful if it begins early in life or soon after the allergy develops for the first time. Recently a sublingual immunotherapy tablet (Grazax) was approved, containing a grass pollen extract, which is similarly effective with injection immunotherapy, with few side effects. This form of immunotherapy can also be used by asthmatic patients who are at high risk for injection-based desensitization [Nasser, 2008; Durham, 2011]. Finally, the anti-IgE antibody, omalizumab, has been shown to be effective in patients with seasonal and perennial allergic rhinitis and moderate-to-severe allergic asthma [Casale, 2001; Corren, 2003].

6. Rhinitis and asthma: A continuum of disease?

The pathology of rhinitis and asthma are similar and the inflammation present in the lungs can also be identified in the nose, even in patients without clinical rhinitis. A similar phenomenon, of bronchial inflammation in rhinitis patients without asthma has also been observed. Inflammatory infiltration, characterized by the presence of eosinophils and CD4+ T cells, was similar in the nasal mucosa of rhinitis patients regardless of the presence of asthma or the allergic status of the patient [Lambrou, 2007]. In another study, asthmatic patients without nasal symptoms exhibited eosinophilic inflammation in the nose [Gaga, 2000]. Djukanovic and colleagues compared biopsies from atopic asthmatics and atopic non-asthmatics and found that atopic non-asthmatics had basement membrane thickening and eosinophilic inflammation resembling asthma. They reported a continuum of severity, with atopic non-asthmatics having milder inflammation and basement membrane thickening compared to atopic asthmatics [Djukanovic, 1992]. Another study in non-asthmatic patients with seasonal AR analyzed bronchial biopsies in and out of pollen season. The results showed that pollen exposure leaded to increased expression of IL-5, increased lymphocytes and eosinophils in the bronchial mucosa [Chakir, 2000]. These results suggest that atopy in general is associated with airway inflammation and that the clinical picture is determined by the severity of inflammation at different airway sites. Several theories have been proposed to explain the links between the upper and lower airways. Proposed mechanisms for the close association between the nasal and bronchial airways include (1) the nasobronchial neural reflex, inducing bronchial obstruction during allergen-specific challenge of the nose [Corren, 1992], (2) pulmonary aspiration of inflammatory material from the nose [Huxley, 1978], (3) loss of protective function of the nose, and (4) allergy as a systemic disease. Mouth breathing caused by nasal obstruction might also be a contributing factor. Regarding the nasobronchial reflex, studies showing bronchoconstriction after nasal exposure to dry, cold air and increased bronchial responsiveness following nasal allergen provocation have long supported this theory [Fontanari, 1997; Braunstahl, 2001; Corren, 1992]. However, there have been studies showing inconsistent results and contradicting this hypothesis [Schumacher, 1986]. Direct drainage of inflammatory or infected material from the nose to the lungs had been considered in the past a straightforward mechanism for inflammatory interaction between the nose and lungs. Aspiration of nasal secretions can occur, especially during sleep and in impaired individuals. However, studies using radiolabeled substances have not shown nasal material draining into the bronchial airways in patients with increased bronchial responsiveness [Bardin, 1990].

7. Microsatellite DNA instability in allergic rhinitis and asthma

Genomic microsatellites (MS) are repetitions of simple 1-6 base pairs nucleotide sequences, present in both coding and non-coding regions of the chromosome. MS are characterized by high levels of polymorphism and although they are mostly considered as evolutionary neutral DNA markers, a small part seems to play significant role in biological phenomena such as gene transcription, translation and other [Samara, 2006]. Genomic MS are associated with high mutational rates, as compared with the rates of mutation at coding chromosome regions [Metzgar, 2000]. The most important genetic alterations in microsatellite markers include microsatellite instability (MSI), which occurs due to frequent errors that appear during the replication of short nucleotide repeats, and loss of heterozygosity (LOH), meaning the loss of genetic material in one allele [De la Chapelle, 2003]. With the use of polymerase chain reaction technology, MS DNA has been converted into a highly versatile genetic marker. Both MSI and LOH have been initially reported in a number of human malignancies and then detected in various benign airway diseases, including chronic obstructive pulmonary disease (COPD), asthma and pulmonary fibrosis [Siafakas, 1999; Paraskakis, 2003; Vassilakis, 2000]. Therefore, MSI and LOH have been proposed as important genetic screening tools. These genetic alterations were successfully detected in sputum cells of patients with asthma, so given the very close relationship between AR and asthma the authors investigated the presence of LOH and/or MI in nasal cytology samples of patients with AR. Nasal brush samples and peripheral blood from 20 patients with allergic rhinitis were analyzed. DNA was extracted and analyzed for MSI and LOH using microsatellite markers D16S289, D4S2394, D4S1651, DXS8039, D3S3606, and D2S2113, harboring potential susceptibility genes for allergic rhinitis and atopy. Microsatellite analysis was also performed in non-atopic control subjects. No MSI and/or LOH were noted in either the allergic rhinitis or the control group. Although MSI and LOH are detectable phenomena in sputum samples of patients with asthma, this seems not to be the case for nasal cytology samples of patients with allergic rhinitis. As already mentioned, remodeling patterns in nasal mucosa of subjects with AR are rather limited and epithelial disruption and desquamation is a feature of bronchial epithelium in asthma and is less marked in the nasal epithelium of patients with rhinitis. Such differences in remodeling between the bronchial and nasal mucosa could be related to the smooth muscle cells interacting with the epithelium and mesenchymal cells. Therefore it makes sense that genetic alterations such as LOH and/or MSI that possibly contribute to the remodeling of the airways would be absent in AR where this phenomenon is far less extensive. Further studies using additional microsatellite markers are needed in order to exclude the presence of LOH and/or MSI in AR [Karatzanis, Am J Rhinol, 2007]. In support of the theory that MSI is a specific finding for the target organ of asthma, i.e. the lungs, despite the fact that inflammation coexists in the nasal mucosa of asthmatic patients, we studied COPD patients and assessed the presence of MSI in nasal cytological samples comparing the results with sputum samples of the same individuals [Karatzanis, Oncol Rep, 2007]. Although MSI was detected in the sputum samples of 7 COPD patients (35%), no instability was found in the nasal cytological samples of the same patients. On the other hand, MSI was successfully detected in nasal samples of patients with nasal polyposis [Karatzanis, 2009]. These studies support the hypothesis that MSI in certain chromosomal loci is not only disease specific as has been previously reported, but is also specific for the target organ of COPD or asthma, i.e. the lung. Microsatellite DNA could have a functional protective role in "shielding" DNA from environmental hazards, as previously hypothesized [Martin, 2005], which is lost through genetic alterations that take place specifically in the lower airways.

8. Conclusion

The relationship between AR and asthma is strongly supported by genetic, epidemiologic, pathophysiologic, and clinical evidence. The one-airway theory underlines the close interaction between upper and lower airways. The majority of asthmatic patients have AR. Both diseases exhibit an array of atopic manifestations all involving IgE-mediated responses leading to release of inflammatory mediators into the nasal and bronchial systems. Genetic predisposition, organ susceptibility, and breathing patterns are likely to be involved in the development of bronchial symptoms in patients with rhinosinusitis. Furthermore, systemic inflammation induced from either the upper or lower airways is postulated to elicit the involvement of both areas. In patients with rhinitis, it is essential to evaluate for asthma, sinusitis, atopic dermatitis, and food allergy as early as possible so that allergen avoidance, diagnostic, and therapeutic approaches can be coordinated. Treatment of allergic rhinitis seems to delay or prevent development of asthma in children. The full appreciation of involvement of upper and lower airway disease in one patient can only be achieved in a multidisciplinary clinical setting, involving doctors being able to examine and interpret clinical abnormalities of upper and lower airways.

9. References

Adams RJ, Fuhlbrigge AL, Finkelstein JA & Weiss ST. Intranasal steroids and the risk of emergency department visits for asthma. *J Allergy Clin Immunol* 2002; 109(4):636- 42.

Almqvist C, Li Q, Britton WJ, et al. Early predictors for developing allergic disease and asthma: examining separate steps in the 'allergic march'. *Clin Exp Allergy* 2007 Sep; 37(9):1296-302.

Arshad SH & Holgate S. The role of IgE in allergen-induced inflammation and the potential for intervention with a humanized monoclonal anti-IgE antibody. *Clin Exp Allergy* 2001; 31:1344–1351.

Bachert C, Vignola AM, Gevaert P, et al. Allergic rhinitis, rhinosinusitis, and asthma: one airway disease. *Immunol Allergy Clin N Am* 2004; 24:19–43.

Baena-Cagnani CE, Berger WE, DuBuske LM, Gurne SE, Stryszak P, Lorber R, et al. Comparative effects of desloratadine versus montelukast on asthma symptoms and use of beta(2)-agonists in patients with seasonal allergic rhinitis and asthma. *Int Arch Allergy Immunol* 2003; 130(4):307– 13.

Bardin PG, Van Heerden BB & Joubert JR. Absence of pulmonary aspiration of sinus contents in patients with asthma and sinusitis. *J Allergy Clin Immunol* 1990; 86(1):82–8.

Beeh KM, Ksoll M & Buhl R. Elevation of total serum immunoglobulin E is associated with asthma in nonallergic individuals. *Eur Respir J* 2000; 16: 609–614.

Boulet LP. Asymptomatic airway hyper-responsiveness: a curiosity or an opportunity to prevent asthma? *Am J Respir Crit Care Med* 2003; 167:371-378.

Bousquet J, Jacot W, Vignola AM, Bachert C, Van Cauwenberge P. Allergic rhinitis: a disease remodeling the upper airways? *J Allergy Clin Immunol.* 2004 Jan; 113(1):43-9.

Bousquet J, Khaltaev N, Cruz AA, Denburg J, Fokkens WJ, Togias A, et al; World Health Organization; GA(2)LEN; AllerGen. Allergic Rhinitis and its Impact on Asthma (ARIA) 2008 update (in collaboration with the World Health Organization, GA(2)LEN and AllerGen). *Allergy*. 2008 Apr;63 Suppl 86:8-160.

Braman SS, Barrows AA, DeCotiis BA, Settipane GA & Corrao WM. Airway hyper-responsiveness in allergic rhinitis. A risk factor for asthma. *Chest* 1987, 91:671-674.

Braunstahl GJ, Overbeek SE, Kleinjan A, et al. Nasal allergen provocation induces adhesion molecule expression and tissue eosinophilia in upper and lower airways. *J Allergy Clin Immunol* 2001; 107(3):469–76.

Broide DH. Allergic rhinitis: Pathophysiology. *Allergy Asthma Proc.* 2010 Sep-Oct; 31(5):370-4.

Burgess JA, Walters EH, Byrnes GB, et al. Childhood allergic rhinitis predicts asthma incidence and persistence to middle age: a longitudinal study. *J Allergy Clin Immunol* 2007 Oct; 120(4):863–9.

Casale TB & Dykewicz MS. Clinical implications of the allergic rhinitis - asthma link. *Am J Med Sci* 2004; 327(3):127–138.

Casale TB, Condemi J, LaForce C, Nayak A, Rowe M, Watrous M, et al. Effect of omalizumab on symptoms of seasonal allergic rhinitis: a randomized controlled trial. *JAMA* 2001; 286(23): 2956–67.

Castro M, Mathur S, Hargreave F, Boulet LP, Xie F, Young J, Wilkins HJ, Henkel T & Nair P; for the Res-5-0010 Study Group. Reslizumab for Poorly Controlled, Eosinophilic Asthma: A Randomized, Placebo-Controlled Study. *Am J Respir Crit Care Med.* 2011 Aug 18.

Celedon JC, Palmer LJ, Weiss ST, Wang B, Fang Z & Xu X. Asthma, rhinitis, and skin test reactivity to aeroallergens in families of asthmatic subjects in Anqing, China. *Am J Respir Crit Care Med* 2001; 163(5):1108–12.

Chakir J, Laviolette M, Turcotte H, et al. Cytokine expression in the lower airways of nonasthmatic subjects with allergic rhinitis: influence of natural allergen exposure. *J Allergy Clin Immunol* 2000; 106:904–10.

Chanez P, Vignola AM, Vic P, et al. Comparison between nasal and bronchial inflammation in asthmatic and control subjects. *Am J Respir Crit Care Med* 1999; 159:588–95.

Corren J, Adinoff AD, Buchmeier AD, et al. Nasal beclomethasone prevents the seasonal increase in bronchial responsiveness in patients with allergic rhinitis and asthma. *J Allergy Clin Immunol* 1992; 90(2):250–6.

Corren J, Adinoff AD, Irvin CG. Changes in bronchial responsiveness following nasal provocation with allergen. *J Allergy Clin Immunol* 1992; 89(2):611 –8.

Corren J, Casale T, Deniz Y & Ashby M. Omalizumab, a recombinant humanized anti-IgE antibody, reduces asthma-related emergency room visits and hospitalizations in patients with allergic asthma. *J Allergy Clin Immunol* 2003; 111(1):87– 90.

Crystal-Peters J, Neslusan C, Crown WH, et al. Treating allergic rhinitis in patients with comorbid asthma: the risk of asthma-related hospitalizations and emergency department visits. *J Allergy Clin Immunol* 2002; 109(1):57–62.

De la Chapelle A. Microsatellite instability. *N Engl J Med* 2003; 349:209–10.

Dixon AE, Kaminsky DA, Holbrook JT, et al. Allergic rhinitis and sinusitis in asthma: differential effects on symptoms and pulmonary function. *Chest* 2006 Aug; 130(2):429–35.

Djukanovic R, Lai CK, Wilson JW, et al. Bronchial mucosal manifestations of atopy: a comparison of markers of inflammation between atopic asthmatics, atopic non-asthmatics, and healthy controls. *Eur Respir J* 1992; 5:538–44.

Durham SR, Walker SM, Varga EM, Jacobson MR, O'Brien F, Noble W, Till SJ, Hamid QA, Nouri-Aria KT. Long-term clinical efficacy of grass-pollen immunotherapy. *N Engl J Med.* 1999 Aug 12; 341(7):468-75.

Durham SR; GT-08 investigators. Sustained effects of grass pollen AIT. *Allergy.* 2011 Jul; 66 Suppl 95:50-2. doi: 10.1111/j.1398-9995.2011.02639.x.

Fontanari P, Zattara-Hartmann MC, Burnet H, et al. Nasal eupnoeic inhalation of cold, dry air increases airway resistance in asthmatic patients. *Eur Respir J* 1997; 10:2250–4.

Foresi A, Pelucchi A, Gherson G, et al. Once daily intranasal fluticasone propionate (200 micrograms) reduces nasal symptoms and inflammation but also attenuates the increase in bronchial responsiveness during the pollen season in allergic rhinitis. *J Allergy Clin Immunol* 1996;98(2):274–82.

Gaga M, Lambrou P, Papageorgiou N, et al. Eosinophils are a feature of upper and lower airway pathology in non-atopic asthma, irrespective of the presence of rhinitis. *Clin Exp Allergy* 2000; 30(5):663–9.

Greisner WA 3rd, Settipane RJ & Settipane GA. Co-existence of asthma and allergic rhinitis: a 23-year follow-up study of college students. *Allergy Asthma Proc* 1998; 19(4):185–8.

Guerra S, Sherrill DL, Martinez FD, et al. Rhinitis as an independent risk factor for adult-onset asthma. *J Allergy Clin Immunol* 2002; 109(3):419–25.

Halpern MT, Schmier JK, Richner R, et al. Allergic rhinitis: a potential cause of increased asthma medication use, costs, and morbidity. *J Asthma* 2004; 41(1):117–26.

Huxley EJ, Viroslav J, Gray WR, Pierce AK. Pharyngeal aspiration in normal adults and patients with depressed consciousness. *Am J Med* 1978; 64(4):564– 8.

Illi S, von Mutius E, Lau S, et al. The pattern of atopic sensitization is associated with the development of asthma in childhood. *J Allergy Clin Immunol* 2001; 108:709–14.

Inman MD. Bone marrow events in animal models of allergic inflammation and hyperresponsiveness. *J Allergy Clin Immunol* 2000; 106:S235–41.

Karatzanis AD, Samara KD, Tzortzaki E, Zervou M, Helidonis ES, Velegrakis GA & Siafakas N. Microsatellite DNA instability in nasal cytology of COPD patients. *Oncol Rep.* 2007 Mar; 17(3):661-5.

Karatzanis AD, Samara KD, Zervou M, et al. Assessment for microsatellite DNA instability in nasal cytology samples of patients with allergic rhinitis.*Am J Rhinol.* 2007 Mar-Apr;21(2):236-40.

Karatzanis AD, Tzortzaki E, Samara KD, Neofytou E, Zenk J, Iro H, Siafakas N & Velegrakis GAl. Microsatellite DNA instability in nasal polyposis. Laryngoscope. 2009 Apr;119(4):751-6.

Kocevar VS, Bisgaard H, Johsson L, et al. Variations in pediatric asthma hospitalization rates and costs between and within Nordic countries. *Chest* 2004; 125:1680–4.

Lambrou P, Zervas E, Oikonomidou E, Papageorgiou N, Alchanatis M & Gaga M. Eosinophilic infiltration in the nasal mucosa of rhinitis patients: is it affected by the presence of asthma or the allergic status of the patients? *Ann Allergy Asthma Immunol.* 2007 Jun;98(6):567-72.

Leynaert B, Neukirch C, Kony S, Guenegou A, Bousquet J, Aubier M & Neukirch F. Association between asthma and rhinitis according to atopic sensitization in a population-based study. *J Allergy Clin Immunol* 2004, 113:86-93.

Leynaert B, Neukirch F, Demoly P & Bousquet J. Epidemiologic evidence for asthma and rhinitis comorbidity. *J Allergy Clin Immunol* 2000; 106(5 Pt 2):201- 5.

Linneberg A, Henrik Nielsen N, Frølund L, et al. The link between allergic rhinitis and allergic asthma: a prospective population-based study. The Copenhagen Allergy Study. *Allergy* 2002; 57(11):1048–52.

Loerbroks A, Apfelbacher CJ, Amelang M & Sturmer T. Obesity and adult asthma: potential effect modification by gender, but not by hay fever. *Annals of epidemiology* 2008 Apr; 18(4):283–9.

Lowe AJ, Hosking CS, Bennett CM, et al. Skin prick test can identify eczematous infants at risk of asthma and allergic rhinitis. *Clin Exp Allergy* 2007 Nov; 37(11):1624–31.

Lundback B. Epidemiology of rhinitis and asthma. *Clin Exp Allergy* 1998;2:3–10.

Marcucci F, Passalacqua G, Canonica GW, et al. Lower airway inflammation before and after house dust mite nasal challenge: an age and allergen exposure-related phenomenon. *Respir Med* 2007; 101(7):1600–8.

Marshall GD. Therapeutic options in allergic disease: antihistamines as systemic antiallergic agents. *J Allergy Clin Immunol* 2000; 106:S303–9.

Martin P, Makepeace K, Hill SA, Hood DW, Moxon ER. Microsatellite instability regulates transcription factor binding and gene expression. *Proc Natl Acad Sci U S A.* 2005; 102(10):3800-4.

Meltzer E, Malmstrom K, Lu S, Brenner B, Wei L, Weinstein S, et al. Concomitant montelukast and loratadine as treatment for seasonal allergic rhinitis: placebo-controlled clinical trial. *J Allergy Clin Immunol* 2000;105(5):917- 22.

Meltzer EO. The relationships of rhinitis and asthma. *Allergy Asthma Proc* 2005; 26:336–40.

Metzgar D, Bytof J & Wills C. Selection against frame shift mutations limits microsatellite expansion in coding DNA. *Genome Res* 2000; 10:72-80.

Moller C, Dreborg S, Ferdousi HA, Halken S, Host A, Jacobsen L, et al. Pollen immunotherapy reduces the development of asthma in children with seasonal rhinoconjunctivitis (the PAT study). *J Allergy Clin Immunol* 2002; 109(2):251–6.

Nasser S, Vestenbaek U, Beriot-Mathiot A, Poulsen PB. Cost-effectiveness of specific immunotherapy with Grazax in allergic rhinitis co-existing with asthma. *Allergy.* 2008 Dec; 63(12):1624-9.

Niggemann B, Jacobsen L, Dreborg S, et al. Five-year follow-up on the PAT study: specific immunotherapy and long-term prevention of asthma in children. *Allergy* 2006; 61(7):855–9.

Paraskakis E, Sourvinos G, Passam F et al. Microsatellite DNA instability and loss of heterozygosity in bronchial asthma. *Eur Respir J* 2003; 22:951-955.

Peat JK, Salome CM & Woolcock AJ. Longitudinal changes in atopy during a 4-year period: relation to bronchial hyperresponsiveness and respiratory symptoms in a population sample of Australian schoolchildren. *J Allergy Clin Immunol* 1990; 85(1 Pt 1):65– 74.

Plaschke PP, Janson C, Norrman E, Bjornsson E, Ellbjar S & Jarvholm B. Onset and remission of allergic rhinitis and asthma and the relationship with atopic sensitization and smoking. *Am J Respir Crit Care Med* 2000; 162(3 Pt 1):920 –4.

Polosa R, Knoke JD, Russo C, et al. Cigarette smoking is associated with a greater risk of incident asthma in allergic rhinitis. *J Allergy Clin Immunol* 2008 Jun; 121(6):1428–34.

Polosa R, Li Gotti F, Mangano G, et al. Effect of immunotherapy on asthma progression, BHR and sputum eosinophils in allergic rhinitis. *Allergy* 2004; 59(11):1224–8.

Porsbjerg C, von Linstow ML, Ulrik CS, Nepper-Christensen S & Backer V. Risk factors for onset of asthma: a 12-year prospective follow-up study. *Chest* 2006, 129:309-316.

Samara K, Zervou M, Siafakas NM & Tzortzaki EG. Microsatellite DNA instability in benign lung diseases. *Respir Med.* 2006 Feb;100(2):202-11.

Schumacher MJ, Cota KA, Taussig LM. Pulmonary response to nasal-challenge testing of atopic subjects with stable asthma. *J Allergy Clin Immunol* 1986; 78(1 Pt 1):30–5.

Settipane RJ, Hagy GW & Settipane GA. Long-term risk factors for developing asthma and allergic rhinitis: a 23-year follow-up study of college students. *Allergy Proc* 1994; 15(1):21–5.

Sherrill DL, Stein R, Halonen M, Holberg CJ, Wright A, Martinez FD, et al. Total serum IgE and its association with asthma symptoms and allergic sensitization among children. *J Allergy Clin Immunol* 1999; 104:28–36.

Siafakas NM, Tzortzaki EG, Sourvinos G, et al. Microsatellite DNA instability in COPD. *Chest* 1999;116:47–51.

Thomas M, Kocevar VS, Zhang Q, et al. Asthma-related health care resource use among asthmatic children with and without concomitant allergic rhinitis. *Pediatrics* 2005; 115: 129–34.

Van-Ganse E, Kaufman L, Derde MP, Yernault JC, Delaunois L & Vincken W. Effects of antihistamines in adult asthma: a meta-analysis of clinical trials. *Eur Respir J* 1997; 10(10): 2216– 24.

Vassilakis DA, Sourvinos G, Spandidos DA, et al. Frequent genetic alterations at the microsatellite level in cytologic sputum samples of patients with idiopathic pulmonary fibrosis. *Am J Respir Crit Care Med* 2000; 162:1115–9.

Walsh GM. Reslizumab, a humanized anti-IL-5 mAb for the treatment of eosinophil-mediated inflammatory conditions. *Curr Opin Mol Ther.* 2009 Jun; 11(3):329-36.

Wright AL, Holberg CJ, Martinez FD, Halonen M, Morgan W & Taussig LM. Epidemiology of physician-diagnosed allergic rhinitis in childhood. *Pediatrics* 1994; 94(6 Pt 1):895 -901.

Yawn BP, Yunginger JW, Wollan PC, et al. Allergic rhinitis in Rochester, Minnesota, residents with asthma: frequency and impact on health care charges. *J Allergy Clin Immunol* 1999; 103:54–9.

5

Clinical Variants of Allergic Rhinitis and Asthma Phenotypes in Patients with or Without a Smoking History

Sanja Popović-Grle
School of Medicine, University of Zagreb,
Zagreb University Hospital Center,
Jordanovac Lung Disease Clinic, Zagreb,
Croatia

1. Introduction

Asthma has been a fascinating disease for millennia, while rhinitis has been recognized only for the last two centuries. Rhinitis has been defined so late in the medical practice because of other medical priorities, such as mortal infectious diseases or wounds. Due to a larger number of doctors in the community, better education, diminished impact of epidemics, better standard and increased lifetime, medical doctors have accomplished to observe and help their patients more than previously. A significant contribution to improving allergy management has been achieved through the ability of physicians to write and publish details about their work, exchange experiences, as well as test various hypotheses and perform various experiments. Despite an enormous increase in scientific work in all parts of the world, we still do not know what asthma and rhinitis are, but in the past few decades we have learned that those conditions are closely associated.

Allergic rhinitis is one of the most common clinical presentations of allergy in human beings. It has been noticed that, during the 1990s, at the end of the past century, the prevalence of rhinitis doubled[1]. Allergic rhinitis is one of the 10 most common reasons for visiting general practitioners[2]. Allergic rhinitis is highly associated with doctor-diagnosed asthma. In an Italian study involving 18.647 subjects, a relative risk ratio (RRR) of 12.48 was obtained concerning the association between asthma and rhinitis[3]. Allergic rhinitis depends on the atopic status of the individual with an allergic reaction to a causative allergen, as well as on allergen exposure.

Asthma is defined as ''a common chronic disorder of the airways that is complex and characterized by variable and recurring symptoms, airflow obstruction, bronchial hyperresponsiveness, and an underlying inflammation[4].' It is estimated that 30 million people in Europe have asthma, with the economic cost of asthma amounting to € 17 billion per year[5]. Among the asthmatic population, those who have allergic rhinitis represent different endotype of the asthma syndrome[6]. Distinct asthma phenotypes can be defined on the basis of the lung function, allergen sensitization, and symptoms characteristic of rhinitis and asthma. The asthma endotypes are defined on the basis of asthma phenotypes and the underlying pathophysiological mechanisms.

Patients with asthma and allergic rhinitis phenotypes have all asthma severity degrees, from intermittent through persistent mild, moderate and severe asthma. Some of them have just an early allergic reaction in bronchial mucosa, resulting in acute bronhchospasm, with recurrent wheezing, but some have a late asthmatic response. Allergic asthma and rhinitis usually respond well to inhaled corticosteroids. They are usually not dangerous in the case of severe asthma attacks, unless the patients show risk behavior. Such risks include: non-compliance with the asthma treatment, exposure to extreme (atmospheric or toxic) conditions, and/or severe respiratory infections. They may be greatly modified depending on whether the patients are active or passive smokers. When an ill person is exposed to continuous toxic gases by his/her own will, such as smoking, the immune response in the airways alters. Acute exposure to cigarette smoke is associated with NF-κB activation and synthesis of IL-8 in the alveolar macrophages. After being translocated into the nucleus, the activated NF-κB binds with the DNA and regulates the expression of numerous genes involved in the inflammatory process[7]. The inflammatory cells are distributed unevenly throughout the bronchial tree, both large and small airways, and can be found both in asymptomatic smokers and in patients with chronic obstructive pulmonary diseases (COPD), whose main disease risk factor is smoking[8]. The only difference between the asymptomatic smokers and patients with a type of COPD was quantitative - the smokers with a COPD had a greater number of inflammatory cells, as shown in our own research[9].

The immunological changes in the airways caused by smoking enhance the functional derangement of the airways. Smoking in adolescence reduces the lung function growth rate, so that the expected value of forced expiratory volume in the first second (FEV_1)[10] is not attained. If adolescents gain a permanent habit of smoking, their decline in FEV_1 starts much earlier than in non-smokers[11]. The pulmonary function is a function of age. This means that after birth the pulmonary function continues to evolve and grow, reaching its maximum in adolescence, followed by a plateau until the late twenties. Persons over 30 have a permanent annual physiological loss of lung volume and flow rate, 20-30 ml FEV_1 per year. Smokers have a greater annual decline in FEV_1 than non-smokers[12 13], 60 ml per year[14] on the average. In adolescents who smoke, the loss begins earlier than in non-smokers, significantly shortening the plateau of constant lung function in adolescence, and the process is even faster in the female population[15], which is more vulnerable to cigarette smoke. A higher prevalence of asthma (OR 1.83) and rhinitis (OR 1.61) has been found in adolescent smokers than in non-smokers. It has been found that people with 1-10 pack years have an odds ratio (OR) of 1:47 for developing more severe types of asthma compared to non-smokers with allergic rhinitis, while those with over 20 pack years have a risk OR of 5:59, also compared to allergic non-smokers. Pack years represent the index of total exposure to tobacco smoke, or the overall smoking history. Pack years are important for the assessment of the risk of developing a disease. It is believed that the quantification of over 10 pack years significantly increases the risk of occurrence of a COPD, while the quantification of over 20 pack years represents a high risk of developing lung cancer and heart attack. Each medical document of a person who smokes, not just pulmonary or cardiac where it is essential, but particularly general practice documents, should contain the data on pack years. Pack years are calculated by using the following formula:

$$\text{Pack years} = \frac{\text{Number of cigarettes per day}}{20} \text{ X years of smoking}$$

An average person is not fully aware of the entire problem of smoking and its impact on human health. Smoking is considered to be the biggest risk factor associated with the global burden of disease in developed countries and amounts to 12.2%, expressed in disability adjusted life years (DALY), according to the World Health Organization (WHO). Every 8 seconds someone in the world dies from smoking related diseases[16]. Smoking is a risk factor associated with six of the eight leading causes of death worldwide[17]. Smoking affects the occurrence of disease, its outcome, and in case the outcome is not death, the success of treatment also depends on whether the person is an active or former smoker. The answer to how this is possible lies in the chemical composition of tobacco smoke. Cigarette smoke has over 4000 chemical substances, 3000 respiratory irritants and about 1000 other noxious chemical substances. The International Agency for Research on Cancer has included more than 60 substances in the group of carcinogens[18]. To improve the effect of smoking on the palate (pH changes from acidic to alkaline and increases potential addiction), tobacco leaves are combined with additives. In the United States of America (USA), these additives are regulated in the form of a list of 599 substances[19]. Tobacco smoke is full of free oxygen radicals (up to the extreme number of 1017) and each radical is an unstable molecule. These radicals damage the tissue by their unpredictable and random binding with any other molecules in the vicinity, thus creating further unstable molecules, new radicals, which cause further tissue damage, up to the DNA level. Oxidants and free radicals cause sequestration and accumulation of neutrophils in the pulmonary microcirculation, as well as accumulation of macrophages in the respiratory bronchioli, with macrophages being a potential reservoir of new oxidants[20].

Another important fact is that there are no less harmful cigarettes with low tar content ('light') or a safe level of smoking. European legislation prescribes limitation of the cigarette tar content to 10 mg, nicotine to 1 mg and carbon monoxide to 10 mg per cigarette, which has been incorporated in the Regulation on Health Safety of General Use Items since January 1, 2005 (Official Gazette 42/2004) in the Republic of Croatia. As far as the so-called light cigarettes are concerned, there is a misconception that they contain smaller quantities of harmful substances. Light cigarettes are made in the way that nicotine is overheated and carbon dioxide (CO_2) is blown into it until it assumes the form of expanding foam used to fill the same cigarette paper as ordinary tobacco. Also, light cigarettes have vent holes in the filters to assure that smoke is diluted with air during inhalation. Therefore, smokers of this type of cigarettes inhale more deeply on the average and actually receive the same amount of tar and nicotine.

There is yet another important fact that the general public is usually not aware of, and that is the influence of passive smoking on health. Passive smoking is defined as involuntary inhalation of tobacco smoke. Cigarette smoke coming from a burning cigarette tip is called *second-hand smoke* (SHS). The smoke remaining after putting the cigarette out is called *environmental tobacco smoke* (ETS). Cigarette smoke remains in the room air for the next 8 hours! [21] Tobacco smoke exhaled by a smoker may be the worst of them all, because the substances in cigarette smoke change after getting in contact with human tissue enzymes. Environmental tobacco smoke (ETS) is a mixture of second-hand smoke and smoke exhaled from the lungs of smokers. Scientific evidence on passive smoking have provided non-smokers with strong arguments in their demands to breathe clean air and prohibit smoking in indoor areas, which is now supported by legislation in most developed countries.

It is believed that passive smoking causes 10% of disease mortality in the world, in children mostly due to lower respiratory tract infections (5,939 million) and asthma (651,000), and in adults due to ischemic heart disease (2,836 million) and also asthma (1,246 million), according to the 2004 data published in the Lancet based on the analysis of results from 192 countries worldwide[22]. It is believed that persons exposed to second-hand smoke have a higher production of immunoglobulin E (IgE), total and specific IgE to certain allergens[23]. Passive smoking has been proved to increase the risk of asthma in children. An epidemiological study of 53,879 children showed that passive smoking, either prenatal or postnatal, significantly increases the probability of asthma in children, as well as the occurrence of respiratory problems such as night time cough and wheezing[24]. Another large nationwide study of 102,000 children in the United States proved the connection between tobacco smoke exposure in children in their homes and prevalence of asthma, with a significance level of $p = 0026$[25]. The quality of atmospheric air or socioeconomic status of the family did not affect this correlation between asthma and household smoking. Since the prevalence of asthma increased three times in the past few decades, there are hypotheses that this increase is at least partly caused by the observed major increase in cigarette consumption in the past century[26]. That increase in cigarette consumption further increases the exposure to second-hand smoke, especially in children, thus also increasing the incidence of childhood asthma. It has been shown that the proportion of exhaled nitric oxide (FENO), which is used as a biomarker of airway inflammation in asthma, is associated with the exposure of children to environmental tobacco smoke at the age of 4[27]. Similar data found with regards to the adult population confirms that exposure to tobacco smoke in the environment increases the occurrence of asthma and its exacerbations[28].

These data imply that exposure to toxic ingredients of cigarette smoke is highly associated with allergic rhinitis and/or asthma, as well as to the probability of developing asthma, especially more severe exacerbations. In this study, we were interested to find out whether smoking poses a risk on the presentation of allergic rhinitis and/or asthma, and on clinical variants of these respiratory allergy diseases in patients with diagnosed allergic rhinitis and asthma phenotypes.

2. Methods

The pulmonologists from the Outpatient Department of the Zagreb University Hospital Center, Jordanovac Lung Disease Clinic, located in the moderate continental climate area of Central and Eastern Europe (Zagreb, Croatia) recruited 120 adult asthma patients in consecutive order for purposes of a study carried out in the period from 2006 to 2009 in which 78 healthy persons constituted the control group, in total 198 subjects. They were considered healthy if they had no previous respiratory diseases, and if they answered negative to all questions from the Screening ECRHS II Questionnaire. The European Community Respiratory Health Survey (ECRHS) was part of the European Commission Quality of Life Programme and a nine-year prospective collaborative study carried out in 14 European countries, which collected data from more than 10 000 young adults[29].

All patients had had doctor-diagnosed asthma for longer than 6 months, based on a detailed interview. The symptoms that were considered asthmatic included: chronic cough, expectoration, wheezing, shortness of breath, chest tightness, exercise impairment, or night awakening. The age at asthma appearance, the number of asthma exacerbations and their severity and frequency were available; and the daily and night symptoms, exercise impairment, and dosing of rescue medication (short-acting β_2 agonists) were obtained. The data on sports and smoking habits were also collected. The severity of asthma was classified

according to the Global Initiative for Asthma (GINA) into intermittent, mild persistent, moderate or severe persistent asthma[30]. The level of asthma control was assessed by applying the Asthma Control Test (ACT)[31]. The symptoms that were considered rhinitic included: sneezing, watery secretion, nasal blockage, and nasal itching[32]. The patients with allergic rhinitis or nasal polyps had ENT specialist-established diagnosis.
After examination, all patients performed spirometry and had to fill out a standardized questionnaire for asthmatic patients (ECRHS). Spirometry was performed at least three times from normal breathing followed by slow inhalation to a maximum, on a MasterLab Pro, version 4.3, an apparatus with a pneumotachograph. The best attempt was selected and forced expiratory volume in the first second (FEV_1) recorded according to the standard spirometric procedure (ATS/ERS)[33] and then compared with the referent values according to the European Community for Coal and Steel[34]. The existence of an obstructive ventilatory disorder was considered if FEV_1 was less than 80% of the predicted value, and the FEV_1/FVC ratio under 0.7. The bronchodilator reversibility was tested with 400 μg of the short acting β_2-agonist (salbutamol) and considered positive if the FEV_1 increased by 12% and/or 200 ml after 15-30 minutes[35,36].
The skin prick tests (SPT) were performed on the forearm, with 15 aeroallergens manufactured by Stalallergen, France (*Dermatophagoides pteronyssinus, Dermatophagoides farinae,* cat dander, dog dander, moulds (*Aspergillus fumigatus, Alternaria alternata, Cladosporium herbarum, Candida albicans*), Latex, hazel tree pollen (*Corylus avellana*), birch pollen (*Betulla verrucosa*), grass pollen mixture (*Phleum pratense, Lolium perenne, Dactylis glomerata, Festuca elatior, Poa pratensis),* rye pollen (*Secale cereale*), short ragweed pollen (*Ambrosia elatior*), mugworth pollen (*Artemisia vulgaris*). Negative (saline solution) and positive (histamine 1 mg/ml) controls were used. After 15 minutes, the diameter was measured in millimeters (mm), the long axis (D) and its perpendicular (d). A particular skin prick test was considered positive when the mean wheal size was greater than 3 mm in relation to the negative control $\{(D+d)/2\}\geq 3$[37]. The patients had not taken any antihistamines, anti-depressives or any other therapy which could influence the results of the SPT for at least a week prior to the testing. Descriptive statistics, correlation, t-tests and chi square tests were used for data analysis by means of standard statistical programs.

3. Results

From among the 198 subjects involved in this study, 120 patients had the asthmatic syndrome, 104 had allergic rhinitis and asthma, while 16 had only allergic asthma (Table 1). The duration of allergic rhinitis (AR) was significantly longer than the duration of asthma, $p<0.001$ (Table 2). As far as gender is concerned, the sample of patients with allergic rhinitis and asthma consisted of significantly more female subjects (Table 3).

	n	(%)
asthma only	16	(8.1)
asthma with AR	104	(52.5)
healthy	78	(39.4)
total	198	(100.0)

Table 1. Share of participants with asthma, allergic rhinitis and healthy participants

	Mean	(SD)	Median	(IQR)	Min	Max	Shapiro-Wilk Test
Age at first onset (in years)							
asthma	32	(17.9)	30	(17-44.5)	1	70	P=0.264
allergic rhinitis	28	(16.2)	30	(14-40)	1	64	P=0.122
Duration of illness (in years)							
asthma	10	(10.1)	5	(2-19)	0	32	P<0.001
allergic rhinitis	13	(10,5)	10	(3-21)	1	40	P=0.005

Abbreviation: Mean = arithmetic mean; SD = standard deviation; IQR = interquartile range; Shapiro Wilk Test for normality of distribution

Table 2. Asthma and allergic rhinitis descriptive parameters

	Male		Female		P
	n	(%)	n	(%)	
Diagnosis					0.368
asthma only	6	(17.6)	9	(11.0)	
asthma with AR	28	(82.4)	73	(89.0)	
total	34	(100.0)	82	(100.0)	

Abbreviations: P = Fisher's Exact Test; level of statistical significance, or probability of type I (alpha)

Table 3. Prevalence of asthma and allergic rhinitis by gender

4. Predictors of AR and asthma

4.1 Smoking and non-smoking as Predictors of AR and asthma

	Group				total		OR (95%CI)
	patients		healthy				
	n	(%)	n	(%)	n	(%)	
never smoked	14	(31)	31	(69)	45	(100)	1
smoked	59	(56)	47	(44)	106	(100)	2.8 (1.3-5.8)

Abbreviations: OR = odds ratio; 95%CI = 95% confidence interval for odds ratio
Fisher Exact Test, P = 0.07

Table 4. Prevalence of patients by their smoking history; base: whole sample (n =151)

Ever-smoking proved to be a statistically significant predictor of developing asthma or allergic rhinitis. The prevalence of respondents with asthma or allergic rhinitis among those who had smoked at least once in their life (or still smoke) was significantly higher, 59/106 (56%), than among the respondents who had never smoked 14/45 (31%). The odds for being diagnosed with allergic rhinitis and asthma was 2.8 times and statistically significantly higher among those who had smoked or still smoke than the odds for the illness among those who had never smoked (binary logistic regression; exposed to smoke B coefficient = 1.02; standard error = 0.38; odds ratio = 2.48 95% CI = 1.3-5.8). The proportion of smokers, former or current, in the whole sample of asthmatic or healthy persons was more than one half (53.5%). In the group of active smokers, the smoking history amounted to 24.18±7.49 pack years, while in the group of former smokers the smoking history amounted to 17.53±4.62 pack years.

	Group						total		LR; df; P
	asthma only		allergic rhinitis and asthma		healthy				
	n	(%)	n	(%)	n	(%)	n	(%)	
never smoked	2	(5)	8	(20)	31	(76)	41	(100)	7.704; 2; 0.02
smoked	8	(9)	38	(41)	47	(51)	93	(100)	

Abbreviations: OR = odds ratio; 95%CI = 95% confidence interval for odds ratio;
LR = likelihood ratio, P = level of statistical significance, or probability of type I (alpha)

Table 5. Prevalence of patients by their smoking history; base: whole sample (n =134)

The patients and healthy respondents differed statistically significantly in terms of whether they had ever smoked in life (likelihood ratio = 7.704, P = 0.02). Among the patients who had smoked or smoke, 8/93 (9%) had asthma, compared to 2/41 (5%) of those who had never smoked. Also, 38/93 (41%) of those who had smoked had asthma and allergic rhinitis, compared to 8/41 (20%) who had never smoked.

	Diagnosis				total		OR (95%CI)
	allergic rhinitis and asthma		no respiratory disease				
	N	(%)	n	(%)	n	(%)	
never smoked	8	(21)	31	(79)	39	(100)	1
smoked	41	(47)	47	(53)	88	(100)	3.4 (1.4-8.2)

Abbreviations: OR = odds ratio; 95%CI = 95% confidence interval for odds ratio
Fisher Exact Test, P = 0.06

Table 6. Prevalence of allergic rhinitis and asthma by their smoking history (at least once or never); base: allergic rhinitis + asthma and healthy (n=127)

Ever-smoking proved to be a statistically significant predictor of allergic rhinitis and asthma. The prevalence of allergic rhinitis and asthma among the respondents who had smoked at least once in their life (or still smoke) was significantly higher, 41/88 (47%), than among the respondents who had never smoked, 8/39 (21%). The odds for being diagnosed with allergic rhinitis and asthma was 3.4 times and statistically significantly higher among those who had smoked or still smoke than the odds for developing these illnesses among those who had never smoked (binary logistic regression; exposed to smoke B coefficient = 1.22; standard error = 0.45; odds ratio = 3.4; 95% CI = 1.4-8.2).

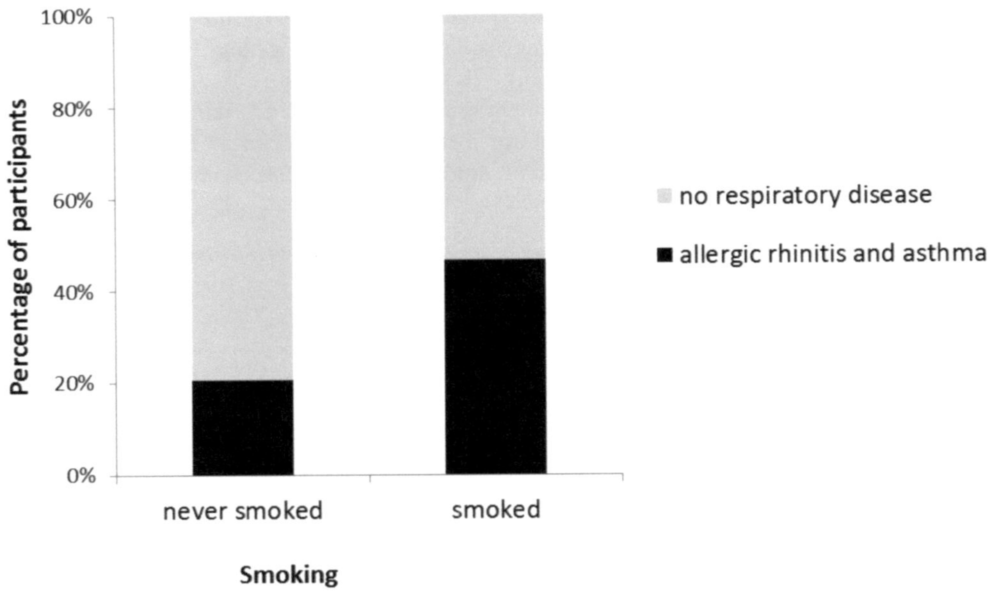

Fig. 1. Prevalence of allergic rhinitis and asthma by smoking history (at least once or never); base: whole sample, (n=127)

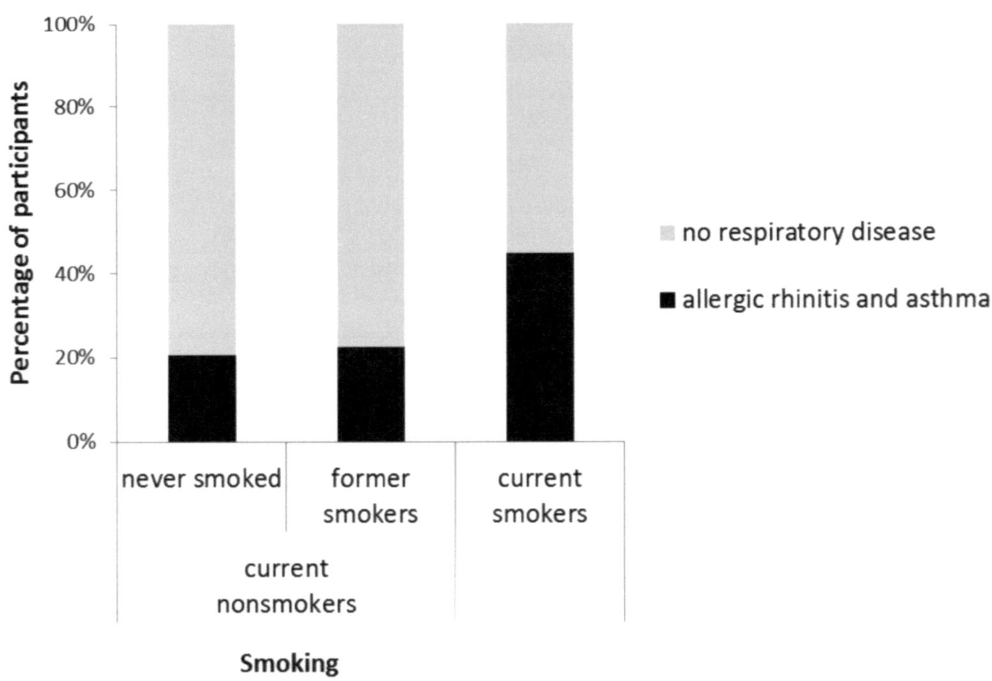

Fig. 2. Prevalence of allergic rhinitis and asthma by current non-smokers, former smokers, and non-smokers; base: whole sample, (n=103)

Current smoking proved to be a statistically significant predictor of allergic rhinitis and asthma in comparison to non-smoking. Current smoking accounted for approximately 7.3% of the variants of allergic rhinitis and asthma (Nagelkerke R squared = 0.073). Current smokers had a 3.1 (310%) time greater chance of developing asthma and allergic rhinitis. 13/29 (45%) current smokers had asthma and allergic rhinitis, compared to 7/34 (21%) people who had never smoked (binary logistic regression, current smokers B coefficient = 1.14; standard error = 0.55; odds ratio = 3.1, 95% CI = 1.0 to 9.5).

4.2 Daily exposure to tobacco smoke and current smoking as predictors of AR and asthma

	Diagnosis				total		OR (95%CI)
	allergic rhinitis and asthma		no respiratory disease				
	n	(%)	n	(%)	n	(%)	
non-smokers							
not exposed to smoke	6	(14)	38	(86)	44	(100)	1
exposed to smoke	10	(33)	20	(67)	30	(100)	3.2 (1.0-10.0)
smokers	13	(45)	16	(55)	29	(100)	5.2 (1.7-15.9)

Abbreviations: OR = odds ratio; 95%CI = 95% confidence interval for odds ratio
Likelihood ratio=9.3; df=2; P=0.01; contingency coefficient = 0.28

Table 7 Prevalence of allergic rhinitis and asthma by current non-smokers' daily exposure to tobacco smoke and current smoking; base: whole sample, (n=103)

Both daily exposure to tobacco smoke among current non-smokers and current smoking proved to be statistically significant predictors of allergic rhinitis and asthma. The prevalence of allergic rhinitis and asthma among the current non-smokers who had been daily exposed to tobacco smoke during the period of 12 months prior to the study, was 10/30 (33%) in comparison to the current non-smokers who had not been daily exposed to tobacco smoke, 6/44 (14%). The odds for being diagnosed with allergic rhinitis and asthma were 3.2 times and statistically significantly higher among the current non-smokers who had been daily exposed to tobacco smoke than the odds for developing these illnesses among the current non-smokers who had not been daily exposed to tobacco smoke (binary logistic regression; exposed to smoke B coefficient = 1.25; standard error = 0.59; odds ratio = 3.2; 95% CI = 1.0-10.0).

The prevalence of allergic rhinitis and asthma among the current smokers, 13/29 (45%), was about three times higher than among those who had not been daily exposed to tobacco smoke, 6/44 (14%). The odds for developing these illnesses were 5.2 times and statistically significantly higher in the case of smokers (binary logistic regression; smokers B coefficient = 1.64; standard error = 0.58; odds ratio = 5.2; 95% CI = 1.7-15.9).

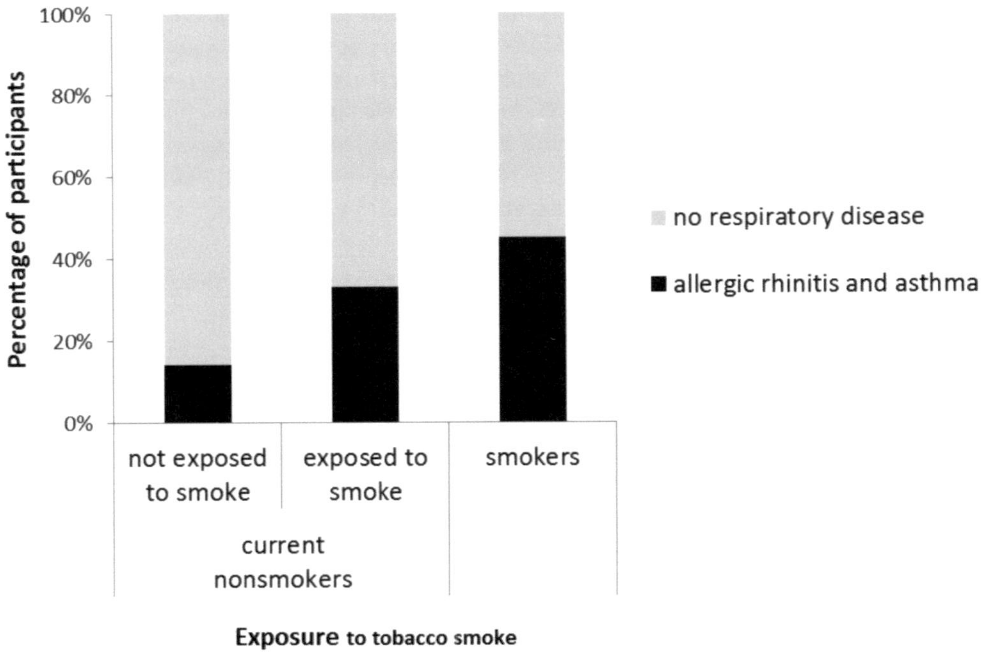

Fig. 3. Prevalence of allergic rhinitis and asthma by current non-smokers' daily exposure to tobacco smoke and current smoking; base: whole sample, (n=97)

4.3 Prevalence of patients who quit or reduced smoking

The healthy respondents and those with allergic rhinitis and asthma did not differ significantly with regard to quitting or reducing smoking (Fisher Exact Test, P = 0.249). Among those with allergic rhinitis and asthma however, the difference between those who quit or reduced smoking and those who didn't was statistically significant (goodness of fit Hi square = 20.83; df = 1; P < 0.01), 88% quit or reduced smoking, while 12% of them still smoke as before.

	Diagnosis				
	allergic rhinitis and asthma		no respiratory disease		P
	n	(%)	n	(%)	
didn't reduce	4	(12)	11	(23)	0.249
reduced	29	(88)	36	(77)	
TOTAL	33	(100)	47	(100)	

Abbreviations: OR = odds ratio; 95%CI = 95% confidence interval for odds ratio
P = Fisher Exact Test; level of statistical significance, or probability of type I (alpha)

Table 8. Prevalence of those who quit or reduced smoking by illness (allergic rhinitis and asthma); base: whole sample (n=70)

5. Allergy diagnostic tests (skin prick tests)

The skin prick tests in the healthy control group were negative in the case of all tested subjects. The patients with allergic rhinitis and asthma endotypes associated with smoking were significantly more sensitized to perennial allergens, mostly to Dermatophagoides pteronyssinus (54% of patients in the ever-smoking group and 39% in the non-smoking group). In the non-smoking group of patients with allergic rhinitis and asthma, greater sensitization was recorded to seasonal allergens, most often to grass pollen (31% of patients in the ever-smoking group and 42% in the non-smoking group).

	$\bar{X}$	*SD*	*Min.*	*Max.*	*SE*
Histamine ever-smokers	6.25	1.38	3	11	0.21
Histamine non-smokers	7.40	1.57	4	12	0.27
Der p ever-smokers	5.69	1.75	3	9	0.19
Der p non-smokers	5.87	1.83	3	14	0.21
Fel d ever-smokers	5.71	1.54	4	13	0.17
Fel d non-smokers	5.92	1.67	3	13	0.16
Alt a ever-smokers	4.91	1.22	3	8	0.12
Alt a non-smokers	5.11	1.34	3	9	0.14
Bet v ever-smokers	7.63	1.68	4	22	0.31
Bet v non-smokers	8.14	1.82	5	25	0.29
Phl p ever-smokers	6.88	1.91	5	18	0.24
Phl p e non-smokers	7.49	1.82	4	27	0.28
Amb e ever-smokers	7.36	1.65	5	19	0.31
Amb e non-smokers	8.10	1.78	5	32	0.34

Abbreviation: $\bar{X}$ = arithmetic mean; SD = standard deviation: Min.= minimal value; Max.= maximal value; SE=standard error; mm=millimeters; Der p=Dermatophagoides pteronyssinus; Fel d=Felis domestica; Alt a= Alternaria alternata, Bet v= Betula verrucosa; Phl p= Phleum pratense; Amb e= Ambrosia elatior.

Table 9. Results of skin prick tests to common inhalation allergens in allergic rhinitis and asthma phenotypes patients with or without a smoking history, reaction by wheal size in mm (positive control: histamine (1 mg/ml), negative control: saline solution).

The wheal reaction to common inhalation allergens (size in mm) in allergic rhinitis and asthma phenotypes patients showed a bigger diameter in patients without a smoking history than in the group of allergic ever-smoking patients (Table 17). The skin wheal reaction to pollen allergens was greater than the reaction to perennial allergens in the case of all patients.

6. Clinical symptom variants in allergic rhinitis and asthma

All subjects in the group of subjects with allergic rhinitis and asthma phenotypes had a few symptoms of their disease, at least three, but most subjects had more than five symptoms. The distribution of their symptoms differed whether they were current or former smokers or lifetime non-smokers. Table 18 shows less histamine-mediated symptoms of allergic rhinitis, such as sneezing or runny nose, in the medical history of non-smoking patients than in the group of smokers, however more blocked nose.

	With a smoking history (ever-smokers) n=59	Without a smoking history (non-smokers) n=45
Sneezing	28 (48%)	27 (61%)
Runny nose	25 (43%)	23 (52%)
Blocked nose	42 (72%)	24 (54%)
Itchy nose	12 (21%)	14 (32%)
Itchy eyes (conjunctivitis)	21 (36%)	12 (27%)

Table 10. Clinical presentation of rhinitic symptoms in patients with allergic rhinitis and asthma phenotypes with or without a smoking history

	With a smoking history (ever-smokers) n=68	Without a smoking history (non-smokers) n=52
Cough	58 (85%)	32 (61%)
Expectoration	52 (76%)	15 (29%)
Wheezing	27 (39%)	30 (57%)
Chest tightness	13 (19%)	21 (41%)
Shortness of breath	22 (32%)	21 (40%)
Exercise impairment	17 (25%)	17 (33%)
Night awakening	14 (21%)	19 (37%)
Asthma exacerbation (moderate/severe)	21 (31%)	14 (26%)
ACT (mean value out of exacerbation)	16	20

Abbreviations: ACT= Asthma Control Test

Table 11. Clinical presentation of asthmatic symptoms in patients with allergic rhinitis and asthma phenotypes with or without a smoking history

The respondents with the ever-smoking habit showed less chest tightness, night awakening and exercise impairment, compared to the non-smoking group, but more moderate or severe asthma exacerbations, with lower asthma control.

	With a smoking history (ever-smokers) n=68	Without a smoking history (non-smokers) n=52
GINA I	3 (04%)	2 (05%)
GINA II	18 (26%)	20 (39%)
GINA III	41 (61%)	26 (49%)
GINA IV	6 (09%)	4 (07%)

Abbreviations: GINA= Global Initiative for Asthma

Table 12. Distribution of diagnosed patients with allergic rhinitis and asthma phenotypes according to the GINA classification, with or without a smoking history

7. Lung fnction (FEV_1)

The distribution of forced expiratory volume in the first second (FEV_1) level did not deviate significantly from the normal distribution among all patients (Shapiro Wilk = 0.994, P =

0.698), among those with asthma only (Shapiro Wilk = 0.962, P = 0.698) or among those with asthma and allergic rhinitis (Shapiro Wilk = 0.982, P = 0.490).

	Mean (SD)	Median (IQR)	Min	Max	Shapiro-Wilk Test
Whole sample	78.7 (19.87)	79.4 (66.3-93.3)	30	140	P = 0.698
Asthma only	77.1 (21.11)	77.2 (62.9-96.7)	39	106	P = 0.816
Asthma and allergic rhinitis	79.9 (21.56)	80.8 (67.3-95.8)	30	124	P = 0.490

Abbreviation: Mean = arithmetic mean; SD = standard deviation; IQR = interquartile range; Shapiro Wilk Test for normality of distribution

Table 13. FEV1 (% of the reference value)

	FEV_1		P
	Mean	SD	
never smoked	15.22	4.97	<0.05
smoked	8.62	5.14	

Abbreviation: Mean = arithmetic mean; SD = standard deviation

Table 14. Difference in the FEV1 average increase (%) after the bronchodilator test with salbutamol by current and ever-smokers, base: only ill (n=47)

The bronchodilator response in the smoking group was statistically significantly lower than in the non-smoking group.

Considering the skin sensitization established on the basis of skin prick tests there were more patients sensitized to perennial allergens in the smoking group (active and former smokers), most to Dermatophagoides pteronyssinus (58%), followed by those sensitized to ragweed pollen (Ambrosia elatior) (34%). In the non-smoking group of patients with allergic asthma, seasonal allergies were more recorded, mostly to grass pollen (42%), while ragweed pollen and tree pollen were similarly distributed (32% and 31%).

The exacerbation rate in both groups did not differ significantly, which may be due to the low number of study groups. Only 4/120 (3.3%) patients were hospitalized due to asthma exacerbations during the observation period. 11/120 (9.2%) ever-smoking patients were hospitalized for asthma exacerbations, some of them even several times. Intensive care treatment was needed in the case of 2/120 (1.7%) patients, however no intubation or mechanical ventilation was necessary.

8. Discussion

Allergic rhinitis and asthma are frequent diseases posing a heavy burden for the society. Allergic rhinitis and asthma presented together are considered to be different asthma phenotype and endotype. The allergic reaction is modified depending on whether the patients are active or passive smokers. A large proportion of patients with allergic rhinitis and asthma are smokers. Our hypothesis was that there were differences in the clinical presentation of allergic rhinitis and asthma phenotypes due to exposure to tobacco smoke.

In the investigated group of patients with allergic asthma, those who also had allergic rhinitis made up a significantly greater number (104/120) compared to the asthmatics without allergic rhinitis. The prevalence of allergic rhinitis in asthmatics in the case of our subjects was 86.7% (Table 1), involving significantly more female subjects (Table 3). Even in children from 6-12 years of age, it was found that 89.7% had moderate to severe rhinitis, which means that they have troublesome sleeping, problems with concentration and diminished learning results[38].

From the total sample of 198 subjects, both in the case of asthmatic and healthy subjects, there were more former or current smokers (106/198) than persons who had never smoked. The proportion of ever-smokers investigated in this study (53.5%) is greater than the proportion of ever-smokers in the general population, according to the epidemiological survey conducted on adults[39] and medical students in Croatia[40]. The mentioned surveys showed there were 27.4% regular daily smokers over 18, of which 34% men and 22% women.

Active smokers had a slightly higher number of pack years than former smokers, however not significantly higher. In the group of active smokers, the number of pack years amounted to 24.18±7.49, while in the group of former smokers the number of pack years amounted to 17.53±4.62. These data show that most smokers smoke for more than a decade or two before starting to consider quitting smoking and before they succeed to do it. Most literature data based on various studies confirm our results. Quitting smoking is a process with several phases preceding the change in behavior, which has been known for a longer period[41]. As smoking produces nicotine addiction, it is not easy to quit smoking due to the abstinence syndrome. Besides a strong motive, some smokers might need a nicotine replacement therapy with pharmacological agents, vareniclin or bupropion, which increases the rate of successful quitters[42].

The odds for being diagnosed with allergic rhinitis and asthma in our study was 2.8 times and statistically significantly higher among those who had smoked or still smoke than the odds for developing these illnesses among those who had never smoked (Table 4). The data from other authors also show that smokers are more likely to develop asthma than non-smokers, although smoking is not believed to cause asthma[43]. Tobacco smoking causes increased bronchial hyperreactivity[44]. After quitting smoking, bronchial hyperreactivity in asthma patients decreases in comparison to the asthma patients who continue to smoke[45].

Among the patients who had smoked, 9% had asthma, compared to 5% of those who had never smoked. Also, 41% of those who had smoked had asthma and allergic rhinitis, compared to 20% of those who had never smoked. These results are statistically significant (p=0.02), with the likelihood ratio of 7.7 for developing allergic asthma and rhinitis if smoking (Table 5).

Ever-smoking proved to be a statistically significant predictor of allergic rhinitis and asthma. The prevalence of allergic rhinitis and asthma among the respondents who had smoked at least once in their life (or still smoke) was significantly higher, 47%, than among the respondents who had never smoked, 21% (Table 6)

Daily exposure to tobacco smoke among current non-smokers and current smokers proved to be a statistically significant predictor of allergic rhinitis and asthma. There were 45% of current smokers in our group with allergic rhinitis and asthma, more than in Northern America where there were 25-35%[46]. The investigated current smokers, in comparison to the investigated former smokers, had a 3.1 time greater chance of developing asthma and allergic rhinitis (Figure 2). The non-smokers who had been exposed to tobacco smoke during the last 12 months prior to the study, had a 3.2 time greater chance of developing asthma and allergic rhinitis (odds ratio = 3.2; 95% CI = 1,0-10,0) in comparison to the non-exposed non-smokers. Also in comparison to the non-exposed non-smokers, the current smokers, daily exposed to cigarette smoke, had a 5.2 time greater chance of developing asthma and allergic rhinitis (odds ratio = 5.2; 95% CI = 1.7-15.9) (Table 7). Daily exposure to tobacco smoke among the former smokers did not prove to be a statistically significant predictor of allergic rhinitis and asthma (odds ratio = 0.9; 95% CI = 0.9-11.2).

The healthy respondents and those with allergic rhinitis and asthma did not differ significantly with regards to reducing the number of cigarettes. Most subjects tried to reduce smoking (77% *vs.* 88%) (Table 8). These results are in concordance with the known fact that more than 70% of smokers want to quit smoking[47].

The bronchodilator response in the smoking group was statistically significantly lower than in the non-smoking group, $p<0.05$. (8.62%±5.14 *vs.*15.22%±4.97, $p<0.01$) (Table 14). As it is known that smokers have higher levels of total immunoglobulin E (IgE)[48] and a greater degree of infiltration of inflammatory cells, especially eosinophils[49], in comparison to non-smokers, it is most likely that inflammatory processes will lead to airways remodeling and fixed bronchial obstruction, with lower reversibility.

As far as skin sensitization established on the basis of skin prick tests is concerned, a greater number of patients from the smoking group (active and former smokers) were sensitized to perennial allergens, while the non-smoking patients with allergic asthma and rhinitis were more sensitized to seasonal allergens. The ever-smoking patients were most usually sensitized to Dermatophagoides pteronyssinus (54%), while the non-smoking allergic patients were more often sensitized to grass pollen (42%). The wheal reaction of the skin to common inhalation allergens in allergic rhinitis and asthma endotypes showed a bigger diameter in patients without a smoking history than in the group of allergic patients who had smoked at least once in their life (Table 9). It seems that smoking diminishes the histamine reaction, which is contrary to most literature data about the increased release of proinflammatory mediators[50].

The distribution of the patients' symptoms differed whether they were current or former smokers or if they were lifetime non-smokers. The allergic rhinitis phenotypes included the clinical variants with nasal blockage as the most frequent symptoms in the smoking group. On the contrary, histamine mediated symptoms of allergic rhinitis, such as sneezing or runny nose, were less expressed in the group of patients with smoking in their medical history than in the group of non-smoking patients (Table 10).

These results could be influenced by different sensitization in the smoking (more to perennial allergens) and the non-smoking group (more to seasonal allergens). Another study revealed more nasal blockage in the group of patients with persistent allergic rhinitis, mainly due to house dust mite allergy[51].

The asthma phenotypes included the clinical variants of more expressed chronic cough (85% vs. 61%) and/or expectoration (76% vs. 29%) in the investigated group of smokers than in the group of non-smokers (Table 11). The asthma phenotypes could be marked by: a) baseline pulmonary function measures: b) specific allergen sensitization by SPT; c) self-reported allergies; d) symptoms characteristic of rhinitis, and e) symptoms characteristic of asthma[52]. The asthma phenotypes were identified as important for the genetic study of asthma and because they might have an impact on the response to asthma therapy[53].

The GINA classification showed more severe degrees of asthma in the investigated group of smokers than in the group of non-smokers (Table 12), mostly in the case of moderate asthma (61% *vs.* 49%). Clinically, smokers with asthma have more severe asthma symptoms than asthmatic non-smokers[54].

During the past years, asthma control has become the most important part of the follow-up of asthmatic patients. The ACT has been recognized as a useful tool for asthma control and validated in numerous countries, including Spain[55] and Croatia[56]. For purposes of one of our previous studies, we recruited 90 consecutive patients with asthma (18-85 years of age, of which 50 women) that filled out the Croatian version of the ACT during their regular visits to the asthma outpatient clinic and during their follow-up visit after 3 months. In the case of the patients who made the second visit (after 3 months), significant correlation between the change in the ACT score and the change in the level of asthma control according to an asthma specialist was recorded ($r^2=0.437$; $P<0.001$). In the current study, we found that the investigated ever-smokers had lower ACT scores in relation to the level of asthma control recorded in the investigated group of non-smokers (16 *vs.* 20), which means that asthma in connection with smoking entails a lower level of asthma control. Other authors also found that asthma in smokers was more difficult to control[57].

The exacerbation rate in the ever-smoking group was bigger than in the non-smoking group (31% *vs.* 26%). In the investigated group, 4/120 (3.3%) patients were hospitalized due to asthma exacerbation during the observation period. 11 (9.2%) of them were ever-hospitalized for asthma exacerbation, some of them a few times. Two patients (1.7%) were treated in the Intensive Care Unit, but neither was mechanically ventilated. According to the literature data, smokers with asthma have more frequent and severe exacerbations of asthma than non-smokers with asthma and are therefore more likely to visit hospital emergency departments, more frequently need to be placed in intensive care units, and more frequently need to be put on invasive ventilation than non-smokers, which results in higher mortality due to asthma in the case of the same[58]. The number of investigated patients with asthma exacerbations was not high. This result confirms the known fact that after the inhaled steroid therapy had been introduced, the number of hospitalized patients with asthma exacerbation declined dramatically.

The lung function analysis in both groups of patients with asthma, smokers and non-smokers, even after being divided in subgroups, current and former smokers, did not show statistically significant differences (Table 13). Based on this particular study, no conclusion can be brought regarding the association of smoking and the FEV_1 level, probably due to the fact that the sample included mainly young population, around 40 years of age.

According to our results, the usual course of a respiratory allergy is that allergic rhinitis precedes the appearance of asthma. The duration of allergic rhinitis (AR) was significantly longer than the duration of asthma, $p<0.001$ (Table 2). Adults with allergic rhinitis who smoke are significantly more likely to develop asthma, which was confirmed by our results and other authors as well. The more a person smokes, the greater is the probability of developing more severe asthma types, thus making the asthma control more difficult[59]. Smoking influences the clinical presentation of allergic asthma and rhinitis, the severity of the disease and the success of the treatment. The success of the treatment is significantly better after the patient quits smoking, not just in the case of patients with asthma and allergic rhinitis, but also in lung cancer patients recording longer survival rates than those who continue to smoke. In asthmatic patients, smoking reduces the effect of drugs, such as inhaled corticosteroids[60], which may lead to increased risk of hospitalization and intubation due to respiratory failure in the case of severe asthma exacerbations[61].

Due to the fact that most patients affected with allergic rhinitis are young, at the beginning of a career, this diagnosis has such a big impact on their life comparable to the impact on the patients with moderate asthma[62]. Allergic rhinitis and asthma phenotyping or, even better, endotyping, is important in terms of personalized medicine, the promising way to an individualized, tailored approach to each allergic patient.

9. Conclusion

Smoking causes clinical differences in patients with allergic rhinitis and asthma phenotypes. Daily exposure to tobacco smoke among the investigated current non-smokers and current smokers proved to be a statistically significant predictor of allergic rhinitis and asthma. The ever-smoking patients have more severe asthma and more moderate to severe exacerbations, but experience less symptoms. Physicians should pay more attention to patients with allergic rhinitis and asthma phenotypes who smoke.

10. References

[1] Ciprandi G, Vizzaccaro A, Ciprillo I, Crimi P, Canonica GW. Increase of asthma and allergic rhinitis prevalence in young Italian men. Int Arch Allergy Immunol 1996; 111:278-83.

[2] Gregory C, Cifaldi M, Tanner LA. Targeted intervention programs: creating a customized practise model to improve the treatment of allergic rhinitis in a managed care population. Am J Manage Care 1999; 5:485-96.

[3] Accordini S, Cappa V, Braggion M, Corsico AG, Bugiani M, Pirina P, Verlato G, Villani S, de Marco R, for the ISAYA Study Group. The Impact of Diagnosed and Undiagnosed Current Asthma in the General Adult Population. Int Arch Allerg Immunol 2011; 155 (4): 403-11.

[4] National Heart, Lung, and Blood Institute, National Institutes of Health, US Department of Health and Human Services. Expert panel report 3: guidelines for the diagnosis and management of asthma. Section 2, p. 1. 2007. Available at: http://www.nhlbi.nih.gov/guidelines/asthma/asthgdln.htm. Accessed June 27, 2011.

[5] European Lung Foundation and European Respiratory Society. European Lung Whitebook, 2008.

[6] Lotwall J, Cezmi AA, Bacharier LB, Bjermer L, Casale TB, Custovic A, Lemanske RF, Wardlaw AJ, Wenzel SE, Greenberger PA. Asthma endotypes: a new approach to classification of disease entities with the asthma syndrome. J Allerg Clin Immunol 2011; 127(2):355-60..

[7] Di Stefano A, Caramori G, Oates T, Capelli A, Lusuardi M, et al. Increased expression of nuclear factor-κ B in bronchial biopsies from smokers and patients with COPD. Eur Respir J 2002;20:556-63.

[8] Isajevs S, Taivans I, Svirina D, Strazda G, Kopieika U. Patterns of inflammatory responses in large and small airways in smokers with and without chronic obstructive pulmonary disease. Respration 2011; aop.10.1159/000322560.

[9] Rumora L, Milevoj L, Popović-Grle S, Barišić K, Čepelak I, Žanić Grubišić T. Level changes of blood leukocytes and intracellular signalling pathways in COPD patients with respect to the smoking attitude. Clin Biochem 2008;41(6):387-94.

[10] Gold DR, Wang X, Wypij D, Speizer FE, Ware JH, Dockery DW. Effects of cigarette smoking on lung function in adolescent boys and girls. N Engl J Med 1996;335:931–937.

[11] Sherrill DL, Lebowitz MD, Knudson RJ, Burrows B. Smoking and symptom effects on the curves of lung function growth and decline. Am Rev Respir Dis 1991;144:17–22.

[12] Fletcher C, Peto R. The natural history of chronic airflow obstruction. BMJ 1977;1:1645–1648.

[13] Popović-Grle S, Pavičić F, Bakran I, Plavec D. Could annual FEV1 decline in smokers predict the development of COPD? ERS Annual Congress Berlin, September 20-24, 1997. Eur Respir J 1997; 10 (suppl. 25): 94s.

[14] Anthonisen NR, Connett JE, Murray RP. Smoking and lung function of Lung Health Study participants after 11 years. Am J Respir Crit Care Med 2002;166:675–679.

[15] Downs SH, Brandli O, Zellweger JP, et al. Accelerated decline in lung function in the smoking women with airway obstruction: SAPALDIA 2 cohort study. Respir Res 2005;6:45.

[16] WHO Report on the Global Tobacco epidemic. 2008. The Mpower package.

[17] Đorđević V, Popović-Grle S. Allergic diseases and smoking. U Lipozenčić J and associates. Allergic and immune diseases. Medicinska naklada, Zagreb, 2011.

[18] International Agency for Research on Cancer. IARC Monographs on the evaluation of carcinogenic risks to humans. Volume 83: Tobacco smoke and involuntary smoking. Lyon, France, 2004.

[19] Wigand JS. Additives, cigarettes design and tobacco product regulation. A Report to the WHO, Tobacco Free Initiative, Tobacco product regulation group, Kobe, Japan 28 Jun-02 July, 2006.

[20] Nishikawa M, Nobumasa K, Ito T, Kudo M, Kaneko T et al. Superoxide mediates cigarette-smoke infiltration of neutrophils into airways through the nuclear factor-κ B activation and IL-8 mRNA expression in guinea pig in vivo. Am J Respir Cell Mol Biol 1999; 20:189-98.

[21] Šimunić M. Why (not to) smoke? 515 Questions and answers. Biblioteka časopisa "Psiha", Zagreb.

[22] Oberg M, Jaakkola MS, Woodward A, Peruga A, Pruss-Ustun A. Worlwide burden of disease from exposure to second-hand smoke: a retrospective analysis od data from 192 countries. Lancet 2011;377(9760):139-46.

[23] Kimata H. Selective induction of total and allergen-specific igE production by passive smoking. Eur J Clin Invest 2003;33811):1024-5.

[24] Pattenden S, Antova T, Neuberger M, Nikiforov B, De Sario M, et al. Parenteral smoking and children's respiratory health:independentent effects of prenatal and postnatal exposure. Tob Control 2006;15(4):294-301.

[25] Goodwin RD, Cowles RA. Household smoking and childhood asthma in the >United States: a state.level analysis. J Asthma 2008; 45(7):607-10

[26] Goodwin RD. Enviromental tobacco smoke and the epidemic of asthma in children: the role of cigarette use. Ann Allergy Asthma Immunol 2007;98(5):447-54.

[27] Perzanowski MS, Divjan A, Mellind RB, Canfield SM, Rosa MJ, Chew GL, Rundle A, Goldstein IF, Jacobson JS. Exhaled NO among inner-city children in New York City. J Asthma 2010;47(9):1015-21.

[28] Eisner MD. Environmental tobacco smoke and adult asthma. Clin Chest med 2002;23(4):749-61.

[29] (Available at: http://www.ecrhs.org. accessed July 08, 2011.)

[30] Global Initiative for Asthma. Global Strategy for Asthma Management and Prevention, Global Initiative for Asthma (GINA) 2010. Available from: http://www.ginasthma.org., accesed May 12, 2011.

[31] Nathan RA, Sorkness CA, Kosinski M. Development of the Asthma Control Test: a survey for assessing asthma control. J Allerg Clin Immunol 2004;113:59-65.
[32] van Cauwenberge P, Bachert C, Passalacqua G, Bousquet J, Canonica GW, Durham SR, Fokkens WJ, Howart PH, Lund V, Malling HJ, Mygind N, Passali D, Scadding GK, Wang DY: Consensus statement on the treatment of allergic rhinitis. European Academy of Allergology and Clinical Immunology. Allergy 2000, 55(2), 116-34.
[33] Miller MR, Hankinson J, Brusasco V, Burgos F, Casaburi R, Coates A et al. Standardization of spirometry. In: ATS/ERS task forse: Standardization of lung function testing. Ed. Brusasco V, Crapo R, Viegi G. Eur Respir J 2005; 26:319-38.
[34] Report of the Working Party of the European Community for Coal and Steel: Standardization of Lung Function Tests. Bull Europ Physiopath Resp 1983, 19 (Suppl 5), 3-38.
[35] Popović-Grle S, Pavičić F, Bićanić V, Radošević Z. Kako procijeniti farmadinamski test pri opstrukciji dišnih putova? Arh hig rada toksikol 1991; 42:239-43.
[36] Tudorić N, Vrbica Ž, Pavičić F, Korolija-Marinić D, Fijačko V, Fistrić T, Gudelj I, Kukulj S, Matanić D, Miculinić N, Plavec D, Popić G, Popović-Grle S, Turkalj M: Smjernice Hrvatskog pulmološkog društva za dijagnosticiranje i liječenje astme u odraslih. Liječ Vjesn 2007, 129, 315-80.
[37] The European Academy of Allergology and Clinical immunology. Subcommitee on skin tests. Dreborg S, Frew A, ed: Allergen standardization and skin tests. Allergy 1993, 48 (Suppl 14), 48-82.
[38] Jáuregui I, Dávila I, Sastre J, Bartra J, Cuvillo A, Ferrer M, Montoro J, Mullol J, Molina X, Valero A. Validation of ARIA (Allergic Rhinitis and its Impact on Asthma) classification in a pediatric population: The PEDRIAL study.Pediatric Allergy and Immunology 2011; 22(4): 388-92.
[39] Kovačić L, Gazdek D, Samardžić S. Hrvatska zdravstvena anketa: pušenje. Acta Med Croat 2007: 61(3); 281-285.
[40] Vrazic H, Ljubicic D, Schneider NK. Tobacco use and cessation among medical students in Croatia - results of the Global Health Professionals Pilot Survey (GHPS) in Croatia, 2005.
[41] Prochaska JO, diClemente CC. Stages and processes of self-change of smoking: Toward an integrative model of change. J Consult Clin Psychol 1983;51(3):390-5.
[42] Popović-Grle S. Farmakološko liječenje prestanka pušenja. U: Popović-Grle S, Krstačić G, ur. Kako i zašto prestati pušiti? Priručnik stalnog medicinskog usavršavanja, poslijediplomski tečaj I. kategorije Medicinskog Fakulteta Sveučilišta u Zagrebu, Zagreb,2011., p.78-84.
[43] Willemse BWM, Postma DS, Timens W, ten Hacken NHT. The impact of smoking cessation on respiratory symptoms, lung function, airway hyperresponsiveness and inflammation. Eur Respir J 2004;23:464–476.
[44] Willemse BWM, Postma DS, Timens W, ten Hacken NHT. The impact of smoking cessation on respiratory symptoms, lung function, airway hyperresponsiveness and inflammation. Eur Respir J 2004;23:464–476.
[45] Thomson NC, Chaudhuri R, Livingston E. Asthma and cigarette smoking. Eur Respir J 2004;24:822–833.

[46] Peters JM, Avol E, Navidi W, et al. A study of twelve Southern California communities with differing levels and types of air pollution: I. Prevalence of respiratory morbidity. Am J Respir Crit Care Med 1999; 159: 760–7.

[47] U.S.Centers for Disease Control. Cigarette Smoking Among Adults - United States 2000. Weekly MMWR July 26 2002. Volume 51(29) Pages 642 -645.

[48] Popović-Grle S. Criteria for allergologic diagnostics of bronchial sensitization in chronic obstructive pulmonary diseases. (Master thesis). Zagreb: Medicinski fakultet; 1989.

[49] Botelho FM, Llop-Guevara A, Trimble NJ, Nikota JK, Bauer CM, Lambert KN, Kianpour S, Jordana M, Stampfli MR. Cigarette smoke differentially impacts eosinophilia and remodeling in a house dust mite asthma model. Am J Respir Cell Mol Biol 2011. epub ahead Feb 11.

[50] Yanbaeva DG, Dentener MA, Creutzberg EC, et al. Systemic effects of smoking. Chest 2007; 131: 1557–66.

[51] Popović-Grle S, Vrbica Z, Janković M, Klarić I. Different phenotypes of intermittent and persistens respiratory allergy in Zagreb, Croatia. Ann Agric Environ Med 2009;16:137-142.

[52] Pillai SG, Tang Y, van den Oord E, Klotsman M, Barnes K et al. Factor analysis in the genetics of asthma International Network family study identifies five major quantitative asthma phenotypes. Clin Exp Allergy 2008;38(3):421-9.

[53] Gonem S, Desai D, Siddiqui S, Brightling CE. Evidence for phenotype-driven treatment in asthma patients. Curr Opin Allergy Clin Immunol 2011;11(4):381-5.

[54] Vesterinen E, Kaprio J, Koskenvuo M: Prospective study of asthma in relation to smoking habits among 14,729 adults. Thorax 1988; 43:534-539.

[55] Rodrigo GJ, Arcos JP, Nannini LJ, Neffren H, Broin MG, Contrera M, Pineyro L. Reliability and factor analysis of the Spanish version of the asthma control test. Ann Allergy Clin Immunol 2008;100(1):17-22.

[56] Popović-Grle S, Plavec D, Lampalo M, Pelicarić D, Pavičić F. Validation of the Croatian version of the asthma control test (ACT). Croat Med J 2011; in press.

[57] Stapleton N, Howard-Thompson A, George C. Hoover RM, Self Th. Smoking and asthma. J Am Board Fam Med 2011; 24(3):313-22.

[58] Silverman RA, Boudreaux ED, Woodruff PG, et al: Cigarette smoking among asthmatic adults presented to 64 emergency departments. Chest 2003; 123:1472-1479.

[59] Polosa R, Russo C, Caponnetto P, Bertino G, Sarva M, Antic T, Mancuso S, Al-Delaimy WK. Greater severity of new onset of asthma in allergic subjects who smoke: a 10-year longitudinal study. Respir Res 2011;24:12(1):16 Epubahead of print 31 Jan. 2011.

[60] Thomson NC, Chaudhuri R, Livingston E. Asthma and cigarette smoking. Eur Respir J 2004;24:822–833.

[61] LeSon S, Gershwin ME. Risk factors for asthmatic patients requiring intubation: a comprehensive review. Allergologia et Immunopathologia 1995; 23:235–247.

[62] Demoly P, Didier P, Mathelier-Fusade P, Drpuet M, David M, Bonnelye G, de Blic J, Klossek JM. Physician and patient survey of allergic rhinitis in France: perceptions on prevalence, severity of symptoms, care management and specific immunotherapy. Allergy 2008; 63(8):1008-14.

6

Cough in Allergic Rhinitis

Renata Pecova and Milos Tatar
Comenius University in Bratislava, Jessenius Faculty of Medicine in Martin
Slovakia

1. Introduction

The diseases of the nose and paranasal sinuses are among the most commonly identified causes of chronic cough (*Pratter, 2006*). Depending on the population studied and the variations in diagnostic algorithm, the diseases of nose and sinuses are reported to contribute to coughing in 20–40% of patients with chronic cough who have normal chest radiograph (*Chung & Pavord, 2008*). The mechanisms of chronic cough in rhinosinusitis are incompletely understood. Several mechanisms have been proposed, single or in combination: upper airway cough syndrome previously postnasal drip (PND), direct irritation, inflammation in the lower airways and the cough reflex sensitization (*Pratter, 2006*).

2. Cough

Cough has been described as the ´watchdog of the lungs´. Its onset is almost always associated with peripheral stimulation; this is indicative of its reflex character (*Korpas & Tomori, 1979*). Cough is mostly an infrequent and physiological act in where its functions are to protect against aspiration and clearing bronchial excretions along with removal of infective and foreign substances that find their way in the respiratory tract. This happens as a reflective act, though cough may also be a voluntary action. When cough occur more frequent and persist, it is usually a cardinal sign of respiratory disease. In this situation protective systems fail or collapse due to overloading of foreign substances or excessive bronchial excretions and to compensate this breakdown cough frequency increases. The action of cough can be divided into three phases: inspiratory, compressive and expulsive (*Coryllos, 1937; Korpas & Tomori, 1979*). Cough is a defensive reflex that protects the airways from inhaling potentially damaging particles, aeroallergens, pathogens, aspirate and secretions accumulated (*Mazzone et al., 2003*). Like any other reflex process, cough is effected by means of a reflex arc, which is composed of five basic links: receptors, an afferent pathway, a centre, an efferent pathway and effectors (*Korpas & Tomori, 1979*).

2.1 Airway afferent and receptors

The airway afferent nerve fibers may be divided into several subtypes based on their physicochemical sensitivity, adaptation to sustained lung inflation, neurochemistry, origin, myelination, conduction velocity and sites of termination in the airways (*Mazzone et al., 2003*). The lack of specificity and characteristics for each of these subgroups has made the study and to define them separately quite difficult. By gross dividing, however, these physiological and morphological attributes can be used to identify at least three broad classes of afferent nerve fibers: rapidly adapting mechanoreceptors (RARs), slowly adapting mechanoreceptors (SARs) and unmyelinated C-fibers (C-fibers) *(Mazzone et al., 2003).*

2.1.1 Rapidly adapting receptors (RARs)

While the anatomical arrangement of RARs termination is unknown, functional studies suggest that these receptors terminate within or beneath the epithelium and are localized to both intra- and extrapulmonary airways (*Bergren & Sampson, 1982; Riccio et al., 1996c, Ho et al., 2001*). RARs, as its name implies, is differentiated from the other airway afferent nerves by their rapid (1-2sec) adaptation to sustained lung inflations (*Armstrong & Luck 1974; Coleridge & Coleridge, 1984; Ho et al., 2001; Sant´Ambrogio & Widdicombe, 2001; Widdicombe, 2001*). Other distinguishing properties of RARs include their sensitivity to lung collapse and/or lung deflation, their responsiveness to alterations in dynamic lung compliance (thus their sensitivity to bronchospasm), and theirs conduction velocity (4-18m/sec), suggestive of small myelinated axons (*Bergren & Sampson, 1982; Jonzon et al., 1986; Riccio et al., 1996; Ho et al., 2001; Widdicombe, 2001*). Analysis has shown that sustained activation of RARs produced by dynamic lung inflation, bronchospasm or lung collapse is not attributable to an electrophysiological adaptation (*Bergren & Sampson 1982; Pack & DeLaney, 1983; McAlexander et al., 1999; Ho et al., 2001).* Maybe a more suitable name for better defining RARs are dynamic receptors that respond to changes in airway mechanical properties (e.g., diameter, length, interstitial pressures).

The dynamic mechanical forces accompanying lung inflation and deflation sporadically activates RARs throughout the respiratory cycle and becomes more active as the rate of lung inflation increase (*Pack & DeLaney 1983; McAlexander et al., 1999; Ho et al., 2001*). This means that the RARs activity during respiration is connected to respiratory rate and is higher in small animals, while in larger animals, it would be almost unmeasurable. In the smaller animals, RARs-dependent reflexes will also require a heightened activity in the already active RARs.

Even though RARs may be insensitive to ´direct´ chemical stimuli, stimuli from bronchospasm or obstruction due to mucus secretion or oedema can increase the RAR activity (*Mohammed et al., 1993; Bonham et al., 1996; Bergren, 1997; Joad et al., 1997; Canning et al., 2001; Widdicombe, 2001*). By preventing the local end-organ effects that is stimulated by substances such as histamine, capsaicin, substance P and bradykinin, activation of RARs can be markedly inhibited or abolished (*Mazzone et al., 2003*). Stimuli that evoke cough react RARs and RARs fullfill many of the accepted criteria for mediating cough *(Sant´Ambrogio et al., 1984; Canning et al., 2000; Sant´Ambrogio & Widdicombe, 2001; Widdicombe 2001*). Studies of vagal cooling have shown further evidence of RARs role in the cough reflex, that block cough at temperatures that selectively abolish activity in myelinated fibers (including RARs) while preserving C-fiber activity (*Widdicombe, 1974; Tatar et al., 1988; Tatar et al., 1994).*

2.1.2 Slowly adapting stretch receptors (SARs)

SARs is equal to RARs in at they also are highly sensitive to the mechanical forces lungs deal with during breathing. SARs, however, differentiate from RARs in that their activity increases sharply during inspiratory phase and peaks just before the initiation of expiration (*Ho et al., 2001; Schelegle & Green, 2001*), while RARs can be activated during both inflation and deflation of the lung (including lung collapse) (*Ho et al. 2001; Widdicombe, 2003*). This makes it likely that SARs are the primary afferent fibers involved in the Hering-Breuer reflex, a reflex which ends inspiration and initiates expiration when the lungs are adequately inflated (*Schelegle & Green, 2001*). SARs also adapt more slowly to stimuli from sustained lung inflations, than, as the name implies, RARs demonstrate rapid adaption (*Ho et al., 2001; Widdicombe, 2003*). SARs may also be differently spread throughout the airways (*Schelegle & Green, 2001*).

Evoking of reflexes is also done differently by SARs and RARs. Activation by SARs results in a reduction in airway tone due to inhibition of cholinergic drive to the airway smooth muscle (*Canning et al., 2001*).

There is suggested after single-unit recordings from the vagus nerve in rabbits that activity of SARs neither increase before or during ammonia-induced coughing (*Matsumoto, 1988*). Even though this means that RARs do not play any big part in the cough reflex, RARs clear influence over the respiratiory pattern indicates that they do have a role in cough reflex. It is suggested that the usage of the loop diuretic frusemide (furosemide) will increase the baseline acitvity of RARs, and thereby account for the reported antitussive effects of this agent in animal and human subjects. Reports have shown that preloading, in contrast, that likely will increase baseline SARs activity, will increase expiratory efforts during cough (*Hanacek & Korpas, 1982; Nishino et al., 1989*). On the contrary, experiments on rabbits inhaling sulfur dioxide have been used in an attempt to selectively block SARs activity show that the cough reflex is coincidentally attenuated (*Hanacek et al., 1984, Sant´Ambrogio et al., 1984*). This selectivity to sulfur dioxide for airway SARs is however questionable since several reports show that sulfur dioxide has an excitatory action on airway C-fibers (*Atzori et al., 1992; Wang et al., 1996*).

Studies done on CNS processing has also suggested that cough may be facilitated by SARs. There is proposed that a central cough network in which SARs facilitate cough via activation of brainstem second-order neurons (pump cells) of the SARs reflex pathway (*Shannon et al., 1998*).

2.1.3 C-fibers

C-fibers are unmyelinated afferent fibres which are similar to the unmyelinated nociceptors of the somatic nerve fibers both physiologically and morphologically, and these C-fibers constitute the majority of afferent nerves innervating the airways (*Coleridge & Coleridge, 1984; Ma & Woolf, 1995; Lee & Pisarri, 2001*). Being unmyelinated differ their conduction velocity compared to RARs and SARs, but their relative insensitivity to mechanical stimulation, lung inflation and their responsiveness to bradykinin and capsaicin is also important differentiations (*Armstrong & Luck, 1974; Riccio et al., 1996; Bergren, 1997; Ho et al., 2001; Canning et al., 2001; Lee & Pisarri, 2001; Widdicombe, 2001*). C-fibers also differ from the RARs in that bradykinin- and capsaicin-evoked activation of their endings in the airways is not inhibited by pre-treatment with bronchodilators. Oppositely, bronchodilators such as prostaglandin E_2, adrenaline and adenosine may enhance excitability of airway afferent C-fibers (*Ho et al., 2000; Lee & Pisarri, 2001*). By this, C- fibers differentiate from RARs in at their bronchopulmonary C-fibers are directly activated by substances like bradykinin and capsaicin.

Studies on C-fibers has been done on many animals, and morphological studies on guinea-pigs and rats have shown that C- fibers innervate the airway epithelium together with effector structures within the airway wall *(Lundberg et al., 1984; Baluk et al., 1992; Riccio et al., 1996; Hunter & Undem, 1999)*. Several studies show a unique neurochemical property of the bronchopulmonary fibers has been used to illustrate the distribution and peripheral nerve terminals of the unmyelinated airway afferent nerve endings. These studies reveal that C-fiber have the ability to synthesize neuropeptides that afterwards are transported to their central and peripheral nerve terminals *(Baluk et al., 1992; Riccio et al., 1996c; Hunter & Undem, 1999; Myers et al., 2002)*. Coleridge & Coleridge *(1984)* described in afferent vagal C-fiber innervations of the lungs and airways and its functional significance, that in dogs C-fibers may be further subdivided into bronchial and pulmonary fibers, a differentiation based on sites of termination and on responsiveness to chemical and mechanical stimuli. Based on this division, pulmonary C-fibers may be unresponsive to histamine, while bronchial C-fibers are activated by histamine. This observation is made on dogs, and in whether the physiologic differences are similar in other species are still unknown, but recent studies have described C-fiber subtypes innervating in the intrapulmonary airways and lungs of mice and guinea pigs (*Kollarik et al., 2003; Undem et al., 2003*). C-fibers are believed to have an important role in airway reflexes. Even with their polygonal shape that made them respond to chemical and mechanical stimulation, compared to RARs and SARs, the threshold for mechanical stimulation is markedly increased *(Matsumoto, 1988; Deep et al., 2001*). As a consequence, C-fibers mostly lie latent throughout the respiratory cycle, but are easily activated by chemical stimuli such as capsaicin, bradykinin, citric acid, hypertonic saline, and sulphur dioxide *(Riccio et al., 1996c; Ho et al., 2001; Widdicombe, 2001; Lee & Pisarri, 2001)*. Increased airway parasympathetic nerve activity and chemoreflex, characterized by apnea (followed by rapid shallow breathing), bradycardia, and hypotension are all reflex responses elicited by C- fiber activation *(Coleridge & Coleridge, 1984; Canning et al., 2001)*. In species like rats and guinea-pigs bronchospasm and neurogenic inflammation by C-fibre activation which elicit peripheral release of neuropeptides via an axon reflex *(Barnes, 2001; Lee & Pisarri, 2001)*.

The function of the C-fibers in the cough reflex is debatable. Many studies have given evidence to the hypothesis that C-fiber activation in the airways precipitate cough. In some cases there is believed that selective stimulants like capsaicin, bradykinin and citric acid evoke cough in conscious animals and humans (*Coleridge & Coleridge, 1984; Forsberg & Karlsson, 1986; Mohammed et al., 1993; Karlsson, 1996; Mazzone et al., 2002)*. In addition, capsaicin is used in pretreatment when needed to selectively deplete C-fibers of neuropeptides, which abrogate cough in guinea-pigs induced by citric acid, but by evoking C-fibers by mechanical probing has no effect on cough *(Forsberg & Karlsson, 1986)*. At last, pharmacological studies that take the advantage of the unique expression of neurokinins by the airway C-fibers, have shown that bradykinin-, citric acid-induced cough in cats and guinea-pigs is attenuated or abolished by neurokinin receptor antagonists *(Bolser et al., 1997)*.

All these evidences above indicate that C-fibers take part in the cough reflex. On the other hand, there are also evidences suggesting that C-fibers do not evoke cough and may instead inhibit cough by stimulation of RARs-fibers. For instance, in studies with anesthetized animals, C-fibre stimulation has consistently failed to evoke coughing, even though cough can be readily induced in these animals by mechanically probing mucosal sites along the airways *(Tatar et al., 1988; Tatar et al., 1994; Canning et al., 2000; Deep et al., 2001)*. Systemic administration of C-fibre stimulants may in fact have been shown to inhibit cough evoked by RARs stimulation in various species *(Tatar et al., 1988; Tatar et al., 1994; Canning et al., 2000)*. Further evidence supports the C-fibers role in inhibition of cough in that vagal cooling to temperatures that can maintain C-fiber-dependent reflexes can abolish cough *(Tatar et al., 1994)*.

The reason for these antagonistic evidences about C-fibers and cough are ambiguous. One reason may be that general anesthesia in animals selectively disrupt the ability of C-fibers to evoke cough without unfavourably affecting cough induced by stimulation of RARs. Nishino et al. (1996) studies of cough and the reflexes on irritation of airway mucosa in man show that general anesthesia has a profound influence over cough reflex. But there is unlikely that C-fibre activation and C-fibre-mediated reflex are entirely prevented by anesthesia *(Roberts et al., 1981; Coleridge & Coleridge, 1984; Bergren 1997; Canning et al., 2001)*. So, action by anesthesias on C-fibers may either work by setting off cough activation by the inhibitory effects of C-fiber or it must selectively inhibit cough-related natural pathways. As an alternative, general anesthesia might actually intervene with the conscious perception of airway irritation and thereby interfere with the subjects urge to cough. One interesting fact of this circumstance is that capsaicin-evoked cough can be consciously suppressed in humans tested *(Hutchings et al., 1993)* Despite a lot of studies, there is still an equally possible hypothesis that C-fibre stimulation alone is too insufficient to evoke cough but are dependent on the airway afferent interactions in both the periphery and the level of CNS *(Canning & Mazzone, 2005)*.

2.2 Central regulation of cough

Studies have come a long way in understanding the central mechanism involved in cough production. Evidence has shown that a single network of neurons seems to mediate cough as well as breathing (*Shannon et al., 1996; Shannon et al., 1997; Shannon et al., 1998; Shannon et al., 2000*).

Though, it is obvious that cough and breathing are two different behaviors. It is a process called reconfiguration, in which the same network produces different behaviors that involve dynamic alteration of the excitability of key elements and/or recruitment of previously silent elements. There is suggested that the excitability of this network is additionally controlled by a ´gating´ mechanism that is sensitive to antitussive drugs (*Bolser et al., 1999*).

2.3 Plasticity

Coughing is connected with both acute and chronic respiratory diseases such as upper respiratory infections, asthma, gastro-oesophageal reflux (GOR), as well as other more seldom causes. It is likely that the cough arises due to production of various tussigenic agents in the wall of the airway, and increased sensitivity of the cough reflex pathway. Though, the structures involved and the molecular mechanism of the sensitivity is still unknown. Afferent nerves are under constantly changing in structure and activity. Neuroplasticity is the general term to the change in structure and function of nerves (*Woolf & Salter, 2000*). Cough plasticity represents the changes in neuronal excitability, receptor expression, transmitter chemistry and the structure of the nerve. Unfortunately, not much is known about the function of vagal nerve plasticity in human disease. Most facts have been collected by using various tissue and animal models in studies on the somatosensory system, and functional and electrophysiological studies of the vagal afferent nerves.

Clinical studies on cough reflex sensitivity show that it can be quantified by several methods (*Pounsford et al., 1985a; Choudry & Fuller, 1992*). Capsaicin and citric acid are the most commonly used tussigenic agent, and their use have expressed that some diseases are associated with an appreciable increase in cough reflex sensitivity. During these studies one must take into consideration that cough reflex hypersensititiy may be stimulus specific, and thereby influence the cough sensitivity.

2.3.1 Molecular mechanisms of increased excitability

Allergic inflammation or various inflammatory mediators have under scientific level shown to both increase cough reflex sensitivity and excitability of afferent nerves of the airway. For example, in humans PGE_2 enhance capsaicin-induced cough (*Choudry et al., 1989*). It has also been done a large amount of clinical studies that have displayed that certain pathological conditions are accompanied by a considerable increase in cough reflex sensitivity in humans. This is also shown in studies done on animals, for example in guinea-pigs, when allergic inflammation or inhalation of bradykinin potentiated cough was evoked by capsaicin and citric acid (*Lii et al., 2001*). Studies done in rats have shown that inhalation of inflammatory mediators (also PGE_2 and eosinophil major basic protein) follow potentiation of capsaicin-induced action potential discharge in nociceptive fibers in the lungs (*Ho et al., 2000*). In addition, inflammatory condition enhances the excitability of RARs fibers. As in studies on sensitized guinea pigs trachea was exposed to antigen causing a substantial increase in the mechanosensitivity of RARs fibers (*Riccio et al., 1996a*). Later, it has been shown that cough may be evoked in all species used in studies by using either chemical stimulation of airway mucosa or by inhalation of acidic saline or capsaicin (*Canning, 2008*).

Besides these studies done, relatively little studies resulting in published articles have occurred relating to the airway afferent excitability and the underlying mechanisms that increases it.

Most of the studies on mechanistic basis of afferent nerve excitability and plasticity have been done on nociceptive-type somatosensory neurons which are isolated from the dorsal root ganglia (*Woolf & Salter, 2000*). Somatosensory- and airways nociceptive fibers share many properties and therefore give useful information on how the excitability on the airway nociceptor works. But, one must not exclude the fact that RARs phenotype fibre is not readily analogous to any type of somatosensory afferent. So, still little is known in how the airway RARs excitability is modulated.

2.3.2 Vanilloid receptor (TRPV1) mechanisms

Vanilloid receptor now referred to as TRPV1 (previously called vanilloid receptor 1 (VR1)), is of the vagal afferent nociceptors (C-fibers and Aδ-fibers) that innervate the airway express the capsaicin receptor, a member of the transient potential family (*Riccio et al., 1996b; Fox, 2002*). Unfortunately, the extent to which capsaicin can lead to RARs activation in vivo is likely trough indirect means because TRPV1 is not expressed by RAR-type fibers in the airways of guinea-pigs (*Myers et al., 2002*).

Membrane depolarization is a result of the TRPV1 which work as an ionotropic receptor that when activated serve as a nonselective cation channel leading to depolarization of membrane (*Caterina & Julius, 2001*). It is important to know that besides being activated by vanilloid compounds, TRPV1 is also activated by endogenous lipid mediators such as ananamide and arachidonic acid metabolites of various lipoxygenase enzymes (*Caterina &*

Julius, 2001; Shin et al., 2002). Some metabotrophic receptors of TRPV1 may also be activated by intracellular signal transduction mechanism. Studies in both airway afferent fibers and somatosensory neurons indicate the hypothesis that bradykinin can, at least partly, activate sensory nerves through production of lipogenase product of arachidonic acid and subsequent activation of TRPV1 (*Shin et al., 2002*). One other important fact is the hydrogen ions ability to activate TRPV1 on airway physiology with pH ~6 at 37°C (*Caterina & Julius, 2001*).

TRPV1 also have a distinct characteristic by its ability to integrate different kinds of stimuli, meaning that the action of one TRPV1 agonist potentiates the action of the other (*Caterina & Julius, 2001*). TRPV1 have the ability to accumulate in the airway wall during different kinds of pathological condition. As in asthma, the inflammation could, by a decrease of pH of airway wall, increase the concentration of hydrogen ions, bradykinin and certain lipid mediators.

Increase of TRPV1 conductance secondary to phosholipase C (PLC) activation and subsequent phosphorylation of TRPV1 by protein kinase C (PKC) can be done by agonists of protein G protein-coupled (Gp-coupled) receptors (*Premkumar & Ahern, 2000*). This indicates that inflammatory mediators that stimulate classical G-protein-coupled receptors can increase conductance through TRPV1. There are evidence showing that PLC may also release TRPV1 from phosphatidylinositol (*Riccio et al., 1996b*) and phosphate inhibition (*Chuang et al., 2001*). This action may take part in increasing the TRPV1 activity after stimulation of nerve growth factor (NFG) of Tyrosine Receptor Kinase A (trk-A) receptors as well as B_2-receptors activation by bradykinin.

Gs-coupled receptors may also increase the amplitude of the TRPV1-mediated generator potential. In rats, rising of cAMP increases capsaicin-induced conductance in their nociceptive neurons, an action that may be inhibited by protein kinase A (PKA)-inhibitors (*Lopshire & Nocol, 1998*). Further studies also show that in rat pulmonary nociceptors capsaicin-induced action potential discharge is increased by prostaglandin E_2 (PGE_2) (*Ho et al., 2000*). It is also proven that there is an increase in expression of TRPV1 in rat sensory neurons by neutrophins like NGF (*Michael & Priestley, 1999*). Even though it is not made any studies in humans concerning healthy or diseased airways, places of airway inflammation is known to be elevated by nerve growth factors (*Virchow et al., 1998*). TRPV1 is not the only mechanism that can affect nociceptor excitability. Decrease of threshold for mechanical stimulation of airway afferent nerves have been shown in various inflammatory mediators (*Ho et al., 2000; Riccio et al., 1996a*). How this is done is still unknown, but studies suggest that it might involve several ion channels and modulation of these.

2.3.3 Sodium channels

Voltage-gated sodium channels have the possibility to affect the threshold for action potential generation and peak frequency of action potential discharge both in number and activity. The mammals have abundant of different sodium channels in nerves, and based on their sensitivity to tetrodotoxin (TTE) we divide them into two groups, the TTX-sensitive and TTX-resistant sodium channels. In airway afferent nerves both groups of channels are found (*Carr & Undem, 2001*). Of extra interest are the TTX-resistant channel and its ability to regulate excitability of modulation by inflammatory mediators (*Gold et al., 1996*). Studies made on guinea-pigs and their jugular ganglia showed that most of these nerves have enough TTX-resistant sodium channels to achieve an action potential generation (*Christian &*

Togo, 1995). Even though there still are some questions about the details of the channels function, there are data proving that airway-specific jugular neuronal cell bodies have enough TTX-resistant current to support formation of action potential (*Carr & Undem, 2001*). Some inflammatory mediators have influence the sodium current. PGE_2, adenosine and 5-hydroxytryptamine (5-HT) are some mediators that have shown to be able to enhance the TTX-resistant sodium current in somatosensory neurons (*Gold et al., 1996*). Though, what impact these mediators have are still not established.

2.3.4 Neurotransmitter plasticity

Neuropeptides are present both in peripheral and central C-fibers innervating the airways, and substance P and related tachykinins are the most common neuropeptides, though other peptide are also found there.

An increased production of different types of neuropeptides in inflammatory disease is a typical action, and is proven in animal models and several inflammatory diseases, such as COPD (*Tomaki et al., 1995*). This action often happens after an increase in expression of preprotachykinin genes in the sensory neurons (*Hunter et al., 1998; Fischer et al., 1996*). How the signalling occurs is still not known, but neutrotrophins are believed to be involved since they are known to interact with tyrosine kinase-linked receptors (trk receptors) to evoke signals in the cell body. Neurotrophin–trk receptor complexes affect transcriptions of different genes, also those involving neuropeptide synthesis and are likely transported via axonal system from nerve terminals to the cell body (*Klesse and Parada, 1999*). In the presence of airway inflammation, neurotrophins such as nerve growth factor (NGF) and brain-derived neurotrophin factor are rarely found, and production may even be increased (*Virchow et al., 1998*).

In inflammatory reactions release of neurokinins may cause vasodilatation, plasma extravasation, and even bronchial smooth cell contraction in some species (*Advenier & Emonds-Alt, 1996*). These actions have shown in indirectly activate RARs nerves in guinea-pigs which further participate in tussigenive activity of these agents (*Advenier & Emonds-Alt, 1996; Joad et al., 1997*). Neuropeptides are synthesized in body cells, transported to peripheral and central terminals and in central terminals in brainstem they are released after action potential release (*Woolf and Salter, 2000*). This release in the central terminals is likely to have an essential role in regulating the cough reflex sensitivity. RARs fibers in central neurons have shown in some cases to have a convergence on the same secondary terminals as nociceptive C-fibers (*Mazzone & Canning, 2002*). This evidence, and adding the fact those electrophysiological effects on neurokinins on postsynaptic membrane provide the abstract model of the process that is called by scientists "central sensitization"(*Woolf & Salter, 2000*). This refers to the action where one type of nerve input, for example nociceptive C-fibre, actually increases the synaptic transmission of another type of input, as in RARs fibers. This may lead to a decrease in the amount of RAR input needed to trigger cough in the CNS.

While older studies suggest that inflammation may cause increase in sensory neuropeptides secondary to induction of preprotachykinin genes in nociceptive neurones, it is now indicated in studies of both somatosensory and vagal sensory systems, that inflammation also may cause phenotypic change in the neuropeptidergic innervation (*Neumann et al., 1996; Carr et al., 2002; Myers et al., 2002*). Studies of airway afferent neurones in guinea pigs with allergen or virus infection showed increased number of sensory neurokinins (*Fischer et al., 1996; Carr et al., 2002; Myers et al., 2002*). In response to inflammation there is also histologically proved that the neuropeptides produced in this case are also transported to central terminals of the RAR neurons (*Myers et al., 2002*). This is an important finding which supports the fact that there is a mechanical activation of RARs fibers leading neurokinin release in the brainstem as a response to inflammation from allergy or respiratory virus infection. A neuropeptide innervation of the somatosensory system has been documented where painful sensation has phenotypically shifted to painless stimuli, an action referred to as allodynia (*Neumann et al., 1996*). From this one could start to wonder if this may have some influence in the extraneous cough sensation that may cause the desire to cough without having any to cough up in the airway.

2.3.5 Change in nerve fibre density and extraneuronal effects

The environment causes change in the density of sensory innervation (*Stead, 1992*). This change due to either growth factor release or tissue damage may lead to nerve fibre growth and fibresprouting, but if this causes an increased sensitivity to cough is still unknown and minimal studies have been done on this topic.

3. Cough in adults

European Respiratory Society recommends two possible definitions of cough *(Morice et al., 2007): 1)* Cough is a three-phase expulsive motor act characterized by an inspiratory effort (inspiratory phase), followed by a forced expiratory effort against a closed glottis (compressive phase) and then by opening of the glottis and rapid expiratory airflow (expulsive phase). 2) Cough is a forced expulsive maneuver, usually against a closed glottis and which is associated with a characteristic sound.
Cough is classified as acute and chronic. This classification is useful clinically, since the etiology of acute cough differs from the etiology of chronic cough. Chronic cough in adults is a cough which persists for over 8 weeks.

3.1 Acute cough in adults

Cough is the commonest symptom for which people seek medical advice *(Irwin et al., 1993)*. Lower airway infections are the most common cause of acute cough. Lower airway infections refer to acute tracheobronchitis, acute bronchiolitis and community acquired pneumonia (CAP). Acute tracheobronchitis is mostly viral in origin. Influenza virus, rhinovirus, parainfluenza virus, Respiratory syncytical virus (RSV), adenovirus and coronavirus are the pathogens most commonly associated with acute cough in patients with acute tracheobronchitis. All these viruses have a short incubation period of between one and four days, and all symptoms including cough usually resolves within three weeks *(Pek & Boushey, 2003)*. Many people with viral cough do not seek medical advice, but treat themselves with over the counter products. This means that there is no sufficient statistical data about the extent of acute cough *(Morice, 2003)*. 5-10% of all cases with acute tracheobronchitis are caused by bacteria. Among the most common bacterial pathogens are Bordetella pertussis, Mycoplasma pneumoniae, Streptococcus pneumoniae and Chlamydia pneumoniae. CAP is a common cause of hospitalization and death from infectious disease in adults. The etiological agent is identified in only 50% of all cases. Streptococcus pneumoniae, Haemophilus influenzae and Staphylococcus aureus are among the most commonly identified microbial pathogens that cause pneumonia *(Pek & Boushey, 2003)*.

The mechanism of cough in lower airway infection is not completely understood. Possible mechanisms have been suggested by *Pek & Boushey (2003): 1)* Irritation of the nerve endings in the larynx and trachea caused by dripping of secretions containing inflammatory mediators from the nasopharynx into larynx or trachea is one possible mechanism. Exposure of the nerve endings (e.g. RARs) caused by damage and destruction of the airway epithelium is thought to decrease the cough threshold to environmental irritants and inflammatory secretions, thus causing cough. 2) The infection of the airways also leads to accumulation of secretions and debris in the airway lumen. As a result the mechanoreceptors in the bronchial mucosa are activated, triggering cough to clear the airways for the excess secretions and foreign material. 3) Cough may also occur because of stimulation of nerve endings by inflammatory mediators released directly from airway epithelial cells or from inflammatory cells attracted to the site of infection. 4) Neuropeptidases degrade neuropeptides released from adjacent afferent nerve endings. Enhanced effect of neuropeptidases because of decrease in the neutral endopeptidase from epithelial cells is also one possible mechanism triggering cough in lower airway infections.

3.2 Chronic cough in adults

The three most common causes of chronic cough are asthma bronchiale, GERD and chronic upper airway syndrome (CUAS) - previously postnasal drip syndrome. Other causes of chronic cough include post viral cough, cough in patients with chronic obstructive pulmonary diseases, cough induced by ACE inhibitor therapy and cough in lung cancer patients *(Chung et al., 2003).*

A single cause of cough in a patient is less common than multiple causes of cough. In a study performed by *Palombini et al. (1999)* they found that asthma, CUAS, GERD either alone or in combination, were responsible for 93.6% of the cases of chronic cough. These three conditions were so frequent that they suggested the use of the term "pathogenic triad of chronic cough". 38.5% of the patients investigated had a single cause of cough, while 61.5 % of the patients had two or more causes of cough.

3.3 Acute cough in children

Some studies of acute cough are old and show systematic reviews on the natural history of the acute cough in children (35-50years). Hay and Wilson (*2002*) did prospective study of the period 1999-2001 of acute cough, which displayed that within 10 days 50% of the children showed recovery, and 90% within 25 days. Also an Australian prospective community study recorded respiratory episodes of 2.2-5.3 year for children aged ≤ 10 years, with results showing a mean duration of 5.5-6.8 days of the episodes *(Leder et al., 2003).* Thereby indicating that acute cough should be defined as cough less then 14 days of duration.

The most common etiology of acute cough in children is due to an uncomplicated viral acute respiratory tract infection, though one must exclude more serious problems as aspiration of foreign material *(Chang et al., 2006).*

3.4 Chronic cough in children

Acute cough in children is defined as cough less than 2 weeks, prolonged acute cough (subacute) 2-4 weeks, chronic cough more than 4 weeks *(Chang et al., 2006*). Definition of cough in adults is subdivided differently. Acute cough duration is of less than 3 weeks, subacute 3-8 weeks and chronic more than 8 weeks *(Pratter el al., 2006; Morice et al., 2007).* Chronic cough may be classified according to its etiology. By this classification cough is divided into ´expected´ cough, non-specific cough and specific cough; its scientific rationale is discussed elsewhere *(Chang, 2005).* In expected cough, the cough is anticipated, such as after an acute respiratory tract infection. In specific cough the cause is clearly definable by usage of history and examination, where coexisting symptoms and sign often help in diagnosing the etiology. These causes are often serious. Nonspecific cough is a dry cough where neither known aetiology nor any respiratory disease has been identified. Chronic cough in children is most commonly due to an upper respiratory tract infection, asthma, gastrointestinal reflux as well as other more uncommon causes.

3.5 Cough reflex sensitivity assessment

The cough reflex sensitivity can be assessed by the inhalation cough challenge test. In this test an acid or a non-acid tussive is used to induce cough experimentally. The most common non-acid tussive is capsaicin, while citric and tartaric acids are the most commonly used acid tussives. Before 2007 standardized methods did not exist, making it impossible to compare data in studies obtained from different institutions. The European Respiratory Society (ERS) developed guidelines in 2007 on the standardization of testing with tussive and non tussive tussives *(Morice et al., 2007).*

During the inhalation cough challenge test, the tussives can be administered either by using single-dose or the dose-response method *(Morice et al., 2001).* In the single-dose method, one concentration of capsaicin or citric acid is administered. In the dose-response method the tussives are administered over a prolonged period. In the dose-response method, variations in respiratory frequency and tidal volume are thought to cause variation in the amount of tussive delivered from individual to individual, and therefore accuracy and reproducibility is poor. The single dose method is the most widely used method, because of the accuracy and reproducibility of the dose delivered *(Morice et al., 2007).*

The inspiratory flow rate affects the pattern of distribution of the tussives in the airways. Variation in the inspiratory flow rate thus will affect the cough challenge test. The lowering the inspiratory flow rate will increase the cough response to citric acid. Controlling the flow rate ensures that the same amount of tussive is delivered to different individuals *(Barros et al., 1991).* To control the inspiratory flow rate, ERS currently recommend the use a compressed air-driven nebulizer controlled by a dosimeter modified by an inspiratory regulatory flow regulator valve *(Morice et al., 2007).*

The patient should be told not to suppress any coughs and not to talk immediately after inhalation of the tussive, since talking suppresses the cough response. The cough induced by capsaicin and citric acid occur immediately and only sustain for a short period. Therefore only coughs that occur within 15 sec after the administration of the tussive should be counted. Any cough occurring after this interval should not be counted, since it is not likely to be induced by the tussive agent. In studies the concentration of the selected tussive agent causing two (C2) and five (C5) coughs are reported. C2 is the concentration first resulting in 2 or more coughs, while C5 is the first concentration resulting in 5 or more coughs. In patient with high cough threshold a C5 value may not be possible to obtain, and ERS recommend that these individuals are excluded from the clinical trials *(Morice et al., 2007).*

During the cough challenge test it is also recommended to use placebo inhalations with physiological saline *(Morice et al., 2001)*. The saline solution should be used randomly between the different concentrations of the tussive agent. This is thought to decrease voluntary suppression of cough *(Morice et al., 2007)*.
Tachyphylaxis is the process in which the effect of a drug is reduced during continuous use or by constantly repeated drug administration. In one study that used continuous inhalation over 1 min with capsaicin, the cough frequency was reduced by one third. In continuous inhalation with citric acid, no coughs were evoked after the 1 min period *(Morice et al., 1992)*. The ERS recommends an interval between cough challenge measurements of minimally 1 hour. The optimal interval is set by the ERS to 2 hours.
No serious adverse effect is associated with cough challenge testing using capsacin as tussive agent. The most commonly reported side effect is transient throat irritation *(Morice et al., 2007)*.
Citric acid inhalation may result in a small reduction of forced expiratory volume (FEV), but this is thought to be without clinical significance *(Laude et al., 1993)*. Capsaicin induces bonchoconstriction, but it is not tough to have clinical significance in healthy individuals or in individuals with asthma bronchiale. However, ERS recommend that bronchodilators should be easily available when a cough challenge test is performed *(Morice et al., 2007)*.

4. Cough in rhinosinusitis

Rhinitis refers to inflammation of the nasal mucosa, while sinusitis means inflammation of the mucosa in one or more of the paranasal sinuses. A continuum exists between rhinitis and sinusitis owing to the anatomical and physiological relationship of the nose and paranasal sinuses. Sinus inflammation generally develops in association with rhinitis and the term rhinosinusitis is applied to these disorders *(Probst et al., 2005)*. Chronic rhinosinusitis is among the commonest causes of chronic cough in adults. In 20-40% of patients with chronic cough who have normal chest x-ray, chronic rhinosinusitis is reported to be the cause of the cough *(Tatar et al., 2009)*.
Chronic rhinosinusitis may be caused by diseases of a chronic inflammatory, allergic, traumatic or neoplastic nature. Chronic rhinosinusitis may also develop as a result of anatomical changes, as seen in e.g. septal deviation or septal spurs. Impaired ventilation of the ostiomeatal unit caused by obstruction or stenosis is the common mechanism for development of rhinosinusistis. The obstruction impairs drainage from the sinus systems. The drainage is further impaired by swelling of the mucosa in the narrow anatomical canal of the ostiomeatal unit. A viscous circle of recurrent acute inflammations that develops into a chronic inflammation is established. In adults the maxillary and ethmoid cells are the sinuses most commonly affected *(Probst et al., 2005)*.
The mechanism of chronic cough in rhinosinusitis is until now not completely understood. Chronic upper cough syndrome, previously postnasal drip, cough reflex hypersensitivity and aspiration of secretions are among the mechanisms thought to be responsible, either alone or in combination *(Tatar et al., 2009)*.
The cough is produced by stimulation of the pharyngeal nerve endings, which are branches of the vagus nerve. The stimulation occur secondary to secretion from the nose and sinuses dripping into the hypopharynx, a process known as postnasal drip *(Palombini & Araujo, 2003)*. However, only some of the patients with postnasal drip complain of cough, and some

patients with chronic cough caused by rhinosinusitis do not experience postnasal drip. Therefore it is unlikely that postnasal drip is the only mechanism responsible for cough in nasal disease *(Tatar et al., 2009)*. Cough reflex sensitization is often observed in patients with chronic cough, including those with nasal diseases. The cough reflex cannot be triggered from the nose, but cough reflex sensitization may occur in nasal diseases. *Tatar et al. (2009)* have suggested that central sensitization of the cough reflex mediated by the nasal trigeminal sensory nerves may be one of the possible mechanisms of chronic cough in patients with nasal diseases. Chronic cough in nasal diseases may also be secondary to aspiration of secretions. The secretions are thought to stimulate the vagal afferents in the lung, thereby mediating cough. However more evidence is needed before this last mentioned mechanism can be accepted as a mechanism of cough in nasal diseases *(Pratter, 2006)*.

The diseases of the nose and paranasal sinuses are among the most commonly identified causes of chronic cough (*Pratter, 2006*). Depending on the population studied and the variations in diagnostic algorithm, the diseases of nose and sinuses are reported to contribute to coughing in 20–40% of patients with chronic cough who have normal chest radiograph (*Chung & Pavord, 2008*). The mechanisms of chronic cough in rhinosinusitis are incompletely understood. Several mechanisms have been proposed, single or in combination: postnasal drip (PND), direct irritation, inflammation in the lower airways and the cough reflex sensitization (*Pratter, 2006)*.

4.1 Cough reflex hypersensitivity

Cough reflex hypersensitivity refers to a condition in which the cough reflex is more readily inducible. Cough reflex hypersensitivity can be demonstrated as 1) the lowered intensity of a stimulus required to trigger cough or 2) enhanced coughing in response to a stimulus with the constant intensity. In clinical and laboratory experiments, the cough reflex hypersensitivity is detected by measuring the cough threshold or by evaluating changes in the number of coughs induced by a stimulus with defined intensity. The cough threshold is measured by a controlled inhalation of increasing concentrations of an aerosolized tussigen, commonly capsaicin or acidic solutions (*Morice et al., 1997*) and (*Choudry & Fuller, 1992*). The cough threshold is defined as the lowest concentration of the tussigen required to induce a predetermined number of coughs (typically 2 and 5 coughs, denoted C_2 and C_5, respectively). The cough reflex hypersensitivity is found when the cough threshold in the patient group is lower than in the appropriate reference group.

The cough reflex hypersensitivity is often reported in patients with chronic cough attributed to disparate causes including nasal diseases (*McGarvey et al., 1998*). It is implied that the cough reflex hypersensitivity contributes to coughing. In patients with a sensitized cough reflex, the environmental and endogenous stimuli are predicted to be more effective to trigger cough. Thus the cough reflex hypersensitivity results in the amplification of cough, similar to the amplification of pain in hyperalgesia. The observations that the cough sensitivity decreases with the successful treatment or natural resolution of cough also support the notion that the cough sensitization contributes to coughing (*McGarvey et al., 1998, O´Connell et al., 1994, O´Connell et al., 1996*).

There is a consensus that the cough reflex cannot be triggered from the nose. There is the mechanistic question whether the cough reflex can be sensitized from the nose. Based on the general concept that the activation of nasal sensory nerves leads to cough reflex hypersensitivity, a series of studies in humans and in animal models were carried out (*Tatar et al., 2009*).

4.2 Sensory nerve activators in the nose sensitize the cough reflex

The hypothesis that the afferent nerve activators applied into the nose sensitize the cough reflex in humans by using sensory activators histamine and capsaicin was aevaluated. Histamine is a prototypic mediator of nasal inflammation that directly stimulates a subset of nasal sensory nerves (*Taylor-Clark et al., 2005*). The TRPV1 selective agonist capsaicin is also an efficient activator of the nasal sensory nerves (*Taylor-Clark et al., 2005*). A large proportion of the TRPV1-positive trigeminal neurons innervating the nose express a variety of receptors relevant for detection of stimuli associated with inflammation. For example, nasal trigeminal neurons functionally express the histamine H1 receptor, the leukotriene cys-LT_1 receptor (*Taylor-Clark et al., 2005; Taylor-Clark et al., 2008a, Taylor-Clark et al., 2008b*). Intranasal administration of capsaicin likely stimulates large proportion of nerves that are also stimulated or modulated by nasal inflammation. Local and reflex consequences of the sensory nerves activation with histamine and capsaicin (such as substance P release from peripheral terminals and reflex vasodilation) may generate additional stimuli that further stimulate nasal sensory nerves (*Tani et al., 1990; Petersson et al., 1989*). In addition, direct effects of histamine on the cells other than sensory nerves likely lead to generation of more endogenous sensory stimuli.

Consistent with the extensive data from human studies (*Philip et al., 1994; Secher et al., 1982*) intranasal administration of histamine and capsaicin failed to trigger cough in healthy subjects (*Plevkova et al., 2004; Plevkova et al., 2006*). The effective activation of nasal sensory nerves by histamine and capsaicin was confirmed by the occurrence of sensations and symptoms typically described after intranasal administration of these agents. The cough was induced by inhalation of a tussigen aerosol during the time window of the most pronounced nasal symptoms evaluated by a composite score.

Both histamine and capsaicin applied into the nose caused sensitization of the cough reflex in healthy subjects (*Plevkova et al., 2004; Plevkova et al., 2006*). Following the intranasal administration of capsaicin or histamine, the number of coughs induced by inhalation of a defined dose of capsaicin was increased by 60–80%. Similarly, intranasal histamine did not trigger cough but sensitized the cough reflex in patients with allergic rhinitis (*Plevkova et al., 2005*). These data are consistent with the hypothesis that the activation of nasal sensory nerves sensitizes the cough reflex (*Tatar et al., 2009*).

4.3 Cough reflex is sensitized in patients with allergic rhinitis

The cough reflex hypersensitivity in patients with allergic rhinitis was evaluated (*Pecova et al., 2005; Pecova et al., 2008*). Chronic nasal symptoms attributable to sensory nerve activation in patients with rhinitis implicate that the inflammation leads to repeated activation of sensory nerves. The repeated activation and mediators associated with inflammation can induce sensitization at multiple levels of sensory pathways. Thus we predicted that the cough reflex is more sensitive in patients with allergic rhinitis than in healthy subjects (*Pecova et al., 2005; Pecova et al., 2008, Tatar et al., 2009).*

The grass pollen-sensitive patients with allergic rhinitis were studied out of pollen season. All patients included in the studies were free of nasal symptoms at the time of investigation. We found that the cough reflex was more sensitive in patients with allergic rhinitis compared to healthy subjects (measured by the capsaicin C_2 cough threshold) (*Pecova et al., 2005*). This finding was reproduced in a separate study in which the capsaicin C_5 threshold was evaluated in another groups of patients and healthy subjects (*Pecova et al., 2008*). In this study, the concentrations of capsaicin causing five coughs (C_5, geometric mean and 95% CI) were 132.4 (41.3–424.5) µM and 13.1 (6.0–28.6) µM in healthy subjects (5 M/7F, mean age 23 yrs) and patients with allergic rhinitis (5 M/7F, mean age 23 yrs), respectively ($P < 0.05$). We conclude that the cough reflex is sensitized in patients with allergic rhinitis (*Pecova et al., 2008*).

Since the symptoms of allergic rhinitis in pollen-sensitive patients are most prominent during the pollen season, we hypothesized that the sensitization of cough is most pronounced in this period. Fifteen patients were evaluated out of pollen season (January–February) and in the grass pollen season (May–June) in a paired study(*Pecova et al., 2005*). The capsaicin cough C_2 threshold was reduced in the pollen season vs. out of the pollen season, 0.11(0.3–0.33) µM vs. 0.84(0.14–5.2) µM, respectively ($P < 0.05$). Thus the cough reflex in patients with allergic rhinitis is further sensitized in the period when the nasal inflammation is more active.

4.4 Sensitized cough reflex and coughing in humans

In a series of studies it was demonstrated that the cough reflex in healthy subjects is sensitized by the intranasal administration of sensory nerve activators (*Plevkova et al., 2004; Plevkova et al., 2006*). These results are consistent with the hypothesis that the activation of nasal sensory nerves sensitizes the cough reflex (*Tatar et al., 2009*). We also show that the cough reflex is sensitized in patients with allergic rhinitis *Pecova et al., 2005; Pecova et al., 2008, Tatar et al., 2009*) and is further sensitized in this group by intranasal sensory activator histamine (*Plevkova et al., 2005*) and during the period of more active nasal inflammation (*Pecova et al., 2005*). Our results may help to explain the mechanisms contributing to chronic cough associated with rhinosinusitis (*Tatar et al., 2009*).

These results are highly indicative that nasal sensory nerves are the neural pathways involved in the sensitization of cough. The wealth of data from the somatosensory (*Jiand & Woolf, 2001*) and vagal (*Mazzone et al., 2005; Mazzone & Canning, 2002*) systems allows for an informed speculation that central cough reflex hypersensitivity mediated by nasal sensory nerves underlies the observed cough sensitization. In this scenario the afferent inputs from the nose feed into the central regulatory circuits of the cough reflex in a manner rendering the cough reflex hypersensitive. It has been demonstrated that the cough reflex triggered from trachea is sensitized by the stimulation of sensory nerves innervating distal parts of the respiratory system (lungs) in animal models (*Mazzone and Canning, 2005*), or even from the esophagus in humans (*Javorkova et al., 2008*). The sensitization of cough by the nasal trigeminal sensory pathways is perhaps more complex than the vagally mediated sensitization, since the trigeminal and the cough-triggering vagal sensory nerves terminate in different areas of the brainstem. Interestingly, the sensitization of cough from the nose can be induced even in anaesthetized animals, suggesting that the cough sensitization does not require intact cortical function.

The situation is more complex in patients with allergic rhinitis. Our data discussed thus far predict that the cough reflex hypersensitivity mediated by acute sensory nerve activation occurs in the symptomatic patients. However, in the patients without symptoms (such as the patients with allergic rhinitis out of the allergen season) the absence of the symptoms indicates limited nasal sensory activity. Yet the cough reflex is strongly sensitized in this group (*Pecova et al., 2005; Pecova et al., 2008, Tatar et al., 2009)*. It seems unlikely that the nasal sensory nerves in patients without symptoms are stimulated in a manner that is sufficient to maintain the cough sensitization but insufficient to trigger the symptoms. Rather, we speculate that the cough sensitization is induced by sensory activation during the period with symptoms and then outlasts the sensory activation. Inflammatory mediators, neurotrophic factors and other signals emanating from the nose during symptomatic period could, in theory, initiate long-lasting neural plastic changes in the circuits regulating the cough reflex (*Chen et al., 2001; Bonham et al., 2006*). Mechanistic studies are needed to evaluate this speculation.

Nasal provocation with histamine induces significantly stronger sneezing responses in subjects with allergic rhinitis compared with healthy subjects - a sensitized sneezing reflex (*Gerth Van Wijk & Dieges, 1987; Sanico et al., 1999*). We noted that intranasal histamine was more effective in reducing the capsaicin cough threshold in patients with allergic rhinitis than in healthy subjects (*Plevkova et al., 2004; Plevkova et al., 2005*). The simplest explanation is that the nasal sensory nerve pathways are sensitized, resulting in increased sensory feeding into the cough and sneeze regulatory areas. It is noteworthy in this context that nasal inflammation induces lasting changes in expression of molecules predicted to positively regulating activation and excitability in nasal afferent nerves (*O´Hanlon et al., 2007; Keh et al., 2008*). However, a separate sensitization of cough and sneezing at the higher regulatory levels of cough and sneezing reflexes is also a viable option.

Another explanation is that the cough reflex is sensitized in patients with allergic rhinitis because of allergic inflammation in the lower airways and lungs. This possibility cannot be excluded. Numerous studies have shown that the inflammation in the lower airways and lungs in patients with allergic rhinitis is in many aspects similar to that in asthmatics (*exemplified by Braunstahl et al., 2003*). However, the studies in asthmatics failed to consistently show lowered capsaicin or citric acid cough thresholds (*Fujimura et al., 1992; Chang et al., 1997; Schmidt et al., 1997*). Since this is in contrast with the dramatic sensitization of cough in allergic rhinitis, this mechanism likely plays only a limited role.

Allergic rhinitis was chosen as a model of a well-defined nasal inflammation allowing for selection of a relatively homogeneous patient population (skin prick test pollen-sensitive patients). Although the cough reflex was sensitized in allergic rhinitis, none of the patients complained about coughing. The increased cough reflex sensitivity is consistently found in patients with chronic cough and the effective treatment of cough is accompanied by normalization of the cough hypersensitivity. These observations advanced the hypothesis that the cough reflex hypersensitivity is the mechanism causing the cough. However, the cough reflex hypersensitivity has been also reported in other groups of patients who do not suffer from chronic cough. For example, the cough reflex sensitivity to capsaicin is increased in the GERD patients who do not complain about cough (*Benini et al., 2000; Ferrari et al., 2005*). Interestingly, the magnitude of the cough threshold reduction in the GERD patients is comparable to that found in chronic coughers, and the cough threshold reduction in allergic rhinitis appears to be even larger. The cough hypersensitivity without cough was also found in other diseases (*Pecova et al., 2003a; Pecova et al., 2003b*).

The observations that the cough reflex hypersensitivity is not always accompanied by cough force the conclusion that the cough reflex hypersensitivity alone is not sufficient for clinical presentation of chronic cough. Rather, the increased cough reflex sensitivity contributes to chronic cough by amplifying the cough triggered by endogenous and, perhaps less likely, environmental stimuli. While the cough reflex sensitivity is predicted to worsen the cough, it is unlikely to be its only causal mechanism (*Tatar et al., 2009*).

4.5 Potential mechanisms triggering cough in patients with rhinosinusitis and cough

The cough reflex hypersensitivity is predicted to amplify cough by increasing the efficiency of endogenous and environmental stimuli to trigger cough but is unlikely to cause chronic coughing by itself. There is an ongoing discussion in the literature whether diseases of the nose actually trigger cough (*Morice, 2004; Sanu & Eccles, 2008*). This confusion is also reflected in the recommendation of the term upper airway cough syndrome (UACS) to be used when discussing cough that is associated with upper airway conditions (*Pratter, 2006*).

One proposed mechanism for triggering cough in rhinosinusitis is the postnasal drip (drainage of secretions from the nose or paranasal sinuses into the pharynx). In this scenario the cough-triggering nerves located in the hypopharynx or larynx are stimulated by secretions emanating from the nose and/or sinuses dripping down into these areas (*Irwin et al., 1984*). The arguments against postnasal drip as a sole cause of cough in rhinosinusitis are twofold. Postnasal drip is a common phenomenon, and only a small fraction of patients with the postnasal drip also complain about cough (*O´Hara & Jones, 2006*). Conversely, a proportion (reported ~20%) of patients with chronic cough attributed to rhinosinusitis do not experience postnasal drip. It seems therefore unlikely that postnasal drip is the exclusive mechanism triggering cough. Cough in rhinosinusitis could be also conceivably triggered by aspirated secretions stimulating cough receptors in the lower respiratory tract; however, there are limited data to support this mechanism (*Pratter, 2006*). As is the case with postnasal drip, the aspiration or inhalation of nasal secretions likely occurs also in patients who do not have chronic cough. Enhanced sensitivity to environmental factors has also been linked to chronic cough in rhinosinusitis (*Millquist & Bende, 2006*).

The analysis of the mechanisms triggering cough in rhinitis is further complicated by the fact that rhinosinusitis often coexists with other common causes of chronic cough such as gastroesophageal reflux disease and eosinophilic airway diseases including asthma. Thus the potential cough triggers may be unrelated to the nasal disease (discussed elsewhere in this issue). Rhinitis is also very often part of the asthma presentation (*Togias, 2003*) and chronic sinusitis and postnasal drip can be caused or worsen by gastroesophageal reflux (*Poelmans & Tack, 2005*) introducing even more complexity into the analysis.

Treatment aimed at rhinosinusitis improves chronic cough in many patients who also present with other conditions potentially causing chronic cough (i.e. asthma or GERD). That the rhinosinusitis causes cough reflex hypersensitivity may explain the beneficial effect of this therapy. We speculate that the cough reflex hypersensitivity in combination with one or more cough triggers results in some unfortunate individuals in clinically relevant coughing termed chronic cough associated with rhinitis (*Tatar et al., 2009*).

5. References

Advenier, C. & Emonds-Alt, X. (1996). Tachykinin receptor antagonists and cough. *Pulm Pharmacol*, Vol.9, No 5-6, pp. 329-33.

Armstrong, D.J. & Luck, J.C. (1974). A comparative study of irritant and type J receptors in the cat. *Respir Physiol*, Vol.21, pp. 47-60.

Atzori, L., Bannenberg, G., Corriga, A.M., Lou, Y.P., Lundberg, J.M., Ryrfeldt, A. & Moldeus, P. (1992). Sulfur dioxide-induced bronchoconstriction via ruthenium red-sensitive activation of sensory nerves. *Respiration*, Vol.59, pp. 272-278.

Baluk, P., Nadel, J.A. & McDonald, D.M. (1992). Substance P-immunoreactive sensory axons in the rat respiratory tract: a quantitative study of their distribution and role in neurogenetic inflammation. *J Comp Neurol*, Vol.319, pp. 586-598.

Barnes P.J. (2001). Neurogenic inflammation in the airways. *Respir Physiol*, Vol.125, pp. 145-54.

Barros, M.J., Zammattio, S.L. & Rees, P.J. (1991) Effect of changes in inspiratory flow rate on cough responses to inhaled capsaicin. *Clin Sci (Lond)*, Vol.81, pp. 539-532.

Benini, L., Ferrari, M., Sembenini, C., Olivieri, M., Micciolo, R., Zuccali, V., Bulighin, G.M., Fiorino, F., Ederle, A., Cascio, V.L. & Vantini I. (2000). Cough threshold in reflux oesophagitis: influence of acid and of laryngeal and oesophageal damage. *Gut*, Vol.46, pp. 762–767.

Bergren, D.R. & Sampson, S.R. (1982). Characterization of intrapulmonary, rapidly adapting receptors of guinea-pigs. *Resp Physiol*, Vol.47, pp. 83-95.

Bergren, D.R. (1997). Sensory receptor activation by mediators of defense reflexes in guinea-pig lungs. *Respir Physiol*, Vol.108, pp. 195-204.

Bolser, D.C., DeGennaro, F.C., O'Reilly, S., McLeod, R.L. & Hey, J.A. (1997). Central antitussive activity of the NK1 and NK2 tachykinin receptor antagonists, CP-99,994 and SR 48968, in the guinea-pig and cat. *Br J Pharmacol*, Vol.121, pp. 165-70.

Bolser, D.C., Hey, J.A. & Chapman R.W. (1999) Influence of central antitussive drugs on the cough motor pattern. *J Appl Physiol*, Vol.86, pp. 1017-24.

Bonham, A.C., Kott, K.S., Ravi, K., Kappagoda, C.T. & Joad, J.P. (1996). Substance P contributes to rapidly adapting receptor responses to pulmonary venous congestion in rabbits. *J Physiol*, Vol.493, pp. 229-38.

Bonham,, A.C., Sekizawa, S., Chen, C. & Joad, J.P. (2006). Plasticity of brainstem mechanisms of cough. *Respir Physiol Neurobiol*, Vol.152, pp. 312–319.

Braunstahl, G.J., Fokkens, W.J., Overbeek, S.E., KleinJan, A., Hoogsteden, H.C. & Prins, J.B. (2003). Mucosal and systemic inflammatory changes in allergic rhinitis and asthma: a comparison between upper and lower airways. *Clin Exp Allergy*, Vol.33, pp. 579–587.

Canning, B.J. & Mazzone, S.B. (2005). Afferent pathways regulating the cough reflex. In: Redington AE, Morice AH(eds). Acute and chronic cough. Taylor & Francis. Boca Raton, USA, 2005, pp. 25-48 ISBN 978-0-8247-5958-2.

Canning, B.J. (2008). The cough reflex in animals: Relevance to human cough research. *Lung*, Vol.186 (suppl 1), pp. 23-28.

Canning, B.J., Reynolds, S.M. & Mazzone, S.B. (2001). Multiple mechanisms of reflex bronchospasm in guinea pigs. *J Appl Physiol*, Vol.91, pp. 2642-2653.

Canning, B.J., Reynolds, S.M., Meeker, S. & Undem, B.J. (2000). Electrophysiological identification of tracheal (T) and laryngeal(LX) vagal afferents mediating cough in guniea-pigs(GP). *Am J Respir Crit Care Med*, Vol.161, p. A434.

Carr, M.J. & Undem, B.J. (2001). Ion channels in airway afferenet neurons. Respir Physiol, Vol.125, No.1-2, pp. 83-97.

Carr, M.J., Hunter, D.D., Jacoby, D.B. & Undem, B.J. (2002). Expression of tachykinin in non-nociceptive vagal afferent neurons during raspiratory tract viral infection in guinea pigs. *Am J Respir Crit Care Med*, Vol.165, pp. 1071-5.

Caterina, M.J. & Julius, D. (2001). The vanilloid receptor: a molecular gateway to the pain pathway. *Annu Rev Neurosci*, Vol.24, pp. 487-517.

Chang, A.B. (2005). Defining the cough spectrum ad reviewing the evidence for treating non-specific cough in children. *Curr Pediatr Rev*; Vol.1, pp. 283-296.

Chang, A.B., Landau, L.I., Van Asperen, P.P., Glasgow, N.J., Robertson, C.F., Marchant, J.M. & Mellis, C.M. (2006). Cough in children: definitions and clinical evaluation, Position statement of the Thoracic Society of Australia and New Zealand. *MJA*, Vol.184, pp. 398-403.

Chang, A.B., Phelan, P.D., Sawyer, S.M., Del Brocco, S. & Robertson, C.F. (1997). Cough sensitivity in children with asthma, recurrent cough, and cystic fibrosis. *Arch Dis Child*, Vol.77, pp. 331–334.

Chen, C.Y., Bonham, A.C., Schelegle, E.S., Gershwin, L.J., Plopper, C.G. & Joad, J.P. (2001). Extended allergen exposure in asthmatic monkeys induces neuroplasticity in nucleus tractus solitarius. *J Allergy Clin Immunol*, Vol.108, pp. 557–562.

Choudry, N.B. & Fuller, R.W. (1992). Sensitivity of the cough reflex in patients with chronic cough. *Eur Respir J*, Vol.5, No.3, pp. 296-300.

Choudry, N.B., Fuller, R.W. & Pride, N.B. (1989). Sensitivity of the human cough reflex:effect of inflammatory mediators prostaglandin E2, bradykinin, and histamine. *Am Rev Respir Dis*, Vol.140, pp. 137-41.

Christian, E.P. & Togo, J.A. (1995). Excitable properties and underlying Na^+ and K^+ currents in neurons from the guinea-pig jugular ganglion. *J Auton Nerv Syst*, Vol.56, No.1-2, pp. 75-86.

Chuang, H.H., Prescott, E.D., Kong, H., Shields, S., Jordt, S.E., Basbaum, A.I. et al. (2001). Bradykinin and nerve growth factor release the capsaicin receptor from PtdIns(4,5)P2-mediated inhibition. *Nature*, Vol.411, pp. 957-62.

Chung, K.F. & Pavord, I.D. (2008). Prevalence, pathogenesis, and causes of chronic cough. *Lancet*, Vol. 371, No.9621, pp. 1364-74.

Chung, K.F. (2003). Measurment and assessment of cough. In Cough: Causes, mechanisms and therapy. Edited by: Chung F, Widdicombe J, Boushey H. UK: Blackwell Publishing, pp. 39-48.

Coleridge, J.C. & Coleridge, H.M. (1984). Afferent vagal C-fibre innervation of the lungs and airways and its functional significance. *Rev Physiol Biochem Pharmacol*, Vol.99, pp. 1-110.

Coryllos, P.N. (1937). Action of the diaphragm in cough. Experimental and clinical study on the human. *Am J Med Sci*, Vol,194, pp. 523-35.

Deep, V., Singh, M. & Ravi, K. (2001). Role of vagal afferents in the reflex effect of capsaicin and lobeline in monkeys. *Respir Physiol*, Vol.125, pp. 155-168.

Ferrari, M., Olivieri, M., Sembenini, C., Benini, L., Zuccali, V., Bardelli, E., Bovo, P., Cavallini, G., Vantini, I. & Lo Cascio, V. (1995). Tussive effect of capsaicin in patients with gastroesophageal reflux without cough. *Am J Respir Crit Care Med*, Vol.151, pp. 557–561.

Fischer,. A, McGregor, G..P, Saria, A., Philippin,. B. & Kummer, W. (1996). Induction of tachykinin gene and peptide expression in guinea pig nodose primary afferent neurons by allergic airway inflammation. *J Clin Invest*, Vol.98, No.10, pp. 2284-91.

Forsberg,. K. & Karlsson, J.A. (1986). Cough induced by the stimulation of capsaicin-sensitive sensory neurons in counsious guinea-pigs. *Acta Physiol Scand*, Vol.128, pp. 319-20.

Fox, A. (2002). Airway nerves: in vitro electrophysiology. Curr Opin Pharmacol, Vol.2, No.3, pp. 278-9.

Fujimura, M., Sakamoto, S., Kamio, Y. & Matsuda, T. (1992). Cough receptor sensitivity and bronchial responsiveness in normal and asthmatic subjects. *Eur Respir J*, Vol.5, pp. 291–295.

Gerth Van Wijk, R. & Dieges, P.H. (1987). Comparison of nasal responsiveness to histamine, methacholine and phentolamine in allergic rhinitis patients and controls. *Clin Allergy*, Vol.17, pp. 563–570.

Gold, M.S., Reichling, D.B., Shuster, M.J. & Levine, J.D. (1996). Hyperalgesic agents increase a tetrodotoxin-resistant Na+current in nociceptors. *Proc Natl Acad Sci USA*, Vol.93, No.3, pp. 1108-12.

Hanacek, J. & Korpas, J. (1982). Modification of the intensity of the expiration reflex during short-term inflation of the lungs in rabbits. *Physiol Bohemoslov*, Vol.31, pp. 169-174.

Hanacek, J., Davis, A. & Widdicombe, J.G. (1984). Influence of lung strech receptors on the cough reflex in rabbits. *Respiration*, Vol.45, pp. 161-8.

Hay, A.D. & Wilson, A.D. (2002). The natural history of acute cough in childeren aged 0-4 years in primary care: a systematic review. *Br J Gen Pract*, Vol.52, pp.401-409.

Ho, C.Y., Gu, Q., Hong, J.L. & Lee, L.Y. (2000). Prostaglandin E(2) enhances chemical and mechanical sensitivities of pulmonary C fibers in the rat. *Am J Respir Crit Car Med*, Vol.162, pp. 528-533.

Ho, C.Y., Gu, Q., Lin, Y.S. & Lee, L.Y. (2001). Sensitivity of vagal afferent endings to chemical irritants in the rat lung. *Respir Pysiol*, Vol.127, pp. 113-24.

Hunter, D.D. & Undem, B.J. (1999). Identification and substance P content of vagal afferent neurons innervating the epithelium of the guinea-pig trachea. *Am J Respir Crit Care Med*, Vol.159, pp. 1943-1948.

Hunter, D.D., Castranova, V., Stanley, C. & Dey, R.D. (1998). Effects of silica exposure on substance P immunoreactivity and preprotachykinin mRNA expression in trigeminal sensory neurons in Fischer 344 rats. *J Toxicol Environ Health*, Vol.53, No.8, pp. 593-605.

Hutchings, H.A., Morris, S., Eccles, R. & Jawad, M.S. (1993). Voluntary suppression of cough induced by inhalation of capsaicin in healthy volunteers. *Respir Med*, Vol.87, pp. 379-382.

Irwin, R.S., French, C.L., Curley, F.J., Zawacki, J.K. & Bennett, F.M. (1993). Chronic cough due to gastroesophageal reflux. Clinical, diagnostic, and pathogenetic aspects. *Chest*, Vol.104, No.5, pp. 1511-7.

Irwin, R.S., Pratter, M.R., Holland, P.S., Corwin, R.W. & Hughes, J.P. (1984). Postnasal drip causes cough and is associated with reversible upper airway obstruction. *Chest*, Vol.85, pp. 346–352.

Javorkova, N., Varechova, S., Pecova, R., Tatar, M., Balaz, D., Demeter, M., Hyrdel, R. & Kollarik M. (2008). Acidification of the oesophagus acutely increases the cough sensitivity in patients with gastro-oesophageal reflux and chronic cough. *Neurogastroenterol Motil*, Vol.20, pp. 119–124.

Jiand, R.R. & Woolf, C.J. (2001). Neuronal plasticity and signal transduction in nociceptive neurons: implications for the initiation and maintenance of pathological pain. *Neurobiol Dis*, Vol.8, pp. 1–10.

Joad, J.P., Kott, K.S. & Bonham, A.C. (1997). Nitric oxide contributes to substance P-induced increase in lung rapidly adapting receptor activity in guinea-pigs. *J Physiol*, Vol.503, No.3, pp. 635-43.

Jonzon, A., Pisarri, T.E., Coleridge, J.C. & Coleridge, H.M. (1986). Rapidly adapting receptor activity in dogs is inversely related to lung compliance. *J Appl Physiol*, Vol.61, pp. 1980-7.

Karlsson, J.A. (1996). The role of capsaicin-sensitive C-fibre afferent nerves in the cough reflex. *Pulm Pharmacol*, Vol.9, pp. 315-21.

Keh, S.M., Facer, P., Simpson, K.D., Sandhu, G., Saleh, H.A. & Anand, P. (2008). Increased nerve fiber expression of sensory sodium channels Nav1.7, Nav1.8, and Nav1.9 in rhinitis. *Laryngoscope* , Vol.118, pp. 573–579.

Klesse, L.J. & Parada, L,F. (1999). Trks:signal transduction and intracellular pathways. *Microsc Res Tech*, Vol.45, No.4-5, pp. 210-6.

Kollarik, M., Dinh, Q.T., Fischer, A. & Undem, B.J. (2003). Capsaicin-sensitive and -insensitive vagal bronchopulmonary C-fibers in the mouse. *J Physiol*, Vol.551, No.3, pp. 869-879.

Korpas, J. & Tomori, Z. (1979). *Cough and other respiratory reflexes*, Karger, ISBN 3-8055-3007-2, Basel, Switzerland.

Laude, E.A., Higgins, K.S. & Morice, A.H. (1993). A comparative study of the effects of citric acid, capsaicin and resiniferatoxin on the cough challenge in guinea-pig and man. *Pulm Pharmacol*, Vol., No.3, pp. 171-5.

Leder, K., Sinclair, M.I., Mitakakis, T.Z., et al. (2003). A community-based study of respiratory episodes in Melbourne, Australia. *Aust N Z J Public Health*, Vol. 27, pp. 399-404.

Lee, L.Y. & Pisarri, T.E. (2001). Afferent properties and reflex functions of bronchopulmonary C-fibers. *Respir Physiol*, Vol.125, pp. 47-65.

Lii, Q., Fujimura, M., Tachibi, H., Myou, S., Kasahara, K. & Yasui, M. (2001). Characterization of increased cough sensitivity after antigen challenge in guinea pigs. *Clin Exp Allergy*, Vol.31, No.3, pp. 474-84.

Lopshire, J.C. & Nocol, G.D. (1998). The cAMP transduction cascade mediates the prostaglandin E2 enhancement of the capsaicin-elicited current in rat sensory neurons: wholecell and single-channel studies. *J Neurosci*, Vol.18, No.16, pp. 6081-92.

Lundberg, J.M., Hokfelt, T., Martling, C.R., Saria, A. & Cuello, C. (1984). Substance P-immunoreactive sensory nerves in the lower respiratory tract of various mammales including man. *Cell Tisse Res*, Vol. 235, pp. 251-261.

Ma, Q.P. & Woolf, C.J. (1995). Involvement of neurokinin receptors in the induction but not maintainance of mechanical allodynia in rat flexor motoneurons. *J Physiol*, Vol.486, pp. 769-777.

Matsumoto S. (1988). The activities of lung strech and irritant receptors during cough. *Neurosci Lett*, Vol.90, pp. 125-129.

Mazzone, S.B. & Canning, B.J. (2002). Synergistic interactions between airway afferent nerve subtypes mediating reflex bronchospasm in guinea pigs. Am J *Physiol Regul Integr Comp Physiol*, Vol.283, No.1, pp. R86-R98.

Mazzone, S.B., Canning, B.J. & Widdicombe, J.G. (2003). Sensory pathways for the cough reflex,. In: Chung, F., Widdicombe, J. & Boushey, H. (eds) Cough: Causes, Mechanisms ans Therapy. Oxford: Blackwell Publishing. pp. 161-171.

Mazzone, S.B., Mori, N. & Canning, B.J. (2002). Bradykinin-induced cough in counscious guinea-pigs. *Am J Respir Crit Care Med*, Vol.165, p. A773.

Mazzone, S.B., Mori, N. & Canning, B.J. (2005). Synergistic interactions between airway afferent nerve subtypes regulating the cough reflex in guinea-pigs. *J Physiol*, Vol.569, pp. 559–573.

McAlexander, M.A., Myers, A.C. & Undem, B.J. (1999). Adaptation of guinea pigs vagal airway afferent neurones to mechanical stimulation. *J Physiol*, Vol.521, pp. 239-247.

McGarvey, L.P., Heaney, L.G., Lawson, J.T., Johnston, B.T., Scally, C.M., Ennis, M., Shepherd, D.R. & MacMahon, J. (1998). Evaluation and outcome of patients with chronic non-productive cough using a comprehensive diagnostic protocol. *Thorax*, Vol.53, pp. 738–743.

Michael, G.J. & Priestley, J.V. (1999). Differential expression of the mRNA for the vanilloid receptors subtype 1 in cells of the adult rat dorsal root and nodose ganglia and its downregulation by axotomy. *J Neurosci*, Vol.19, No.5, pp. 1844-54.

Millqvist, E. & Bende, M. (2006). Role of the upper airways in patients with chronic cough. *Curr Opin Allergy Clin Immunol*, Vol.6, pp. 7–11.

Mohammed, S.P., Higenbottam, T.W. & Adcock, J.J. (1993). Effects of aerosol-applied capsaicin, histamine and prostaglandin E2 on airway sensory receptors in anaesthetized cats. *J Physio,l* Vol.469, pp. 51-66.

Morice, A.H. (2003). Epidemiology of cough. In Cough: Causes, mechanisms and therapy. Edited by: Chung F, Widdicombe J, Boushey H. UK: Blackwell;2003, pp. 11-16.

Morice, A.H. (2004). Post-nasal drip syndrome–a symptom to be sniffed at?. *Pulm Pharmacol Ther*, Vol.17, pp. 343–345.

Morice, A.H., Fontana, G.A., Belvisi, M.G., Birring, S.S. et al. (2007). ERS guidelines on the assessment of cough. *Eur Respir J*, Vol.29, pp. 1256-1276.

Morice, A.H., Higgins, K.S. & Yeo, W.W. (1992). Adaptation of cough reflex with different types of stimulation. *Eur Respir J*, Vol.5, No.7, pp. 841-7.

Morice, A.H., Kastelik, J.A. & Thompson, R. (2001). Cough challenge in the assessment of cough reflex. *Br J Clin Pharmacol*, Vol.52, pp. 365-375.

Myers, A.C., Kajekar, R. & Undem, B.J. (2002). Allergic inflammations-induced neuropeptide production in rapidly adapting afferent nerves in guniea pig airways. *Am J Physiol Lung Cell Mol Physiol*, Vol.282, pp. L775-L781.

Neumann, S., Doubell, T.P., Leslie, T. & Woolf, C.J. (1996). Inflammatory pain hypersensitivity mediated by phenotypic switch in myelinated primary sensory neurons. *Nature*, Vol.384, pp.360-4.

Nishino, T., Sugimori, K., Hiraga, K. & Hond, Y. (1989). Influence of CPAP on reflex responses to tracheal irritation in anesthetized humans. *J Appl Physiol*, Vol.67, pp.954-958.

Nishino, T., Tagaito, Y. & Isono, S. (1996). Cough and the reflexes on irritation of airway mucosa in man. *Pulm Pharmacol*, Vol.9, pp. 485-493.

O'Connell, F., Thomas, V.E., Pride, N.B. & Fuller R.W. (1994). Capsaicin cough sensitivity decreases with successful treatment of chronic cough. *Am J Respir Crit Care Med*, Vol.150, pp. 374–380.

O'Connell, F., Thomas, V.E., Studham, J.M., Pride, N.B. & Fuller R.W. (1996). Capsaicin cough sensitivity increases during upper respiratory infection. *Respir Med*, Vol.90, pp. 279–286.

O'Hanlon, S., Facer, P., Simpson, K.D., Sandhu, G., Saleh, H.A. & Anand, P. (2007). Neuronal markers in allergic rhinitis: expression and correlation with sensory testing, *Laryngoscope*, Vol.117, pp. 1519–1527.

O'Hara J. & Jones N.S. (2006). "Post-nasal drip syndrome": most patients with purulent nasal secretions do not complain of chronic cough. *Rhinology*, Vol.44, pp. 270–273.

Pack, A.I. & DeLaney, R.G. (1983). Response of pulmonary rapidly adapting receptors during lung inflation. *J Appl Physiol*, Vol.55, pp. 955-963.

Palombini, B.C. & Araujo, E. (2003). Cough in postnasal drip, rhinitis and rhinosinusitis. In Cough: Causes, mechanisms and therapy. Edited by: Chung F, Widdicombe J, Boushey H. UK: Blackwell;2003, pp. 107-114.

Palombini, B.C., Villanova, C.A., Araujo, E., Gastal, O.L., Alt, D.C., Stolz, D.P. & Palombini, C.O. (1999). A pathogenic triad in chronic cough: asthma, postnasal drip syndrome, and gastroesophageal reflux disease. *Chest*, Vol.116, No.2, pp. 279-84.

Pecova, R., Frlickova, Z., Pec, J. & Tatar M. (2003a). Cough sensitivity in localized scleroderma with no clinical symptoms from lower airways. *J Physiol Pharmacol*, Vol.54 (Suppl. 1), pp. 25–28.

Pecova, R., Frlickova, Z., Pec, J. & Tatar M. (2003b). Cough sensitivity in atopic dermatitis. *Pulm Pharmacol Ther*, Vol16, pp. 203–206.

Pecova, R., Vrlik, M. & Tatar M. (2005). Cough sensitivity in allergic rhinitis. *J Physiol Pharmacol*, Vol.56 (Suppl. 4), pp. 171–178.

Pecova, R., Zucha, J., Pec, M., Neuschlova, M., Hanzel, P. & Tatar, M. (2008). Cough reflex sensitivity testing in seasonal allergic rhinitis patients and healthy volunteers. *J Physiol Pharmacol*, Vol.59(Suppl 6), pp. 557-564.

Pek, W.Y. & Boushey, H.A. (2003). Cough in lower airway infections. In Cough: Causes, mechanisms and therapy. Edited by: Chung F, Widdicombe J, Boushey H. UK: Blackwell;2003, pp. 83-96.

Petersson, G., Malm, L., Ekman, R. & Hakanson, R. (1989). Capsaicin evokes secretion of nasal fluid and depletes substance P and calcitonin gene-related peptide from the nasal mucosa in the rat. *Br J Pharmacol*, Vol.98, pp. 930–936.

Philip, G., Baroody, F.M., Proud, D., Naclerio, R.M. & Togias, A.G. (1994). The human nasal response to capsaicin. *J Allergy Clin Immunol*, Vol.94, pp. 1035–1045.

Plevkova, J., Brozmanova, M., Pecova, R. & Tatar M. (2006). The effects of nasal histamine challenge on cough reflex in healthy volunteers. *Pulm Pharmacol Ther*; Vol.19, pp. 120–127.

Plevkova, J., Brozmanova, M., Pecova, R. & Tatar M. (2005). Effects of intranasal histamine on the cough reflex in subjects with allergic rhinitis. *J Physiol Pharmacol*, Vol.56 (Suppl. 4), pp. 185–195.

Plevkova, J., Brozmanova, M., Pecova, R. & Tatar, M. (2004). Effects of intranasal capsaicin challenge on cough reflex in healthy human volunteers. *J Physiol Pharmacol*, Vol.55 (Suppl. 3), pp. 101–106.

Poelmans, J. & Tack, J. (2005). Extraoesophageal manifestations of gastro-oesophageal reflux. *Gut*, Vol.54, pp. 1492–1499.

Pounsford, J.C., Birch, M.J. & Saunders, K.S. (1985). Effect of bronchodilators on the cough response to inhaled citric aid in normal and asthmatic subjects. *Thorax*, Vol.5, pp. 296-300.

Pratter, M.R. (2006). Chronic upper airway cough syndrome secondary to rhinosinus diseases (previously referred to as postnasal drip syndrome): ACCP evidence-based clinical practice guidelines. *Chest*, Vol.129(Suppl 1), pp. S63-71.

Pratter, M.R., Brightling, C.E., Boulet, L.P. & Irwin, R.S. (2006). An empiric integration approach to the management of cough: ACCP evidence-based clinical practice guidelines. *Chest*, 129, pp. 222-231.

Premkumar, L.S. & Ahern, G.P. (2000). Induction of vanilloid receptor channel activity by protein kinase C. *Nature*, Vol.408, pp. 985-90.

Probst, R., Grevers, G. & Iro, H. (2005). Basic Otorhinolaryngology: A Step-by-Step Learning Guide. 1st edition. Thieme; 2005, 430 p.

Riccio, M.M., Kummer, W., Biglari, B., Myers, A.C. & Undem, B.J. (1996c). Interganglionic segregation of distinct vagal afferent fibre phenotypes in guinea-pig airway. J *Physiol*, Vol.496, pp. 521-530.

Riccio, M.M., Kummer, W., Biglari, B., Myers, A.C., Undem, B.J., Pride, N.B. & Fuller, R.W. (1996b). Interganglionic segregation of distingct agal afferent fibre phenotypes in guinea-pig airways. *J Physiol*, Vol.496, No.2, pp. 521-30.

Riccio, M.M., Myers, A.C. & Undem, B.J. (1996a). Immunomodulation of afferent neurons in guinea-pig isolated airways. *J Physiol*, Vol.491, No.2, pp. 499-509.

Roberts, A.M., Kaufman, M.P., Baker, N.G., Brown, J.K., Coleridge, H.M. & Coleridge, J.C. (1981). Reflex tracheal contraction induced by stimulation of bronchial C-fibers in dogs. *J Appl Physiol*, Vol.51, pp. 485-93.

Sanico, A.M., Koliatsos, V.E., Stanisz, A.M., Bienenstock, J. & Togias, A. (1999). Neural hyperresponsiveness and nerve growth factor in allergic rhinitis. *Int Arch Allergy Immunol*, Vol.118, pp. 154–158.

Sant´Ambrogio, G. & Widdicombe, J.G. (2001). Reflexes from airway rapidly adapting receptors. *Respir Physiol*, Vol.125, pp. 33-45.

Sant´Ambrogio, G., Sant´Ambrogio, F.B. & Davis, A. (1984). Airways receptors in cough. *Bull Eur Physiopathol Respir*, Vol.20, pp. 43-47.

Sanu, A. & Eccles, R. (2008). Postnasal drip syndrome. Two hundred years of controversy between UK and USA. Rhinology, Vol.46, pp. 86–91.

Schelegle, E.S. & Green, J.F. (2001). An overview of the anatomy and physiology of slowly adapting pulmonary strech receptors. *Respir Physiol*, 125, pp. 17-31.

Schmidt, D., Jorres, R.A. & Magnussen, H. (1997). Citric acid-induced cough thresholds in normal subjects, patients with bronchial asthma, and smokers. *Eur J Med Res*, Vol.2, pp. 384–388.

Secher, C., Kirkegaard, J., Borum, P., Maansson, A., Osterhammel, P. & Mygind, N. (1982). Significance of H1 and H2 receptors in the human nose: rationale for topical use of combined antihistamine preparations. *J Allergy Clin Immunol*, Vol. 70, pp. 211–218.

Shannon, R., Baekey, D.M., Morris, K.F. & Lindsey, B.G. (1997). Brainstem respiratory networks and cough. *Pulm Pharmacol*, Vol.9, pp. 343-7.

Shannon, R., Baekey, D.M., Morris, K.F. & Lindsey, B.G. (1998). Ventrolateral medullary respiratory network and a model of cough motor pattern generation. *J Appl Physiol*, Vol.84, pp. 2020-2035.

Shannon, R., Baekey, D.M., Morris, K.F., Li, Z. & Lindsey, B.G. (2000). Functional connectivity among ventrolateral medullary respiratory neurons and responses during fictive cough in the cat. *J Physiol*, Vol.525, pp. 207-24.

Shannon, R., Bolser, D.C. & Lindsey, B.G. (1996). Neural control of coughing ans sneezing. In: Miller AD, Bianchi AL, Bishop BP, eds. Neural Control of Breathing. Boca Raton: CRC Press, 1996, pp. 215-24.

Shin, J., Cho, H., Hwang, S.W., Jung, J., Shin, C.Y., Lee, S.Y. et al. (2002). Bradykinin-12-lipoxygenase-VR1 signaling pathway for inflammatory hyperalgesia. *Proc Natl Aced Sci USA*, Vol.99, No.15, pp. 10150-5

Stead, R.H. (1992). Nerve remodelling during intestinal inflammation. *Ann N Y Acad Sci*, Vol.664, pp. 443-55.

Tani, E., Senba, E., Kokumai, S., Masuyama, K., Ishikawa, T. & Tohyama M. (1990). Histamine application to the nasal mucosa induces release of calcitonin gene-related peptide and substance P from peripheral terminals of trigeminal ganglion: a morphological study in the guinea pig. *Neurosci Lett*, Vol.112, pp. 1–6.

Tatar, M., Plevkova, J., Brozmanova, M., Pecova, R. & Kollarik, M. (2009). Mechanisms of the cough associated with rhinosinusitis. *Pulm Pharmacol Ther*, Vol.22, pp. 121-6.

Tatar, M., Sant´Ambrogio, G. & Sant´Ambrogio, F.B. (1994). Laryngeal and tracheobronchial cough in anesthetized dogs. *J Appl Physiol*, Vol.76, pp. 2672-2679.

Tatar, M., Webber, S.E. & Widdicombe, J.G. (1988). Lung C-fibre receptor activation and defensive reflexes in anaethetized cats. *J Physiol*, Vol.402, pp. 411-420.

Taylor-Clark, T.E., Kollarik, M., MacGlashan, D.W. Jr. & Undem B.J. (2005). Nasal sensory nerve populations responding to histamine and capsaicin. *J Allergy Clin Immunol*, Vol.116, pp. 1282–1288

Taylor-Clark, T.E., Nassenstein, C. & Undem B.J. (2008a). Leukotriene D4 increases the excitability of capsaicin-sensitive nasal sensory nerves to electrical and chemical stimuli. *Br J Pharmacol*, Vol.154, pp. 1359–1368.

Taylor-Clark, T.E., Undem, B.J., Macglashan, D.W. Jr., Ghatta, S., Carr, M.J. & McAlexander, M.A. (2008b). Prostaglandin-induced activation of nociceptive neurons via direct interaction with transient receptor potential A1 (TRPA1). Mol *Pharmacol*, Vol.73, pp. 274–281.

Togias, A. (2003). Rhinitis and asthma: evidence for respiratory system integration. *J Allergy Clin Immunol*, Vol.111, pp. 1171–1183.

Tomaki, M., Ichinose, M., Miura, M., Hirayama, Y., Yamauchi, H., Nakajima, N. et al. (1995). Elevated substance P content in induced sputum from patients with asthma and patients with chronic bronchitis. *Am J Respir Crit Care Med*, Vol.151, pp. 613-7.

Undem, B.J., Oh, E.J., Lee, M. & Weinreich, D. (2003). Subtypes of vagal nociceptive C-fibers in guinea pig lungs. *Am J Respir Crit Care Med*, Vol.167, Suppl., p. A708.

Virchow, J.C., Julius, P., Lommatzsch, M., Luttmann, W., Renz, H. & Braun, A. (1998). Neurotrophins are increased in bronchoalveolar lavage fluid after segemental allergen provocation. *Am J Respir Crit Care Med*, Vol.158, No.6, pp. 2002-5.

Wang, A.L., Blackford, T.L. & Lee, L.Y. (1996). Vagal bronchopulmonary C-fibers and acute ventilatory response to inhaled irritants. *Respir Physiol*, Vol.104, pp. 231-239.

Widdicombe, J.G. (1974). Pathophysiology of lung reflexes. *Bull Physiopathol Respir (Nancy)*, Vol.10, No.1, pp. 65-9.

Widdicombe, J.G. (2001). Airways receptors. *Respir Physiol*, Vol.125, pp. 3-15.

Widdicombe, J.G. (2003). Overview of neural pathways in allergy and asthma. *Pulm Pharmacol Ther*, Vol.16, No.1, pp. 23-30.

Woolf, C.J. & Salter, M.W. (2000). Neuronal plasticity: increasing the gain in pain. *Science*, Vol.288, pp. 1765-9.

7

Allergic Rhinitis and Its Impact on Sleep

J. Rimmer[1] and J. Hellgren[2]
[1]*Woolcock Institute and University of Sydney, Department of ENT, Sydney*
[2]*Head & Neck Surgery, Sahlgrenska Academy, Göteborg*
[1]*Australia*
[2]*Sweden*

1. Introduction

Allergic rhinitis affects a fifth of the population in industrialised countries and sleep disturbance has emerged as one of the major impacts of allergic rhinitis on patients. Sleep disturbances and its consequences on daytime sleepiness and fatigue affects the health related quality of life negatively and contributes significantly to patients'suffering and major health economic costs. Experimental studies have shown that sleep disturbances are induced when the nose is blocked with adhesive tape or petroleum jelly during sleep in healthy individuals. Nasal obstruction is the most commonly reported symptom by patients with allergic rhinitis and it causes an increased number of microarousals (short awakenings). Nasal obstruction is believed to be the most important mechanism behind poor sleep and daytime sleepiness in allergic rhinitis. Relieving nasal obstruction with nasal steroids significantly improves subjective sleep compared to placebo. Allergic rhinitis is present in a majority of patients with asthma. Identifying and treating allergic rhinitis improves sleep and the health related quality of life which reduces patient suffering and potentially saves significant health economic health costs. The present chapter reviews the current literature of allergic rhinitis and its impact on sleep and the health related quality of life.

1.1 Abbreviations

AR: allergic rhinitis
PAR: perennial allergic rhinitis
SAR: seasonal allergic rhinitis
SDB: sleep disordered breathing
RDS: rhinitis disturbed sleep

1.2 Prevalence

The prevalence of allergic rhinitis has steadily increased in developed countries since the industrial revolution and now affects 20-40% of the population (1,2). Studies suggest that allergic rhinitis and conjunctivitis are rare in infants but are estimated to affect around one in six children aged 6-7 years, one in ten children aged 13-14 years, 18% of those aged 15-34 years and 10% of older adults aged 35-54 years. AR is more common than asthma and chronic rhinosinusitis. Symptoms generally persist for at least ten years, often longer (3). Sleep disordered breathing has been recorded in 68% of PAR patients and 48% with SAR (4).

1.3 Costs

More than $6 billion was spent on prescription medications for AR in 2000 (5) in the USA. A specifically commissioned report in Australia estimated the total costs costs of Allergic disease (not asthma) including prescription medication to be $349 million in Australia in 2007 (3).

1.4 Symptoms

Symptoms of AR include nasal blockage or congestion occurring in up to 85%, and this tends to be the dominant symptom in children (5). It is generally most troublesome in the early morning on waking which may relate to the circadian rhythm for cortisol although the peak in symptoms is delayed compared to that of nocturnal asthma (6am versus 4am) (6). Nasal obstruction is the symptom that relates most to impaired quality of life (7). In addition there is a direct relationship between sleep impairment and symptom severity (5, 8). Nasal obstruction has been shown to be an independent risk factor for OSAS (obstructive sleep apnoea syndrome) (9). Other symptoms include sneezing, pruritis, anterior rhinorrhoea, post nasal drip and these may also contribute to SDB.

Numerous studies have shown that AR results in impaired QOL and affects numerous activities eg work productivity and attendance, physical activity, exam performance. How much of this is due to the disease itself or the accompanying SDB or both is unclear.

Interestingly many patients report dissatisfaction with the effectiveness of therapy (10).

1.5 Children and AR

SDB is well documented to occur in children and adolescents with AR (5, 11) The most common symptom is nasal obstruction. In children there are typical appearances associated with AR including mouth breathing, allergic shiners, allergic crease, allergic facies and these may be reversed by treatment of the rhinitis. Rhinitis has frequently been considered to be a benign condition in children and one that does not need treating. However more recent data indicates that in addition to symptoms there may be deleterious effects of the condition on their performance. Specifically in children studies have shown reduced examination performance in the spring season and reduced participation in skill based, social and informal activities (12, 13). Habitual snoring is increased in children with AR (14)

2. Sleep problems in AR

Sleep disordered breathing is reported by subjects with allergic rhinitis versus controls including difficulty getting to sleep (24% versus 8%), waking during the night (31% versus 13%) and poor sleep (26% versus 11%) (5, 15) Leger et al additionally noted early wakening in 29% of AR , feeling of lack of sleep in 63%, snoring 40%, insomnia 36%, OSAS 4% and also that there was a greater use of sedatives in the AR group (16). Poor sleep is associated with negative effects on mood, cognition and motor performance. A large epidemiological study of over 4900 subjects showed that AR subjects who reported nocturnal nasal congestion ≥ 5 nights/month were more likely to be habitual snorers, experience excess daytime sleepiness or nonrestorative sleep (17). SDB is felt to relate to nasal obstruction but can also be caused by other symptoms eg rhinorrhea, pruritis and sneezing occurring during the night and also by the effects of inflammatory mediators. In addition commonly co-existing diseases such as asthma in which nocturnal asthma can be a significant symptom can disturb sleep. Nocturnal asthma is attributed to a circadian variation in airway physiology as well as the effects of cytokine changes on sleep (see below).Eczema may also contribute to SDB with symptoms of pruritis often worse at night (18).

Sleep impairment in AR has been demonstrated by means of questionnaires, actigraphy (19,20) and polysomnography (17, 21)

The presence of abnormal sleep in association with AR categorises the disease as moderate to severe according to the ARIA classification of AR (Allergic Rhinitis and its Impact on Asthma) guidelines (Fig 1) (22)

Intermittent symptoms		**Persistent symptoms**
• <4 days per week		• >4 days per week
• Or < 4 weeks		• And > 4 weeks
Mild		**Moderate - severe (≥ 1 item)**
• Normal sleep		• Abnormal sleep
• Normal daily activities		• Impairment of daily activities, sport, leisure
• Normal work and school		• Problems caused at school or work
• No troublesome symptoms		• Troublesome symptoms

Fig. 1. ARIA classification of AR

The average sleep duration of healthy adults is about 7 hours but surveys show that a significant % of the population (43%) achieve less than this (23) and that these subjects felt tired, performed inefficiently and reported feeling drowsy while driving. It has been estimated that 20% of all traffic accidents in industrialised societies are related to sleep disorders.

Sleep disorders refers to a range of disorders including insomnia, OSAS, narcolepsy and idiopathic hypersomnolance, periodic limb disorders of sleep and restless leg syndrome. All of these primary sleep disorders are associated with excess daytime fatigue. SBD in AR includes insomnia and OSAS although recently a separate classification of RDS (rhinitis disturbed sleep) has been postulated (24).

Insomnia is a subjective perception of the amount or quality of sleep. It can comprise delayed initiation of sleep, difficulty with sleep maintenance and early awakening. It is associated with impaired QOL as demonstrated by reduced daytime alertness, lethargy, reduced cognitive functioning and altered emotional states. The 2008 NSF Sleep in America Poll found that 11% of the population described insomnia (26% difficulty falling asleep, 42% waking during the night, 29% woken early and unable to return to sleep)(25). Subjects with insomnia have a higher rate of traffic accidents: 5% versus 2% of normal sleepers.

OSAS in the general population is estimated at 2-4% and results in snoring, severe daytime sleepiness and increased risk of traffic accidents. The risk of RTA for OSAS is 12 times greater than controls and also higher than insomniacs. There is a direct relationship between the apnoea-hypopnoea index and crash risk.

However despite the documented impaired cognition and presence of SDB in AR no studies of driving crash risk have been performed.

RDS is a term that has been suggested to separate the effects of nasal obstruction and pharyngeal obstruction on SDB (24). It has frequently been observed by ourselves and others that the effect of INCS improves nasal related symptoms more consistently and effectively than sleep related objective measures such as the apnoea-hyponoea index and actigraphy measurements (unpublished data,20,24). Therefore effects of INCS on nasal inflammation may result in improvements in subjective sleep indices without improvements in objective sleep measures, supporting the concept of two co-existing conditions. One study undertook polysomnography pre and post pollen season in 25 subjects SAR and 25 normals Subjects with SAR showed a significant increase in symptoms (overall symptoms score 1.08 $\pm$ 2.7 at baseline compared with 21.3$\pm$13.1 in season) and also subjective increases in daytime sleepiness which only occurred in the moderate and severe SAR subjects. Objective sleep parameters showed an increase in objective sleep abnormalities, but the differences occurred within the normal range and were not felt to be of clinical relevance (26). This study tends to support the fact that RDS may be more significant in AR than other causes of SDB such as OSAS and insomnia.

3. Mechanisms of sleep impairment in AR

3.1 Nasal anatomy and physiology

Introduction: The nose is an integrated part of the combined upper and lower airways both in function and inflammatory airways disease such as allergic rhinitis and asthma. There has been an increased focus on the significance of nasal breathing and it´s effect on health related quality of life and sleep during the last decade. Though easily accessible for examination, still little is known about how the regulation of nasal function is disturbed during inflammatory nasal disease.

George Catlin, a famous American painter, who spent years living with the native north American Indians, found that the Indians did not sleep with an open mouth and he described the relationship between a patent nose and good sleep in his book "Shut your mouth and save your life" in 1832. Respiratory function during sleep is a dynamic process involving changes in respiratory drive, airway patency and in airway muscular tone during REM and non REM sleep which makes the relationship between nasal function and poor sleep complex and difficult to assess. Most studies addressing nasal patency in inflammatory airways disease have been performed in awake subjects sitting in the upright position. In reality the nasal mucosa is highly reactive and responds almost instantly to changes in temperature, humidity and a change in body position. In the evaluation of patients with sleep disturbances and allergic rhinitis several aspects of nasal anatomy and physiology thus have to be taken into account.

External nose: The external nose protrudes from the bone aperture and is mainly composed of cartilage, muscle and subcutaneous fat apart from the two nasal bones at the top. The inside of the nasal openings and the anterior part of the nose is covered with skin and thus unaffected by nasal inflammation. The isthmus, is the narrow opening on the inside of the nose corresponding to the insertion of the nasal wings (alae) and the naso labial crest on the outside. More than half of the airway resistance is under normal conditions located here. During inspiration, the nasal openings tends to collapse as the passage of air through the narrow isthmus area put a suction force on the airway walls, the so called Bernouille effect. Patients with narrow nasal openings and weak alae are more prone to alar collapse especially when it combines with other abnormalities such as a septal deviation, turbinate hypertrophy or inflammatory nasal disease. An activation of muscles in the anterior part of the nose help to counteract this tendency to collapse. When air is passed through the narrow isthmus with a high flow rate into the much larger nasal cavity where the flow rate is lower, the air flow becomes turbulent and disperses in a similar fashion to when water is expelled through a garden hose spray nozzle. Through this design the contact area between the air and the walls of the nasal cavity increases and enables the nose to effectively condition the inhaled air.

The nasal cavities: The contact surface between the inhaled air and the mucous membrane is further enhanced by the folded structures on the lateral wall of the nasal cavity called the turbinates. There are three sets of turbinates in each nasal cavity. Most of the nasal cavity is encased in the skull bone and from an anterior view it is pyramid shaped. The inferior turbinates protrude into the airway at the base of the pyramid and an increase in the swelling of the mucosa covering the inferior turbinate can thus effectively obstruct the main nasal air flow like a cork seals a bottle neck.

The nasal mucosa: The nasal respiratory mucosa replaces the skin starting at the head of the inferior turbinate and goes all the way to the nasopharynx. The nasal mucosa has major similarities with the respiratory mucosa of the bronchi and is today considered to be a linked functional organ with the lower respiratory tract which becomes evident in asthma and allergic inflammatory disease. The main difference is the presence of smooth muscle in the bronchi and the presence of sinusoids in the nose. Smooth muscle contraction can cause airway narrowing in the lungs which can be relieved with β-agonists, but these drugs have no effect in the nose. Nasal patency is mainly regulated by variation of blood content in the erectile capacitance vessels called the sinusoids located in the sub mucosa. The regulation of nasal patency in the sinusoids is mediated through a neurovascular mechanism with different triggers such as air temperature, posture and physical exercise (27). Blood can be shifted in and out of the sinusoids through a rich capillary network equipped with artery-venous shunts. Nasal patency is maintained by a continuous sympathetic tone that can be up or down regulated. Increased sympathic activity during physical exercise or addition of adrenergic agonists increase nasal patency while a decrease in sympathetic activity decrease nasal patency as in Horner´s syndrome. In a third of the population “the nasal cycle” causes an alternating congestion and decongestion of the two nasal cavities going from one side to the other, a few hours apart. Nasal patency can also be changed by the application of pressure to the body surface. Unilateral pressure to the axillary region in the sitting position results in nasal congestion on the ipsilateral side and decongestion on the contralateral side, mediated via pressure sensitive receptors in the skin (28). A change in body position from sitting to supine also changes nasal patency, which may be important in regulating nasal patency during sleep as will be discussed in detail further down.

Nasal function: Breathing through the nose conditions the inhaled air which increases in humidity and temperature. Particles are cleared and the immune system is activated against inhaled bacteria and viruses to protect the lungs. Nitric oxide from the nasal and sinus mucosa is added to the inhaled air which promotes the gas exchange in the lungs by enhancing the ventilator-perfusion ratio. During nasal exhalation humidity and energy is effectively recovered from the air compared to the oral route (29). Nasal function also includes the sense of smell and a loss of this function has a marked effect on both the ability to smell and taste. Nasal breathing is the preferred breathing route at rest for most people, but there is a shift to oral breathing at some point when developing nasal obstruction that varies individually. Oral breathing, apart from being less effective than the nose in air conditioning, also promotes airway collapse in oropharynx due to increased upper airway resistance (30).

Assessing nasal patency: Objective measurements of changes in nasal patency can be obtained either as alterations in nasal air flow and resistance or as changes in intranasal diameter and volume. Rhinomanometry, nasal peak flow and nasal spirometry are examples of methods that give a good perception of the overall nasal air flow resistance but are less reliable to predict specific changes in the mucosa. Acoustic rhinometry or rhinostereometry are preferred when studying the variations in the nasal cavity dimensions due to swelling and decongestion at specific sites in the nasal cavity. For instance it has been shown that the minimal cross sectional area at 4 cm from the nostril is where the nasal mucosa decongests the most (31). Acoustic rhinometry, introduced by Hilberg in the 1980`s is by far the most widely used of the 2 methods and is quick to perform (32). Audible sound is lead into the nasal cavity and reflected back to generate a description of nasal cross sectional areas and volumes at different levels. Attempts have been made to correlate intranasal dimensions in healthy subjects to the subjective sensation of nasal patency, age, gender, BMI and head circumference without success. When used to compare changes in the same individual before and after an intervention, acoustic rhinometry has, however, proven accurate with a high reproducibility (33). In a recent review, Eccles found evidence for the benefit of septoplasty in studies using acoustic rhinometry, before and after surgery (34).

3.2 Nasal function and sleep

Nasal obstruction is considered the most important factor that links nasal inflammation to poor sleep but other factors such as the presence of inflammatory mediators affecting the CNS may also contribute. Nasal obstruction due to nasal inflammation is probably multi factorial including altered neurovascular control of the sinusoids, formation of sub mucous edema, secretion of excessive nasal secretions and cicardian changes following the serum cortisol cycle with a peak of nasal congestion in the morning. How these factors interact in nasal obstruction and how it affects sleep still remains unclear. This was recently reviewed by Craig and in summary, most studies showing a relationship between allergic rhinitis and poor sleep have focused on symptoms of nasal congestion rather than objective measurements of nasal patency during sleep (21). In a large north European multicentre study study we also found rhinitis to be an independent risk factor for sleep disturbances in asthma specifically in subjects reporting nasal symptoms every day (35). Studies looking at objective measures of nasal function are rare but Lavie et al found a an increased number of micro arousals during sleep in patients with allergic rhinitis during sleep (36)

When regarding nasal congestion as a cause to poor sleep, one has to consider several options. If the nasal congestion is severe enough it leads to a shift into oral breathing and thus the effect on sleep is due to a change in breathing route. Effects of oral breathing on airway collapse and it´s relationship to OSAS goes beyond the focus of this chapter and will not be discussed here. If, however, nasal breathing is maintained during recumbent body position and sleep, it is necessary to consider both an increased airway resistance and changes to the neurovascular control of the nasal mucosa in relation to nasal inflammation. A relationship between nasal obstruction and sleep disordered breathing has been observed mainly on subjects with oro pharyngeal narrowing in the awake situation and not in all patients with nasal obstruction, underlining that nasal obstruction is a co-factor affecting sleep in a complex way (37). With regard to the neurovascular regulation of the nasal mucosa, interesting data have emerged recently. Objective measurements of nasal patency during sleep are difficult to obtain without interfering with the sleep pattern. Lebowitz has described a study on 10 subjects doing consecutive acoustic rhinometry measurements during sleep while monitoring sleep stage. The results showed that nasal patency varies with sleep stage exhibiting a marked congestion during REM-sleep and decongestion during non-REM sleep (38). Variable nasal obstruction has been found to play a greater role in the pathophysiology of obstructive sleep apnea syndrome, than conditions associated with a fixed obstruction (39). In healthy subjects the nasal patency is typically reduced when going from sitting to supine body position measured with acoustic rhinometry (40). It has been suggested that this alteration of nasal patency supine is due to an increased hydrostatic pressure in the nasal vasculature supine and thus a passive mechanism (41). Ko measured heart rate variability as a measure of activity in the autonomic nervous system simultaneously with rhinomanometry between sitting and supine in 12 healthy subjects and found a significant correlation between decreased sympathetic activity supine followed by decreased nasal patency indicating an active regulation of nasal patency supine (42). In studies of patients with snoring and OSAS without rhinitis nasal geometry changes less or remain unchanged supine compared to healthy controls (43, 44). This could be related to an increased sympathic activity seen in this patient group (45). In fact an increased nasal obstruction or symptoms of nasal obstruction when lying down has been observed in patients with seasonal allergic rhinitis compared to controls, indicating an inflammatory up regulation of the neurovascular control of the nasal mucosa (46 47).

We recently found no response with acoustic rhinometry to a change between sitting and supine in 19 patients with asthma and allergic rhinitis at inclusion, but a normalized reaction (with significantly decreased nasal patency supine) after 6 weeks treatment with a nasal steroid compared to placebo (unpublished data). Disturbances in the neurovascular control of the nasal mucosa supine is thus present in allergic rhinitis along with nasal obstruction and could interfere with nasal function during sleep but this has to evaluated further.

4. Is there a definite relationship between nasal congestion and SDB?

The relationship between subjective and objective measures of nasal obstruction are often poor which can confound studies in this area. Nasal obstruction is an independent risk factor for OSAS (9) but this is not confirmed in all studies. In normal subjects occlusion of the nose during the night causes an increase in sleep apnoea and transient arousals (50) suggesting that nasal obstruction irrespective of cause is an important cause of OSAS. In AR there is a general relationship between the presence and degree of nasal obstruction and obstructive sleep apnoea (8,50,51). This has also been confirmed in population studies (17). Anatomical deformities such as nasal septal deviation, adenoidal hypertrophy, nasal polyps are associated with SDB. However there are also other important predisposing factors for OSAS such as obesity, craniofacial abnormalities and male sex.

4.1 Does reversal of nasal obstruction also reverse the sleep disorder?

Physical modalities of reversal of nasal obstruction include surgery to correct nasal septal deformity, removal of nasal polyps and adenoidectomy. The results of septoplasty in a randomised control trial (52) showed that only a subgroup (15%) benefited in terms of improved OSAS. This is consistent with other studies which often show improvements in some indices eg less sleepiness, better QOL but no changes in the apnoea-hypopnoea index (53). This suggests that OSAS is multifactorial and alleviation of nasal obstruction is only a partial solution. Tonsillectomy and adenoidectomy in children with OSAS can result in complete resolution of symptoms but results are variable between studies with success rates of 27-87% reported (54, 55).

The use of nasal dilators has been examined in 5 studies and has provided equivocal results. Breathe Rite nasal strips: these increase PNIF by a mean of 26L/min and also significantly improve the respiratory index (56)

4.2 Medical treatment for nasal congestion as treatment for SDB

Antihistamines (oral or topical) have less effect on nasal congestion than INCS or decongestants but have been shown to be helpful in improving sleep in some studies (57)

Oral decongestants do reduce nasal congestion but this is not accompanied by improvements in sleep quality probably due to the side effects of pseudoephedrine (58).

Topical decongestants also reduce nasal obstruction and improve sleep but are never recommended for long term use due to the risk of developing rhinitis medicamentosa (59)

Leukotriene receptor antagonists are an effective treatment for SAR providing improvements in nasal congestion and also some improvements in sleep impairment (60).

The first line of treatment when treating nasal obstruction in allergic rhinitis with or without concomitant asthma according to the evidence based guidelines Allergic rhinitis and its impact on asthma (ARIA) is intranasal steroids (48). The evidence is 1A for alleviating nasal congestion but nasal steroids also reduce other symptoms of nasal inflammation such as itching, sneezing and secretion along with a reduction of ocular symptoms (49). This is accompanied by improved QOL. In allergic rhinitis patients treated with nasal steroids improved significantly in self reported quality of sleep but not in objective sleep measured with polysomnography and actigraphy (19,24).

5. Results of current research

We recently conducted a study utilising objective measures of nasal patency (PNIF, acoustic rhinometry) and sleep parameters (actigraphy) in subjects with mild asthma and PAR. The effect of INCS was also determined.

Nineteen patients with asthma and allergic rhinitis were assessed before and after 6 weeks treatment with an intranasal steroid spray (fluticasone propionate) versus 6 weeks of placebo nasal spray in a double blind cross over design (unpublished data). Nasal patency was measured with acoustic rhinometry sitting and supine and objective quality of sleep was measured with actigraphy. Actigraphy measures limb movements during sleep and has been validated against polysomnography. While actigraphy failed to show any improvement in sleep quality after nasal steroid treatment, there was a significant improvement in rhinitis specific health related quality of life measured with the rhinitis quality of life questionnaire (RQLQ). More importantly we found no change in nasal patency between sitting and supine at baseline, indicating an impaired neurovascular control. After 6 weeks treatment with a nasal steroid the nasal reactivity between sitting and supine returned to normal, showing a significant decrease supine compared to sitting. According to ARIA the evidence shows that even though oral antihistamines and leukotriene antagonists have an effect on several symptoms of allergic rhinitis, nasal steroids are the most effective in treating nasal congestion. Our data suggest that nasal steroids also restore neurovascular control in the nasal mucosa, a mechanism that is involved in the adaptation of nasal patency between sitting and supine and in the variation of nasal congestion during sleep. Larger studies are still needed to establish how neurovascular control is affected during wakefulness and during sleep and how nasal obstruction and impaired nasal function interact in patients with allergic rhinitis.

6. Summary

Nasal inflammation in allergic rhinitis adversely affects sleep. Nasal congestion is believed to be one of the more important factors based on self reported data and a limited number of studies evaluating nasal function before and after anti inflammatory treatment. Neurovascular dysfunction in the regulation of nasal patency and circulating inflammatory mediators may also contribute to disturbed sleep along with other rhinitis symptoms such as itching and sneezing. Nasal steroids are effective in treating allergic rhinitis and contribute to reducing symptoms of poor sleep. The causes of SDB in Ar are likely to be multifactorial and include a newly named entity RDS. The specific mechanisms behind allergic rhinitis and poor sleep warrant further examination.

7. References

[1] Salib RJ, et al Allergic rhinitis: past,present and future. Clin Otolaryngol 2003;28:291-303

[2] Lunn M, Craig T Rhinitis and Sleep. Sleep Medicine Reviews 2011; xxxx:1-7

[3] The Economic Impact of Allergic Disease in Australia: not to be sneezed at. Report by Access Economics for ASCIA 2007. Available on the ASCIA website: www.allergy.org.au

[4] Blaiss M et al A study to determine the impact of rhinitis on sufferers' sleep and daily routine. JACI 2005;115:S197

[5] Meltzer EO et al Burden of allergic rhinitis: results from the Paediatric Allergies in America survey. JACI 2009;124:S124

[6] Sutherland ER Nocturnal Asthma Journal of Allergy and Clinical Immunology; 2005:116:1179-1186

[7] Stull DE et al Relationship of nasal congestion with sleep, mood and productivity. Curr Med Res Opinion 2007;23:811-819

[8] Santos CB et al Allergic rhinitis and its effect on sleep, fatigue, and daytime somnolence Ann All Asthma Immunol 2006;97:579-586

[9] Staevska MT et al Rhinitis and sleep apnoea. 2004 Curr All Asthma Rep 4:193-199

[10] Meltzer EO 2 et al Sleep, quality of life and productivity impact of nasal symptoms in the United States: findings from the Burden of Rhinitis in America Survey. Allergy Asthma Proc 2009;30: 244-254

[11] Gupta N et al Allergic rhinitis and Inner-City Children – is there a relationship to sleep disordered breathing? JACI 2007 abstract 606.

[12] Jauregui I et al Allergic rhinitis and school performance J Invest Allergology & Clin Immunol 2009;19S:32-39

[13] Engel-Yeger B et al Differences in leisure activities between children with allergic rhinitis and healthy peers. Int J of Ped Otorhinolaryngology 2010;74:1415-1418

[14] Sogut A et al Prevalence of habitual snoring and symptoms of sleep disordered breathing in adolescents. Int J of Ped Otorhinolaryngology 2009;73:1769-1773.

[15] Storms W et al The Nasal Allergy Survey Assessing limitations (NASL) 2010 survey: Allergic rhinitis associated with substantial sleep disturbances. JACI 2011;127:abstract 836.

[16] Leger D et al Allergic rhinitis and its consequences on quality of sleep. An unexplored area Arch Int Med 2006;166:1744-1748.

[17] Young T et al Chronic nasal congestion at night is a risk factor for snoring in a population-based cohort study. Arch Int Med 2001; 161: 1514-1519.

[18] Bender BG and Leung DYM Sleep disorders in patients with asthma, atopic dermatitis and allergic rhinitis. JACI 2005; 116:1200-1201

[19] Rimmer J et al Sleep disturbance in persistent allergic rhinitis measured using actigraphy. Ann Allergy Asthma and Immunol. 2009;103:190-194

[20] Yuksel H et al Sleep actigraphy evidence of improved sleep after treatment of allergic rhinitis.Ann Allergy Asthma and Immunol 2009; 103: 290-294

[21] Craig T, Sherkat A, Safaee S. Congestion and sleep impairment in allergic rhinitis. 2010 Curr Allergy Asthma Rep 10:113-121

[22] Bousquet J et al World Health Organisation: GA(2)LEN;Allergen. Allergic rhinitis and its impact on asthma. (ARIA) 2008 update. Allergy 2008; 63(suppl 86) 8-160.

[23] Smolensky MH et al Sleep disorders, medical conditions, and road accident risk 2011 Accident Analysis and Prevention 43: 533-548

[24] Meltzer EO et at Intranasal mometasone furoate therapy for allergic rhinitis symptoms and rhinitis-disturbed sleep. Ann All Asthma Immunol 2010;105:65-74

[25] National Sleep Foundation: Sleep In America Poll 2008: www.sleepfoundation.org

[26] Stuck BA et al Changes in daytime sleepiness, quality of life, and objective sleep patterns in seasonal allergic rhinitis: A controlled clinical trial. J or Allergy and Clin Immunol:2004: 113:663-8.

[27] Baraniuk J Neural Regulation of Mucosal Function. 2008 Pulm Pharmacol Ther 21(3): 442–448.

[28] Davies AM, Eccles R Reciprocal changes in nasal resistance to air flow caused by pressure applied to the axilla. 1985 Acta Otolaryngol 99:154–159

[29] Svensson S, Hellgren J. PH in Nasal Exhaled Breath Condensate in healthy adults. 2007 Rhinology 45:214-217.

[30] Fitzpatric M, McLean H, Urton A, Tan A, O´Donnell D, Driver H. Effect of nasal and oral breathing route on upper airway resistance during sleep. 2003 Eur Respir J 22:827-832

[31] Grymer LF, Hilberg O, Acoustic rhinometry; values from adults with subjective normal nasal patency. 1991 Rhinology 29(1):35-47.

[32] Hilberg O.Objective measurement of nasal airway dimensions using acoustic rhinometry:methodological and clinical aspects. 2002 Allergy 57 Suppl 70:5-39

[33] Clement PA, Gordts F Standardisation Committee on Objective Assessment of the Nasal Airway, IRS, and ERS. Consensus report on acoustic rhinometry and rhinomanometry. 2005 Rhinology Sep 43(3):169-179
[34] Moore M, Eccles R. Objective evidence for the efficacy of surgical management of the deviated septum as treatment for chronic nasal obstruction: a systematic review. 2011 Clin Otolaryngol 36:106-113
[35] Hellgren J, Omenaas E, Gíslason T, Jögi R, Franklin K, Lindberg E, Janson C, Torén K. Perennial non-infectious rhinitis-an independent risk factor for sleep disturbances in asthma. 2007 Respir Med. May;101(5):1015-20. Epub 2006 Oct 16.
[36] Lavie P, Gertner R, Zomer J, Podoshin L. Breathing disorders in sleep associated with microarousals in patients with allergic rhinitis. 1981 Acta Otolaryngol 92:529–33.
[37] Pevernagie D, De Meyer M, Claeys S. Sleep breathing and the nose. 2005 Sleep Medicine Reviews 9:437-451
[38] Luc G.T. Morris, MD, Omar Burschtin, MD, Jennifer Setlur, MD,Claire C. Bommelje, MD, Kelvin C. Lee, MD, Joseph B. Jacobs, MD, and Richard A. Lebowitz, MD REM-associated nasal obstruction: A study with acoustic rhinometry during sleep 2008 Otolaryngology–Head and Neck Surgery 139, 619-623
[39] McNicholas WT The nose and OSA: variable nasal obstruction may be more important in pathophysiology than fixed obstruction. 2008 Eur Respir J 32:3-8
[40] Devyani Lal, M.D., Melissa L. Gorges, B.S., Girapong Ungkhara, M.D., Patrick M. Reidy, M.D.,and Jacquelynne P. Corey, M.D. Physiological change in nasal patency in response to changes in posture, temperature, and humidity measured by acoustic rhinometry. 2006 Am J Rhinol 20, 456–462.
[41] Rundcrantz H Postural variations of nasal patency. 1969 Acta Otolaryngol 68:435–443
[42] Ko JH, Kuo TB, Lee GS Effect of postural change on nasal airway and autonomic nervous system established by rhinomanometry and heart rate variability analysis. 2008 Am J Rhinol 22:159-165
[43] Virkkula P, Maasilta P, Hytönen M, Salmi T, Malmberg H Nasal obstruction and sleep-disordered breathing: the effect of supine body position on nasal measurements in snorers. 2003 ActaOtolaryngol 123:648–654
[44] Hellgren J, Yee BJ, Dungan G, Grunstein RR. Altered positional regulation of nasal patency in patients with obstructive sleep apnoea syndrome. 2009 Eur Arch Otorhinolaryngol. Jan;266(1):83-7. Epub 2008 May 14
[45] Phillips CL, Yang Q, Williams A, Roth M, Yee BJ, Hedner JA, Berend N, Grunstein RR The effect of short-term withdrawal from continuous positive airway pressure therapy on sympathic activity and markers of vascular inflammation in subjects with obstructive sleep apnoea. 2007 J Sleep Res 16:217–225
[46] Hasegawa M, Saito Y Postural variations in nasal resistance and symptomatology in allergic rhinitis. 1979 Acta Otolaryngol. 88(3-4):268-72.
[47] Roithmann R, Demenghi P, Faggiano R, Cury A Effects of posture change on nasal patency. 2005 Rev Bras Otorrinolaringol 4:478–484
[48] Brozek JL, Bousquet J, Baena-Cagnani CE, Bonini S, Canonica GW, Casale TB, van Wijk RG, Ohta K, Zuberbier T, Schünemann HJ Allergy and Asthma European Network; Grading of Recommendations Assessment, Development and Evaluation Working Group. Allergic Rhinitis and its Impact on Asthma (ARIA) guidelines: 2010 revision. J Allergy Clin Immunol Sep;126(3):466-760

[49] Craig T, Hanks CD, Fisher L. How do topical nasal corticosteroids improve sleep and daytime somnolence in allergic rhinitis? 2005 J Allergy Clin Immunol 116:1264-1266
[50] Canova CR et al Increased prevalence of perennial allergic rhinitis in patients with obstructive sleep apnoea. Respiration 2004; 71: 138-141.
[51] Nathan RA et al Objective monitoring of nasal patency and nasal physiology in rhinitis. JACI 2005; 115: S442-59
[52] Koutsourelakis I et al Randomised trial of nasal surgery for fixed nasal obstruction in OSA. Eur Resp J 2008;32:110-117.
[53] Roscow DE et al Is nasal surgery an effective treatment for obstructive sleep apnoea? The Laryngoscope 2010;120:1496-1497.
[54] Ye J et al Outcome of adenotonsillectomy for OSAS in children. Ann Otol Rhinol & Laryngol 2010;119:506-513.
[55] Bhattacharjee R et al Adenotonsillectomy outcomes in the treatment of OSA in children: a multicentre retrospective study. Am J Resp and Crit Care Med 2010;182:676-683.
[56] Rupp MR et al Breathe Rite Strips improve Respiratory index in patients with rhinitis and OSA. JACI 2006;abstract 291
[57] Murray JJ et al Comprehensive evaluation of cetirizine in the management of seasonal allergic rhinitis: impact on symptoms, quality of life, productivity and activity impairment. All Asthma Proc 2002;23:391-398.
[58] Sherkat AA et al The role of pseudoephedrine on daytime sleepiness in patients suffering from perennial allergic rhinitis. Ann Allergy Asthma Immunol 2011;106:97-102
[59] McLean HA et al Effect of treating severe nasal obstruction on the severity of obstructive sleep apnoea. Eur Resp J 2005; 25: 521-527.
[60] Rodrigo GJ, Yanez A. The role of antileukotriene theray in seasonal allergic rhinitis: A systemic review of randomised trials. Ann Allergy Asthma Immunol. 2006;96:779-786.

8

Allergic Rhinitis and Sports

Silva Diana, Moreira André and Delgado Luís
Department of Immunology, Faculty of Medicine, University of Porto,
Immunoallergology, Hospital São João, Porto
Portugal

1. Introduction

Rhinitis is an inflammation of the mucosal lining of the nose and is characterized by one or more of the following symptoms: nasal congestion, anterior and posterior rhinorrhea, sneezing, and itching (Bousquet, Khaltaev et al. 2008; Wallace, Dykewicz et al. 2008). It can be associated with eye symptoms (rhinoconjuntivitis) and ear or throat complains (Bousquet, Khaltaev et al. 2008). Rhinitis can be classified etiologically in two types: Allergic Rhinitis (AR) and Nonallergic Rhinitis (Table1) (Bousquet, Khaltaev et al. 2008; Wallace, Dykewicz et al. 2008).

The most common type is AR, and its prevalence has increased over the last decades (Bousquet, Khaltaev et al. 2008). Associated risk factors, such as atopy, family history of allergy, and exposure to allergens and pollution, might explain this fact (Bousquet, Khaltaev et al. 2008; Scadding, Durham et al. 2008). AR is a multifactorial disease influenced by genetic and environmental interaction (Davila, Mullol et al. 2009). Despite that 30-50% of rhinitis patients have non-allergic triggers, 44 to 87% might have a combination of allergic and non-allergic rhinitis mechanism (Dykewicz and Hamilos 2010).

Allergic inflammation is the basic mechanism of this disease, and classically is considered to result from an IgE mediated reaction (Bousquet, Khaltaev et al. 2008). Allergic response can be biphasic, mediated by an early and a late phase (Durham 1998). Early phase response, occurs within the first 0-60 min following allergen exposure, and is mediated by mast cell degranulation and mediator release (Durham 1998; Bousquet, Khaltaev et al. 2008; Scadding, Durham et al. 2008). The late phase reaction involves inflammation, mediated by recruitment of several inflammatory cells, specifically Th2 mediated cell response (Durham 1998). Clinically, AR appears as nasal sneezing, itching of the nose, rhinorrhoea and nasal blockage, in the first minutes after allergen contact. Symptoms like chronic obstruction, hyposmia, post-nasal mucous discharge and nasal hyper-reactivity occur in the late-phase response (Scadding, Durham et al. 2008; Lim and Leong 2010).

World Health Organization (WHO) through the working group Allergic Rhinitis Impact on Asthma (ARIA), changed the classification from time of exposure point of view (*seasonal, perennial and occupational*) to a symptomatic definition (*intermittent allergic rhinitis and persistent allergic rhinitis*) and severity characterization *(mild or moderate-severe).* The seasonal and perennial rhinitis classification is still useful for diagnosis and immunotherapy treatment decision and can be used alongside with ARIA classification (Bousquet, Khaltaev et al. 2008).

I- Allergic rhinitis
II- Nonallergic rhinitis
A.Vasomotor rhinitis (triggered by irritant, cold air, exercise, undeterminated trigger)
B. Gustatory rhinitis
C. Infectious rhinitis
III- Occupational rhinitis
A. IgE mediated (protein or chemical allergens)
B. Uncertain immune mechanism (chemical respiratory sensitizers)
C. Work agravated rhinitis
IV- Rhinitis syndromes
A. Hormonal induced (pregnancy or menstrual cicle induced)
B. Drug induced
1. Rhinitis *medicamentosa*
2. Nonsteroidal anti-inflammatory drugs
3. Oral contraceptives
4. Antihypertensive and cardiovascular agents
C. Atrophic rhinitis
D. Rhinitis associated with inflammatory-immunologic disorders
1. Granulomatous infection
2. Wegener granulomatous
3. Sarcoidosis
4. Midline granuloma
5. Churgh-Strauss syndrome
6. Relapsing polychondritis
7. Amyloidosis

Table 1. Rhinitis classification (adapted from *Dykewicz and Hamilos 2010*)

The most frequent allergic triggers are inhalant allergens, namely mites, pollens, animals and fungi. According to different triggers they can cause perennial or seasonal symptoms. Pre-existing rhinitis can be aggravated by work-place irritants like smoke, cold air and pollutants (Scadding, Durham et al. 2008).

Rhinitis has debilitating consequences, significantly interfering with patients quality of life and activity, namely in sports practice (Katelaris, Carrozzi et al. 2003). It has negative impact on cognitive functions, school performance, sleep, quality of life and even in behaviour, which can significantly impair athletics performance (Katelaris, Carrozzi et al. 2003). This is particularly important, as a higher prevalence of rhinitis has been reported in athletes than general population (Delgado, Moreira et al. 2006). Excluding exercise-induced rhinitis, idiopathic rhinitis and nasal symptoms related to physical, cold air, and chemical contact factors, allergic rhinitis can account for prevalences up to 30% in an athlete population. This chapter deals with allergic rhinitis in sports.

2. Allergic rhinitis in athletes

Exercise induces modulation in innate and adaptive immune system, dependent on host defence, activity level and disease susceptibility (Walsh, Gleeson et al. 2011). This might explain why in some cases there seems to be a possible susceptibility of elite athletes to infection, namely in the upper respiratory tract infection (Moreira 2009; Dijkstra and

Robson-Ansley 2011). In a recent position statement regarding immune function and exercise, *Walsh and colleagues* (Walsh, Gleeson et al. 2011) proposed that in young healthy subjects, who already possess excellent immune responses, an increase in physical activity might not be beneficial to the immune system response, and might induce immune-disease susceptibility, like auto-immune disease or allergy. In fact, self-reported episodes of infection may not be related with infection *per se*, but with allergy-related symptoms (Dijkstra and Robson-Ansley 2011). On other side, the positive effects of exercise training on immune function are more frequently seen when immune function is sub-optimal like in elderly people (Walsh, Gleeson et al. 2011).

There is also immunological data that exercise training can lead to a polarization of T-helper lymphocytes toward the Th2 phenotype, which is known to mediate allergic response (Dijkstra and Robson-Ansley 2011). Athletes and people who regularly exercise in the outdoor urban environment are a specific population in risk for allergic rhinitis (Delgado, Moreira et al. 2006). There is evidence indicating an increased incidence of exercise-induce bronchospasm and atopy in highly trained athletes compared with nonathletic controls (Carlsen, Anderson et al. 2008).

2.1 Nasal physiology and pathophysiology

The upper airways, that include nasal cavity and its tissues, lie in a bony structure that, unlike the lower airways structure, cannot change shape (Dahl and Mygind 1998). Upper airways comprise an epithelium with a basement membrane and a submucosal layer, which is full of venous sinusoids (Dahl and Mygind 1998). These vessels and mucosa glands are responsible for filtration, humidification and warming of inhaled air before it reaches the lower respiratory tract. They are regulated by autonomic nervous system reflexes (Delgado, Moreira et al. 2006) and swelling of the venous sinusoids can lead to upper airway obstruction (Dahl and Mygind 1998). Activation of local nerve reflexes causes sneezing, watery discharge and vasodilation, symptoms associated with rhinitis(Dahl and Mygind 1998).

During exercise, autonomic reflexes improve nasal efficiency (Bonini, Bonini et al. 2006). In dynamic exercise training due to an increase of nasal sympathetic activity, venous sinusoids constrict. The same does not happen with isometric exercise types (Dahl and Mygind 1998; Bonini, Bonini et al. 2006). A watery discharge can also be produced, because cold air induces glandular hyper secretion (Dahl and Mygind 1998; Bonini, Bonini et al. 2006).

During training athletes are repeatedly exposed to several risk factors (allergens, cold air and pollutants) increasing rhinitis symptoms in susceptible individuals (Delgado, Moreira et al. 2006). Some experience improvement with exercise, mediated by nasal sympathetic tone, others may have their symptoms worsen (Valero, Serrano et al. 2005). In fact, weather conditions, like cold or dry air, inhalation of irritants in outdoor exercise exposure can explain the worsening symptoms in some athletes (Schwartz, Delgado et al. 2008). In swimmers chlorine inhalation (an irritant) induces nasal congestion in a more pronounced way in subjects with allergic rhinitis than in nonrhinitic. Some authors explained this fact by nasal mucosa damage mediated by chlorinated products, which could facilitate the penetration of aeroallergens increasing the risk of allergic manifestation (Shusterman, Murphy et al. 1998; Shusterman, Balmes et al. 2003; Shusterman, Murphy et al. 2003). This hypothesis was not supported by a more recent study showing that swimmers had worse rhinitis symptoms, but independently of their atopic status (Alves, Martins et al. 2010).

2.2 Epidemiology

Allergic rhinitis affects 10-20% of general population, and in a higher percentage elite competitive athletes (Katelaris, Carrozzi et al. 2006; Bousquet, Khaltaev et al. 2008). A study in 291 German athletes found a significative increased prevalence of hay fever (25% versus 17% in general population), with the highest prevalence in endurance athletes (Thomas, Wolfarth et al. 2010). These data are concordant with previous data, namely a Canadian study of 698 athletes who practiced different sports under antagonist conditions (dry, cold, humid or mixed air conditions) - a 21% prevalence of allergic rhinitis was found in all participants, except in subjects training in dry air conditions (17%) (Langdeau, Turcotte et al. 2004). In 162 Finish swimmers, 29% had a positive skin test reaction to pollen associated with rhinoconjunctivitis symptoms during spring or summer (Helenius and Haahtela 2000). During the 1990`s, several epidemiological studies of athletes in different sports were made using larger samples. Two studies with 2060 (Helbling, Jenoure et al. 1990) and 1530 Swiss athletes (Kaelin and Brandli 1993) showed a prevalence of rhinoconjunctivitis of respectively 16,8 and 19,7%. In several studies published in the last two decades a prevalence range between 13.3-48.6% was found (Delgado, Moreira et al. 2006) Table 2.

Reference	Design and methods	Year of study, subjects (n)	Rhinitis/SARC* Prevalence (%)
Fitch KD, J Allergy Clin Immunol 1984;73:72-7	Retrospective; medical records analysis	1976, Australian Olympics (185)	8.6
		1980, Australian Olympics (106)	7.5
Helbling A, Schweiz Med Wochenschr 1990;120(7):231-6	Cross-sectional; questionnaire	1986, Swiss athletes (2,060)	16.8*
Kaelin M, Schweiz Med Wochenschr 1993; 123(5): 174-82	Cross-sectional; questionnaire	1990, Swiss athletes (1530)	19.7%*
Potts J, Sports Med 1996; 21:256–261	Cross-sectional; questionnaire	1995, Canadian swimmers (738)	19.0*
Helenius I, J Allergy Clin Immunol 1998; 101(5):646-52	Cross-sectional; skin prick tests with medical diagnosis	1996, Finnish summer athletes (162)	29.6*
Weiler J, J Allergy Clin Immunol 1998; 102:722-6	Cross-sectional, questionnaire (USOC-MHQ)	1996, US summer Olympics (699)	16.9
Weiler J, J Allergy Clin Immunol 2000; 106:267-1	Cross-sectional, questionnaire (USOC-MHQ)	1998, US winter Olympics (699)	13.3
Katelaris CH, J Allergy Clin Immunol 2000; 106:260-6	Cross-sectional; skin prick tests with medical diagnosis	1997/8, Australian summer Olympics (214)	41.0/29.0*
Katelaris CH, Clin J Sport Med 2006; 16(5):401-5	Cross-sectional; skin prick tests with medical diagnosis	1999, Australian Olympics/Paralympics (977)	37.0/24.0*

Lapucci G, J Allergy Clin Immunol 2003; 111:S142	Cross-sectional; skin prick tests with medical diagnosis	2000, Italian summer Olympics (265)	25.3*
Bonadonna P, Am J Rhinol. 2001; 15(5):297-301.	Cross-sectional, questionnaire on cold-induced rhinitis	2001, Italian skiers (144)	48.6
Alaranta A, Med Sci Sports Exerc 2005 ; 37, 5, 707–11	Cross-sectional; self reported medical diagnosis	2002, Finnish Olympic athletes (446);	26.5
		Subgroup of endurance athletes (108)	36.1
Randolph C. Med Sci Sport Exerc 2006:2053–7	Cross-sectional; questionnaire (USOC-MHQ)	2003/4, US recreational runners (484)	34.7
Moreira A. Respir Med 2007;101(6):1123–31	Cross-sectional; self reported medical diagnosis	2003, Finnish marathon runners (141)	17.3
Bonini M, Allergy 2007: 62: 1166-70	Cross-sectional; medical diagnosis	2006, Italian preOlympics (98)	34.7
Macucci F, J Sports Med Phys Fitness. 2007 ; 47(3):351-5	Cross-sectional; medical diagnosis	2006, Italian young athletes (352)	22.2
Salonen RO, Environ Int. 2008; 34(1):51-7	Cross-sectional; self reported medical diagnosis	2007, Finnish young hockey players (793)	18.3
Thomas S; Allergy Asthma Clin Immunol. 2010 Nov 30;6(1):31.	Cross-sectional; questionnaire	2008, German athletes candidates for Summer Olympic Games (291)	25*

Table 2. Prevalence (%) of rhinitis or seasonal allergic rhinoconjunctivitis (SARC) in athletes adapted and updated from *Schwartz, Delgado et al. 2008*..

Allergic rhinitis and asthma frequently co-exist and it seems to be a higher prevalence of asthma in athletes than in the general population (Thomas, Wolfarth et al. 2010). The prevalence of asthma in both the Summer and Winter Olympic athletes has been progressively increasing over recent years (Li, Lu et al. 2008). The prevalence of asthma reported in elite athletes ranged between 3.7-22.8% depending on athletes population (Bonini, Bonini et al. 2006). An evidence-based review of Joint Task Force of the European Respiratory Society (ERS) and the European Academy of Allergy and Clinical Immunology (EAACI) in cooperation with GA2LEN concluded that top athletes are at increased risk of asthma and bronchial hyperactivity, especially with endurance sports practice (Carlsen, Anderson et al. 2008).
The allergic response causes nasal and conjunctival congestion, tearing, breathing difficulties, pruritus, fatigue, and mood changes, which might affect athletic performance (Komarow and Postolache 2005). *Kateralis* showed over spring season a negative effect of allergic rhinoconjuntivitis on performance scores (ability to train and compete). Also a resolution of those symptoms, namely eye symptoms, and improvement on quality of life and performance scores, was seen after treatment with intranasal corticosteroids (Katelaris, Carrozzi et al. 2002).

2.3 Risk factors and exposure

During exercise ventilation increases in power athletes for a short period of time and for longer periods in resistance athletes (Bonini, Bonini et al. 2006). Most of this exercise is practiced in outdoor environments; therefore, athletes are strongly and repeatedly exposed to large amounts of aeroallergens and pollutants, including smoke. This contact in training or in competition periods may increase the likelihood of exercise-induced respiratory symptoms (Delgado, Moreira et al. 2006). The climate conditions, namely the inhaled air temperature and humidity also affect these patients. In swimmers it is also important to consider the contact with chlorine derivatives (Bonini, Bonini et al. 2006; Alves, Martins et al. 2010).

2.3.1 Allergens

Athletes involved in outdoor sports frequently exercise during or just after peak allergen seasons. In fact, major sports events frequently occur at the end of spring and beginning of the summer, and in urban settings (Delgado, Moreira et al. 2006). The Sydney Olympic Games were the second games in the last century to be held in springtime (Katelaris, Carrozzi et al. 2006). Kateralis monitored the pollen levels at Olympic Sydney facilities, and performed a study on Australian elite athletes in order to ascertain the prevalence of allergic conjunctivitis, sensitization and quality of life effect. They found that 41% had allergic rhinoconjunctivitis and, in those with pollen allergy (29%), a significant increase in nasal symptoms with a decreased quality of life score were found (Katelaris, Carrozzi et al. 2000). Aquatic sports athletes were more prone to be symptomatic.

Aerobiological records of pollens are frequently used to monitor the pollen levels and it is important for athletes to prepare themselves, particularly if they are symptomatic to some allergen. An example was the set up of an aerobiological network for the Athens summer Olympic Games (Gioulekas, Damialis et al. 2003).

Indoor allergens, namely mites, are not usually studied, due to the decreased frequency of contact and the specific association of more severe symptoms with endurance outdoor exercise. However, in some more indoor sports persistent rhinitis symptoms can occur and it may be relevant to control this environmental exposure in order to achieve the highest performance levels.

2.3.2 Air pollution

Urban type pollution, automobile and factory exhausts, tobacco smoking and occupational exposures are of great concern globally. Pollutants seem to interact with allergens in inducing sensitization and triggering symptoms in allergic patients (Bonini, Bonini et al. 2006). Increased reactivity to irritants is a phenotypic characteristic of both allergic and non-allergic rhinitis (Bousquet, Khaltaev et al. 2008). There are several studies pointing to adverse effects of outdoor air pollution, caused by carbon monoxide, nitric oxide and ozone among others (Delgado, Moreira et al. 2006). The two agents that most frequently affect upper respiratory airways and rhinitis are: particulate matter, namely diesel exhaust particles (DEP), which result from incomplete combustion of fuels and lubricants (Bousquet, Khaltaev et al. 2008) and volatile organic compounds, whose secondary pollutant is ozone formed through sun-light dependent reaction of volatile compounds. Their peak production is from April to September in the Northern Hemisphere, and a large percentage (40%) is completely absorbed by nasal mucosa (Bousquet, Khaltaev et al. 2008). They enhance the

production of oxygen's derivatives, increasing the permeability of epithelial cells (Bonay and Aubier 2007). Ozone increases the late-phase response to nasal allergens, increasing the eosinophilic influx after exposure and, in nasal mucosa, the histamine containing and inflammatory cells are increased in number (Delgado, Moreira et al. 2006).
In several studies it has been shown that patients living in traffic congested areas have more severe rhinitis and conjunctivitis symptoms (D'Amato and Cecchi 2008). A recently published study in Beijing, using questionnaires in 31,829 individuals and monitoring PM10, SO2 and NO2 air levels, found a significant association between outpatient visits for allergic rhinitis and increasing air pollutant levels (Zhang, Wang et al. 2011). DEP have pro-allergic effects and, associated with pollen exposure, might induce an allergic breakthrough in atopic patients and increase allergic reactions in already symptomatic ones (Delgado, Moreira et al. 2006; Lubitz, Schober et al. 2010). This finding is particularly relevant in athletes who train or compete in outdoor urban environments. So, at the Olympic Games in China, besides allergen monitoring air quality was also monitored to certify air quality, in order athletes could perform their sports safely (Li, Lu et al. 2008). In fact, elite athletes practice sport around the world under different conditions and should be informed to what environment exposure they will be submitted, to adapt themselves and have appropriate preventive measures, namely their allergic symptoms fully controlled.
Besides nasal symptoms, lower airway pathways can also be severely affected, with increasing bronchial hyperactivity and asthma (Bonay and Aubier 2007).
Tobacco smoke is not advised in all populations, and especially in sports practice. Despite this, some athletes smoke or are exposed to passive smoke. Nasal symptoms, rhinorrea and nasal obstruction can occur under tobacco exposure, but not always these are consistent with increased total and specific IgEs (Bousquet, Khaltaev et al. 2008).

2.3.3 Climate exposure

The exposure to different environmental conditions, that are specific to a particular sport, definitely contribute to rhinitis symptoms. Rhinorhea and nasal congestion after exposure to cold air, known as "skier´s nose", can occur in normal individuals, through parasympathetic reflex. This mechanism of rhinitis is not associated with a particular allergic aetiology. In fact, cold dry air is frequently used for determining the presence and degree of nasal hyperreactivity in nonallergic non-infectious perennial rhinitis (Braat, Mulder et al. 1998). In high performance athletes, namely skiers, long distance runners and swimmers with long term exposure to cold, the repeated cooling and drying of mucosa results in an inflammatory infiltration of the airway mucosa, and these effects are reversed after stopping the high performance exercise (Koskela 2007).
In runners, an initial decongestion of mucosa occurs and it is maintained nearly 30 minutes after stopping exercise. This reduction of nasal resistance can lead to mucosa dehydration and a rebound increase in nasal secretion to compensate it. This "runner`s nose" is also integrated in differential diagnosis of allergic rhinitis (Bonini, Bonini et al. 2006). Swimmers are also a specific population of athletes. Their long term and high exposure to chlorine derivatives during regular trainings and competition at increased ventilation can induce mucosal inflammation which facilitate the responsiveness to airborne allergens and induces bronchial hyper responsiveness. *Kateralis* found confirming data in a group of swimmers that were more likely to have rhinitis symptoms and allergic sensitization than those active

in other sports (Katelaris, Carrozzi et al. 2000). In a recent study evaluating the nasal response to exercise in competitive swimmers compared with runners, although swimmers experienced worsening of nasal function after training, these data were independent of the atopic status of the athlete (Alves, Martins et al. 2010), which imposes the question of the swimmers environment as a risk factor for rhinitis.

2.3.4 Infections

Upper respiratory infections, namely acute viral rhinosinusitis, are extremely common in general population. It seems that athletes have an increased incidence, although a comprehensive explanation of this phenomenon was not yet found (Moreira 2009). A recent position statement questions the infectious aetiology of these respiratory symptoms, as few of them had no infectious agent identified. So these symptoms might be due only to an increased inflammation state (Walsh, Gleeson et al. 2011).

2.4 Effects of allergic rhinitis on exercise performance

Allergic rhinoconjunctivitis may be associated with a significant morbidity and a negative impact on life quality. In the general population, cognitive functions, school performance, sleep and even behavioural effects were described, namely in children with attention-deficit hyperreactivity disorders (Borres 2009). In a questionnaire of quality of life performed at spring-time, *Kateralis* showed poorer results in the allergic group, although the sample number was small (18 athletes) (Katelaris, Carrozzi et al. 2003). In another study with a larger sample, 145 athletes with allergic rhinitis who agreed to be treated, had a significant improvement of their quality of life scores under budesonide therapy (Katelaris, Carrozzi et al. 2002). Until now it was not possible to confirm the association of poorly treated rhinitis and a bad exercise performance (Dijkstra and Robson-Ansley 2011). It seems probable that altered airflow dynamics and ventilation caused by allergic rhinitis and nasal obstruction can potentially have a negative effect, mainly in high-intensity activities (Dijkstra and Robson-Ansley 2011). Any factors affecting sleep, decreasing the ability to concentrate or reducing physical fitness, have an easy understandable impact on sports performance. So, despite a direct association has not been proven yet, an indirect one is easily extrapolated (Dijkstra and Robson-Ansley 2011).

The cognitive impact (learning ability and memory) of rhinitis has been particularly studied in children and it seems that patients on anti-histaminic therapy have worse outcomes than patients on placebo (Borres 2009). In a recent study, children with allergic rhinitis on second generation anti-histaminic drugs had a greater treatment satisfaction (Ferrer, Morais-Almeida et al. 2010). Learning disability is a consequence of the frequent sleep disturbances, resulting in daytime sleepiness. Impaired sleep is secondary to nasal congestion which causes micro-arousal and irregular breathing, with snoring and apnea. A secondary effect of all this is school and work absenteeism and training capacity disability (Borres 2009). Correct diagnosis and management of allergic rhinitis can reduce the disease impact.

2.5 Diagnosis

Diagnosis of allergic rhinitis in athletes is based in the concordance of a suggestive history of allergic symptoms and physical examination, supported by diagnostic tests. (Bousquet, Khaltaev et al. 2008; Scadding, Hellings et al. 2011).

2.5.1 History and physical examination

A thorough allergic history remains the best diagnostic tool available (Wallace, Dykewicz et al. 2008; Scadding, Hellings et al. 2011). It is essential for an accurate diagnosis of rhinitis and for assessment of its severity and treatment response (Bousquet, Khaltaev et al. 2008). The patient, in this case the athlete, may present with a variety of symptoms and signs associated with allergic rhinitis such as sneezing, anterior rhinorrhoea and bilateral nasal obstruction (Dijkstra and Robson-Ansley 2011). Frequently, ocular symptoms are concomitant with tearing, burning and itching. Other symptoms include significant loss of smell (hyposmia or anosmia), snoring, post nasal drip or chronic cough, itching ears, nose and throat (Bousquet, Khaltaev et al. 2008; Dijkstra and Robson-Ansley 2011). In athletes, clinical presentation is frequently more subtle and might include poor-quality sleep, fatigue, reduced exercise performance and difficulty to recover after more demanding exercise sessions (Dijkstra and Robson-Ansley 2011). An effective evaluation should include symptoms characterization pattern, chronicity, seasonality and triggers of nasal and related symptoms, medications response, presence of coexisting conditions and the relation with training practice. It is also very important to include assessment of quality of life (Wallace, Dykewicz et al. 2008).

Physical examination of all organ systems potentially affected by allergies should be performed. Further attention should be given for upper respiratory tract system, namely nasal and oropharyngeal examination. Usually in patients with mild intermittent allergic rhinitis, a nasal examination is normal. In other patients, the nasal examination can show bluish-grey discoloration and edema or erythema of mucosa with clear watery rhinorrhoea (Scadding, Hellings et al. 2011). Infectious complications of rhinitis to which athletes seem to be more prone, like otitis and sinusitis, should be discarded during this examination (Lim and Leong 2010). It is important to explore, during clinical investigations, the differential diagnosis for similar symptoms, like non-allergic ones.

2.5.2 Investigations

In an athlete with persistent symptoms or when an allergic aetiology for upper respiratory symptoms is suspected, skin prick testing (SPT) with standardized allergens and/or measurement of allergen-specific IgE in serum should be used. Further investigation of other allergic diseases, namely asthma or exercise-induced bronchospasm should be considered and studied accordingly (Carlsen, Anderson et al. 2008).

Skin prick tests are relevant markers of the IgE-mediated allergic reaction (Bousquet, Khaltaev et al. 2008; Scadding, Durham et al. 2008). They should be carried out in all cases of suspected allergic rhinitis (Scadding, Durham et al. 2008) because there is a high degree of correlation between symptoms and provocative challenges (Bousquet, Khaltaev et al. 2008). The skin reaction is, however, dependent on several variables, namely the quality of the allergen extracts, age, seasonal variation of the sensitization, medications, and even the test interpretation can vary between individuals (Bousquet, Khaltaev et al. 2008; Scadding, Hellings et al. 2011). False positives mostly occur due to dermographism or irritant substances and false negatives are secondary to poor potency extracts, suppressed skin reaction due to antihistamines, tricyclic antidepressants or topical steroids, or an improper technique (Bousquet, Khaltaev et al. 2008; Scadding, Durham et al. 2008).

Using a radioimmunoassay or enzyme immunoassay it is possible to measure serum-total IgE and serum-specific IgE. These can be requested when skin tests are not possible, such as patients under therapy suppressing skin reactivity or when SPT in association with the clinical exam are not concordant (Bousquet, Khaltaev et al. 2008; Scadding, Durham et al. 2008; Wallace, Dykewicz et al. 2008). An isolated total IgE measurement alone should not be used for screening allergic diseases, but may aid the interpretation of specific IgE tests (Bousquet, Khaltaev et al. 2008; Scadding, Durham et al. 2008). The sensitivity of serum specific IgE measurements compared with SPT can vary with the immunoassay technique used (Wallace, Dykewicz et al. 2008). Other *in vitro* tests used are peripheral blood activation markers, through the evaluation of blood basophiles response of degranulation and mediators release (histamine, CysTL, CD63/ CD203c expression) after stimulation with specific allergens. These tests are still just used for investigation (Bousquet, Khaltaev et al. 2008).

Nasal challenge tests are not necessary to confirm diagnosis. They are usually used for research. (Bousquet, Khaltaev et al. 2008; Scadding, Durham et al. 2008)

Imaging of the nose and sino-nasal cavity is used to differentiate the source of sino-nasal symptoms, relation of sino-nasal problem with surrounding structures and the extent of the disease (Scadding, Hellings et al. 2011). Plain sinus radiographs are not indicated in allergic rhinitis or rhinosinusitis diagnosis (Bousquet, Khaltaev et al. 2008). Computerized tomography scan is actually the main radiological investigation for sino-nasal disorders. It is indicated for differential diagnosis purposes, to exclude chronic rhinosinusitis, eliminate rhinitis complication and to evaluate non-responders to treatment (Bousquet, Khaltaev et al. 2008; Scadding, Hellings et al. 2011). It can be particularly useful in athletes to exclude traumatic lesions, which occur frequently in close-contact sports, like box or soccer. It can also be used for monitoring allergic rhinitis disease complications. Magnetic resonance imaging is rarely indicated.

2.5.3 Evaluation tests for severity and allergic rhinitis control

To evaluate severity in an objective way measurements of nasal obstruction and smell are used (Bousquet, Khaltaev et al. 2008). These tests are not made in routine clinical practice but can be useful when allergen challenges are undertaken or septal surgery is contemplated (Scadding, Durham et al. 2008).

Nasal patency can be monitored objectively using nasal peak inspiratory and expiratory flow, acoustic rhinometry, that measures the nasal cavity volume, and rhinomanometry that measures nasal airflow and pressure (Scadding, Hellings et al. 2011). In clinical practice the most frequently used is peak nasal inspiratory flow because it is simple, cheap, fast, available and it can be used for disease home monitoring (Wallace, Dykewicz et al. 2008). Olfactory tests are subjective test that measure odour threshold, discrimination and identification (Bousquet, Khaltaev et al. 2008; Scadding, Durham et al. 2008).

Nasal nitric oxide measurement may be a useful tool in diagnosis, management and to alert for possible mucociliary defects, but its utility in allergic rhinitis needs to be further evaluated (Bousquet, Khaltaev et al. 2008; Scadding, Hellings et al. 2011).

Rhinitis control is frequently monitored with control questionnaires and visual analogue scales (Bousquet, Khaltaev et al. 2008). There are several questionnaires, and some are being proposed for validation, but none is specific for the athletic population. The Rhinitis Control Assessment Test, a 6-item patient completed instrument, and Control of Allergic Rhinitis and Asthma Test (CARAT), which uses 10 questions, are such examples (Fonseca, Nogueira-Silva et al. 2010; Schatz, Meltzer et al. 2010). Specific questionnaires for athletes are also available, such the Allergy Questionnaire for Atheletes (AQUA) that was developed by Bonini, adapting the European Community Respiratory Health Survey Questionnaire (Bonini, Braido et al. 2009).

2.6 Management allergic rhinitis in athletes

Management of allergic rhinitis encompasses patient education, environmental control, pharmacotherapy and allergen-specific immunotherapy. Surgical options may be used in highly selected cases (Bousquet, Khaltaev et al. 2008). Appropriate management requires an "evidence-based medicine" approach, as it is recommended on 2008 and 2010 guidelines of Allergic Rhinitis and its Impact on Asthma (ARIA)(Bousquet, Khaltaev et al. 2008; Brozek, Bousquet et al. 2010). For the elite athlete, it is also important to minimise the potential detrimental effects of allergic symptoms and treatment on performance (Katelaris, Carrozzi et al. 2003).

Treatment requires careful planning to comply to the "anti-doping" regulations and avoid detrimental influences of treatment adverse effects (Katelaris, Carrozzi et al. 2003). Specific aims for the athlete population are outlined in table 3.

Management Plan
Early recognition and diagnosis to avoid exposure to peak levels of relevant allergens and pollutants
Reduction of symptoms and improvement of nasal function to minimize negative effects on sport performance and the risk of exercise-induced asthma
Use therapies complying with World Anti-Doping Agency, not affecting athletic performance

Table 3. Allergic rhinitis in athletes management plan adapted from (Delgado, Moreira et al. 2006)

2.6.1 Environmental control

Reducing allergen exposure has proven to result in improving the severity of the disease and reducing the need for drugs (van Cauwenberge, Bachert et al. 2000). The beneficial effect may take weeks or months to be fully perceived (van Cauwenberge, Bachert et al. 2000). In most cases, and specifically in athletes, complete avoidance is unfeasible (Moreira, Kekkonen et al. 2007). Nevertheless, measures aiming to reduce relevant allergens should be promoted, and are considered as a first step in management. As far as house-dust-mites are concerned, there are some measures like removing carpets from the bedroom, careful and daily cleaning, and regular change of bed linen. Another inhalant allergen, quite important for athletes seasonal activity, are pollens. For athletes it is often impossible to avoid this stimuli due to its ubiquitous presence, but following pollen forecasts and adapting training venues, time of day and training using appropriate face equipment may minimize exposure, at least to peak pollen levels (Wallace, Dykewicz et al. 2008; Dijkstra and Robson-Ansley 2011). Irritants reported to cause nasal symptoms include tobacco smoke, pollution, chlorine and cold air (Wallace, Dykewicz et al. 2008). To prevent high level exposure to these agents some control of the training environment can be achieved improving ventilation systems of swimming pools and ice arenas (Delgado, Moreira et al. 2006) and taking measures to reduce global pollution, such as the one taken in the Chinese Olympic Games (Zhang, Wang et al. 2011). Allergic athletes should avoid outdoor training during pollen, ozone or air pollution alert periods.

2.6.2 Pharmacologic therapy of rhinitis in athletes

The selection of treatment for a patient depends on multiple factors: type of rhinitis, symptom severity, patient age and job (Wallace, Dykewicz et al. 2008). There is limited medical-evidence to what treatment options should be used in elite athletes. Management of allergic rhinitis should be adapted to accommodate factors that may hazard the athlete performance, and the balance between efficacy and safety should be addressed before prescribing. In elite athletes the drug must be accepted by the World Anti-Doping Agency (WADA) rules.

2.6.2.1 H1 anti-histamines

H-1 receptor antagonists or H1 anti-histamines are drugs that block histamine at H1-receptor level (neutral antagonists or inverse agonists). They are effective in symptoms mediated by histamine, namely rhinorrhoea, sneezing, nasal and eye itching (Bousquet, Khaltaev et al. 2008). The recommended treatment in the most updated guidelines for allergic rhinitis patients is the second-generation oral H1-anti-histamines (e.g. rupatadine, ebastine, azelastine, levocetirizine or desloratadine), that do not have anti-cholinergic and sedative, cognitive and psychomotor effects (Brozek, Bousquet et al. 2010). Athletes benefit the most with these choices, namely endurance athletes, since first generation H1 anti-histamines may reduce psychomotor skills by their sedative effect and, by their anticholinergic activity, cause mucosal drying and reduce sweating and temperature regulation (Delgado, Moreira et al. 2006; Dijkstra and Robson-Ansley 2011). Some authors even propose a cautious approach in the prescription of any anti-histamines 24-48h before a major competition (Dijkstra and Robson-Ansley 2011).
Intranasal H1-antihistamine (azelastine and levocabastine) are locally effective reducing itching, sneezing, runny nose and nasal congestion (Bousquet, Khaltaev et al. 2008). Due to their rapid and topical effects they can be used on demand by athletes to treat acute unexplained symptoms in the sport field (Delgado, Moreira et al. 2006). Ocular medication with anti-histamine compounds, using for example olopatadine (with a dual effect of mast cell stabilization), is quite effective in eye symptoms (van Cauwenberge, Bachert et al. 2000)

2.6.2.2 Decongestants

Decongestants, as vasoconstrictor drugs, act on the adrenergic receptor reducing nasal obstruction. Their side effects (increased blood pressure, heart rate, central nervous system stimulation) limit their use (van Cauwenberge, Bachert et al. 2000). Their clinical use should be limited to a short-term (<5 days) in order to avoid rhinitis *medicamentosa* and should not be used isolated (Brozek, Bousquet et al. 2010). Oral use should be carefully considered or avoided in the elite athletes because some of them are forbidden by WADA 2011. For example ephedrine and methylephedrine are prohibited when its concentration in urine is greater than 10 micrograms per milliliter, and pseudoephedrine when its urine concentration is greater than 150 micrograms per milliliter; doses under 150 micrograms per milliliter in urine are now being monitored in order to detect patterns of misuse (WADA 2011).

2.6.2.3 Corticosteroids

Intranasal glucocorticosteroids are the most efficacious medication available for allergic and non-allergic rhinitis treatment (Bousquet, Khaltaev et al. 2008; Scadding, Durham et al. 2008). These medications are safe to be used in athletes and effective in all symptoms of allergic rhinitis as well as ocular symptoms (Bousquet, Khaltaev et al. 2008). It is supported by high quality of evidence (Brozek, Bousquet et al. 2010) and meta-analysis (Weiner, Abramson et al.

1998) that intranasal glucocorticoids are more effective over oral and topical H1-antihistamines (Brozek, Bousquet et al. 2010), and can be used during competition. In a cross-sectional survey in 446 athletes, treatment with corticosteroids was associated with significantly improved nasal symptoms and quality of life (Alaranta, Alaranta et al. 2005). They have slow onset of action (12h) and maximum efficacy over weeks (van Cauwenberge, Bachert et al. 2000). A recent review of *Laekeman* concluded that inhaled corticosteroids require continuous therapy, at least for the symptoms duration (Laekeman, Simoens et al. 2010).

Systemic corticosteroids are indeed the last resort for allergic rhinitis treatment (van Cauwenberge, Bachert et al. 2000). They are prohibited by WADA when administered orally, rectally or by intravenous or intramuscular administration(WADA 2011). If these formulations are indeed necessary for disease treatment, a Therapeutic Use Exemption may give that athlete the authorization to take the needed medicine (WADA 2011).

2.6.3 Allergen immunotherapy

Allergen vaccines (specific immunotherapy; IT) are very effective in controlling symptoms of allergic rhinitis, can potentially modify the disease, and their clinical benefits may be sustained years after discontinuing treatment (Wallace, Dykewicz et al. 2008; Brozek, Bousquet et al. 2010). It is a valuable option, as stated in the 2010 ARIA guidelines, and indicated in symptomatic patients, with proven allergy (demonstrated by IgE antibodies or positive skin prick tests), with a significant and unavoidable exposure and whose symptoms are not controlled with pharmacological therapy (Wallace, Dykewicz et al. 2008). Athletes are frequently included in this group, namely in the case of pollen-allergic athletes who train and compete in outdoor environment, and with symptoms that affect their performance (Delgado, Moreira et al. 2006). This treatment when performed should be done by trained allergist and the athlete warned not to train in a few hours after immunotherapy injection, to reduce the risk of systemic reactions. Subcutaneous immunotherapy (SIT) is recommended in adults and children with seasonal and persistent allergic rhinitis caused by house dust mites (Brozek, Bousquet et al. 2010). In some cases sublingual specific immunotherapy (SLIT) can be used, namely in adults with rhinitis caused by pollens or house dust mites and in children in pollen-mediated allergy (Scadding, Durham et al. 2008; Brozek, Bousquet et al. 2010). Other forms of immunotherapy might be introduced, namely intranasal allergen specific immunotherapy in adults (Brozek, Bousquet et al. 2010)

2.6.4 Other potential treatment options

Other pharmacological treatments can be used in athletes, as a second line approach. Antileukotrienes inhibit inflammatory mediators produced in both allergic and nonallergic rhinitis, particularly after cold, allergen and exercise challenge (Delgado, Moreira et al. 2006). Recent guidelines recommend its use in seasonal allergic rhinitis in adults and children and only in children in the persistent form of rhinitis (Brozek, Bousquet et al. 2010).

Disodium cromoglycate and sodium nedocromil are used in allergic rhinitis as intranasal and ocular preparations. They are effective in some patients, have excellent safety profile, but its use 4 times a day compromises compliance (Scadding, Durham et al. 2008). Comparing to antihistamines they seem less effective (Brozek, Bousquet et al. 2010). They have a specific role in the prophylactic treatment of allergic conjunctivitis (Bousquet, Khaltaev et al. 2008)

Intranasal ipatropium bromide decreases rhinorrea inhibiting parasympathetic stimulation, but does not act in any other rhinitis symptoms (Bousquet, Khaltaev et al. 2008). For this, it

has a small role in allergic rhinitis, but may be useful in winter sports ("skiers nose") increasing the ability of the nose to warm and humidify the air, reducing watery rhinorrhoea caused by exposure to cold dry air (Katelaris, Carrozzi et al. 2003).
Topical saline is beneficial in chronic rhinorrhea and rhinosinusitis, when used as sole modality or in association with inhaled corticosteroids (Wallace, Dykewicz et al. 2008).
Anti-IgE (Omalizumab) use in allergic rhinitis is not proved cost-effective (Bousquet, Khaltaev et al. 2008). A possible indication for this therapy is in asthmatic patient with concomitant allergic rhinitis, with a clear IgE-dependent allergic component, and uncontrolled despite treatment (Kopp 2011).
Other options like homeopathy, acupuncture, herbal medicines and even physical techniques have not proven their efficacy (Brozek, Bousquet et al. 2010).

2.7 Allergic rhinitis as a risk factor for asthma in athletes

Asthma and allergic rhinitis frequently coexist (Bousquet, Khaltaev et al. 2008). The prevalence of asthma in patients with rhinitis varies between 10-40% and rhinitis seems to be an independent factor in the risk of asthma (Bonini, Bonini et al. 2006). It is not still clear whether allergic rhinitis is an earlier clinical manifestation of allergic disease in atopic patients who will develop asthma, or the nasal disease itself is a causative for asthma (Bousquet, Khaltaev et al. 2008). A very recent study with a 4 decades follow-up of nearly 2000 children found that childhood eczema and rhinitis in combination predicted both new-onset atopic asthma by middle age and the persistence of childhood asthma to adult atopic asthma (Martin, Matheson et al. 2011). *Ciprandi* in several studies evaluated the impact of allergic rhinitis in spirometry, bronchodilation and bronchial hyperreactivity results and found a persistent association (Ciprandi, Cirillo et al. 2008; Cirillo, Pistorio et al. 2009; Ciprandi, Cirillo et al. 2011).
Allergic rhinitis and asthma have some strong similarities on inflammation mechanisms. An eosinophilic type of inflammation is present in both upper and lower airways in rhinitic patients. In these patients, nasal allergen challenge can induce increased bronchial hyperresponsiveness, which might represent a sign of common inflammatory features (Bonini, Bonini et al. 2006). In fact, on nasal and bronchial mucosa a similar inflammatory infiltrate is seen, including eosinophils, mast cell, T lymphocytes, and monocytes with similar proinflammatory mediators (histamine, CysLT), Th2 cytokines and chemokines (Bousquet, Khaltaev et al. 2008). Perhaps the inflammation magnitude in these diseases, which represent the systemic response to allergy, may be different resulting in different manifestations (Bousquet, Khaltaev et al. 2008).
The management of allergic rhinitis also improves asthma control and reduces asthma severity (Bousquet, Khaltaev et al. 2008). Intranasal steroids seem to prevent seasonal increase in nonspecific bronchial hyperreactivity and asthma symptoms associated with pollen exposure, and reduce asthma symptoms, exercise-induced bronchospasm and bronchial responsiveness to methacoline (Bonini, Bonini et al. 2006). Three post-hoc studies described in the ARIA guidelines showed that allergic rhinitis treatment reduced potential utilization of healthcare for co-morbid asthma (Bousquet, Khaltaev et al. 2008).
Elite athletes commonly use drugs to treat asthma, exercise-induced bronchial symptoms and rhinitis. They should be adapted accordingly to WADA, and Therapeutic Use Exemptions should be made with appropriate diagnostic approach, namely medical history, physical examination, spirometry and beta-2 agonist reversibility bronchoconstrition and, if

necessary, bronchial provocation test to establish the presence of airway hyperresponsiveness.
Exercise-induced asthma (EAI) also occurs with allergic rhinitis patients, but frequently goes undiagnosed in children and athletes, because of normal spirometry and negative history (Bonini, Bonini et al. 2006). Every athlete should be screened for asthma or exercise-induced-asthma, including resting spirometry with bronchodilator response and, if not conclusive, bronchial provocation with methacoline or exercise challenge in the usual sports field environment or in a controlled environment in the laboratory (Delgado, Moreira et al. 2006).

3. Conclusion

Allergic rhinitis is a very common disease that in athletes may negatively impact athletic performance. Early recognition, diagnosis and treatment are crucial for improving nasal function and reduce the risk of asthma during exercise and competition. This population represents a diagnostic challenge for allergic conditions and are submitted to several risk factors. So, in order to avoid these risks, all elite athletes should be screened for atopy with skin prick tests and/or specific IgE blood tests, and allergic symptoms evaluated using validated and adapted questionnaires. Proper and accurate treatment will allow athletes to compete at the same level as the non allergic ones. For treatment, inhaled corticosteroids represent the first line of treatment in association with second-generation anti-histamines accordingly to the severity of symptoms. All athletes with rhinitis should be evaluated for asthma and exercise-induced asthma, in accordance to their association and the potential risk of allergic rhinitis for asthma.

4. References

Alaranta, A., H. Alaranta, et al. (2005). "Allergic rhinitis and pharmacological management in elite athletes." Medicine and Science in Sports and Exercise 37(5): 707-711.

Alves, A., C. Martins, et al. (2010). "Exercise-induced rhinitis in competitive swimmers." Am J Rhinol Allergy 24(5): e114-117.

Bonay, M. and M. Aubier (2007). "Pollution atmosphérique et maladies respiratoires allergiques." Med Sci (Paris) 23(2): 187-192.

Bonini, M., F. Braido, et al. (2009). "AQUA: Allergy Questionnaire for Athletes. Development and validation." Med Sci Sports Exerc 41(5): 1034-1041.

Bonini, S., M. Bonini, et al. (2006). "Rhinitis and asthma in athletes: An ARIA document in collaboration with GA2LEN." Allergy: European Journal of Allergy and Clinical Immunology 61(6): 681-692.

Borres, M. P. (2009). "Allergic rhinitis: more than just a stuffy nose." Acta Paediatr 98(7): 1088-1092.

Bousquet, J., N. Khaltaev, et al. (2008). "Allergic Rhinitis and its Impact on Asthma (ARIA) 2008 update (in collaboration with the World Health Organization, GA(2)LEN and AllerGen)." Allergy 63 Suppl 86: 8-160.

Braat, J. P., P. G. Mulder, et al. (1998). "Intranasal cold dry air is superior to histamine challenge in determining the presence and degree of nasal hyperreactivity in nonallergic noninfectious perennial rhinitis." Am J Respir Crit Care Med 157(6 Pt 1): 1748-1755.

Brozek, J. L., J. Bousquet, et al. (2010). "Allergic Rhinitis and its Impact on Asthma (ARIA) guidelines: 2010 revision." J Allergy Clin Immunol 126(3): 466-476.
Carlsen, K. H., S. D. Anderson, et al. (2008). "Exercise-induced asthma, respiratory and allergic disorders in elite athletes: epidemiology, mechanisms and diagnosis: part I of the report from the Joint Task Force of the European Respiratory Society (ERS) and the European Academy of Allergy and Clinical Immunology (EAACI) in cooperation with GA2LEN." Allergy 63(4): 387-403.
Ciprandi, G., I. Cirillo, et al. (2008). "Impact of allergic rhinitis on asthma: effects on spirometric parameters." Allergy 63(3): 255-260.
Ciprandi, G., I. Cirillo, et al. (2011). "Impact of allergic rhinitis on bronchi: An 8-year follow-up study." Am J Rhinol Allergy 25(2): 72-76.
Cirillo, I., A. Pistorio, et al. (2009). "Impact of allergic rhinitis on asthma: effects on bronchial hyperreactivity." Allergy 64(3): 439-444.
D'Amato, G. and L. Cecchi (2008). "Effects of climate change on environmental factors in respiratory allergic diseases." Clin Exp Allergy 38(8): 1264-1274.
Dahl, R. and N. Mygind (1998). "Mechanisms of airflow limitation in the nose and lungs." Clin Exp Allergy 28 Suppl 2: 17-25.
Davila, I., J. Mullol, et al. (2009). "Genetic aspects of allergic rhinitis." J Investig Allergol Clin Immunol 19 Suppl 1: 25-31.
Delgado, L., A. Moreira, et al. (2006). "Rhinitis and its impact on sports." Allergy and Clinical Immunology International 18(3): 98-105.
Dijkstra, H. P. and P. Robson-Ansley (2011). "The prevalence and current opinion of treatment of allergic rhinitis in elite athletes." Current Opinion in Allergy and Clinical Immunology(11): 103–108.
Durham, S. R. (1998). "Mechanisms of mucosal inflammation in the nose and lungs." Clin Exp Allergy 28 Suppl 2: 11-16.
Dykewicz, M. S. and D. L. Hamilos (2010). "Rhinitis and sinusitis." Journal of Allergy and Clinical Immunology 125(2 SUPPL. 2): S103-S115.
Ferrer, M., M. Morais-Almeida, et al. (2010). "Evaluation of treatment satisfaction in children with allergic disease treated with an antihistamine: an international, non-interventional, retrospective study." Clin Drug Investig 30(1): 15-34.
Fonseca, J. A., L. Nogueira-Silva, et al. (2010). "Validation of a questionnaire (CARAT10) to assess rhinitis and asthma in patients with asthma." Allergy 65(8): 1042-1048.
Gioulekas, D., A. Damialis, et al. (2003). "15-year aeroallergen records. Their usefulness in Athens Olympics, 2004." Allergy 58(9): 933-938.
Helbling, A., P. Jenoure, et al. (1990). "[The incidence of hay fever in leading Swiss athletes]." Schweiz Med Wochenschr 120(7): 231-236.
Helenius, I. and T. Haahtela (2000). "Allergy and asthma in elite summer sport athletes." J Allergy Clin Immunol 106(3): 444-452.
Kaelin, M. and O. Brandli (1993). "[Exertional asthma in Swiss top-ranking athletes]." Schweiz Med Wochenschr 123(5): 174-182.
Katelaris, C. H., F. M. Carrozzi, et al. (2003). "Allergic rhinoconjunctivitis in elite athletes: Optimal management for quality of life and performance." Sports Medicine 33(6): 401-406.

Katelaris, C. H., F. M. Carrozzi, et al. (2000). "A springtime Olympics demands special consideration for allergic athletes." Journal of Allergy and Clinical Immunology 106(2): 260-266.

Katelaris, C. H., F. M. Carrozzi, et al. (2002). "Effects of intranasal budesonide on symptoms, quality of life, and performance in elite athletes with allergic rhinoconjunctivitis." Clinical Journal of Sport Medicine 12(5): 296-300.

Katelaris, C. H., F. M. Carrozzi, et al. (2006). "Patterns of allergic reactivity and disease in Olympic athletes." Clin J Sport Med 16(5): 401-405.

Komarow, H. D. and T. T. Postolache (2005). "Seasonal allergy and seasonal decrements in athletic performance." Clinics in Sports Medicine 24(2): e35-e50.

Kopp, M. V. (2011). "Omalizumab: Anti-IgE therapy in allergy." Curr Allergy Asthma Rep 11(2): 101-106.

Koskela, H. O. (2007). "Cold air-provoked respiratory symptoms: the mechanisms and management." Int J Circumpolar Health 66(2): 91-100.

Laekeman, G., S. Simoens, et al. (2010). "Continuous versus on-demand pharmacotherapy of allergic rhinitis: evidence and practice." Respir Med 104(5): 615-625.

Langdeau, J. B., H. Turcotte, et al. (2004). "Comparative prevalence of asthma in different groups of athletes: a survey." Can Respir J 11(6): 402-406.

Li, J., Y. Lu, et al. (2008). "Chinese response to allergy and asthma in olympic athletes." Allergy: European Journal of Allergy and Clinical Immunology 63(8): 962-968.

Lim, M. Y. and J. L. Leong (2010). "Allergic rhinitis: evidence-based practice." Singapore Med J 51(7): 542-550.

Lubitz, S., W. Schober, et al. (2010). "Polycyclic aromatic hydrocarbons from diesel emissions exert proallergic effects in birch pollen allergic individuals through enhanced mediator release from basophils." Environ Toxicol 25(2): 188-197.

Martin, P. E., M. C. Matheson, et al. (2011). "Childhood eczema and rhinitis predict atopic but not nonatopic adult asthma: A prospective cohort study over 4 decades." J Allergy Clin Immunol 127(6): 1473-1479 e1471.

Moreira, A., R. Kekkonen, et al. (2007). "Allergy in marathon runners and effect of Lactobacillus GG supplementation on allergic inflammatory markers." Respir Med 101(6): 1123-1131.

Moreira, A. D., L. ; Moreira, P. ; Haahtela, T. (2009). "Does exercise increase the risk of upper respiratory tract infections?" British Medical Bulletin(90): 111-131.

Scadding, G., P. Hellings, et al. (2011). "Diagnostic Tools In Rhinology EAACI position paper." Clinical and Translational Allergy 1(1): 2.

Scadding, G. K., S. R. Durham, et al. (2008). "BSACI guidelines for the management of allergic and non-allergic rhinitis." Clin Exp Allergy 38(1): 19-42.

Schatz, M., E. O. Meltzer, et al. (2010). "Psychometric validation of the rhinitis control assessment test: a brief patient-completed instrument for evaluating rhinitis symptom control." Ann Allergy Asthma Immunol 104(2): 118-124.

Schwartz, L. B., L. Delgado, et al. (2008). "Exercise-induced hypersensitivity syndromes in recreational and competitive athletes: a PRACTALL consensus report (what the general practitioner should know about sports and allergy)." Allergy 63(8): 953-961.

Shusterman, D., J. Balmes, et al. (2003). "Chlorine inhalation produces nasal congestion in allergic rhinitics without mast cell degranulation." Eur Respir J 21(4): 652-657.

Shusterman, D., M. A. Murphy, et al. (2003). "Influence of age, gender, and allergy status on nasal reactivity to inhaled chlorine." Inhal Toxicol 15(12): 1179-1189.

Shusterman, D. J., M. A. Murphy, et al. (1998). "Subjects with seasonal allergic rhinitis and nonrhinitic subjects react differentially to nasal provocation with chlorine gas." J Allergy Clin Immunol 101(6 Pt 1): 732-740.

Thomas, S., B. Wolfarth, et al. (2010). "Self-reported asthma and allergies in top athletes compared to the general population - results of the German part of the GA2LEN-Olympic study 2008." Allergy Asthma Clin Immunol 6(1): 31.

Valero, A., C. Serrano, et al. (2005). "Nasal and bronchial response to exercise in patients with asthma and rhinitis: the role of nitric oxide." Allergy 60(9): 1126-1131.

van Cauwenberge, P., C. Bachert, et al. (2000). "Consensus statement on the treatment of allergic rhinitis. European Academy of Allergology and Clinical Immunology." Allergy 55(2): 116-134.

WADA (2011). "World Anti-Doping Code- The 2011 prohibited list international standard."

Wallace, D. V., M. S. Dykewicz, et al. (2008). "The diagnosis and management of rhinitis: An updated practice parameter." Journal of Allergy and Clinical Immunology 122(2, Supplement 1): S1-S84.

Walsh, N. P., M. Gleeson, et al. (2011). "Position statement. Part one: Immune function and exercise." Exerc Immunol Rev 17: 6-63.

Weiner, J. M., M. J. Abramson, et al. (1998). "Intranasal corticosteroids versus oral H1 receptor antagonists in allergic rhinitis: systematic review of randomised controlled trials." BMJ 317(7173): 1624-1629.

Zhang, F., W. Wang, et al. (2011). "Time-series studies on air pollution and daily outpatient visits for allergic rhinitis in Beijing, China." Science of The Total Environment 409(13): 2486-2492.

9

Occupational Allergic Rhinitis in the Czech Republic – Situation in South Moravia Region

Petr Malenka
Department of Occupational Diseases, St. Anne´s Hospital and Masaryk University, Brno
Czech Republic

1. Introduction

The author will describe in this chapter the definition, pathophysiology, ethiopathogenesis, complex diagnostic procedure and treatment of occupational allergic rhinitis. Then there will be provided an analysis of cases of occupational rhinitis which were diagnosed and notified as an occupational disease in southern Moravia from January 2004 to December 2006.

Allergic rhinitis can occur due to exposure to different allergens in the working environment. Occupational rhinitis symptoms occur during repeated exposure to an offending allergen. Symptoms of occupational rhinitis are the same as those associated with other types of rhinitis and include sneezing, itching, clear rhinorrhea, nasal congestion and nonpurulent discharge.

Criteria for evaluating rhinitis as an occupational disease: positive work history, there had been no nasal allergic disease before obtaining a job, proof of specific sensibilisation existence - exposure test, prick skin testing, IgE, nasal provoking test etc.

Worker with established occupational disease is not able to perform jobs in which he/she would be exposed to either the chemicals which he/she is proven to be hypersensitive or to respiratory pathogenic agents of any origin.

Allergic rhinitis often represents the initial phase of more serious disease such as asthma.

2. Allergic rhinitis

Allergic rhinitis is characterized by the International Consensus on the treatment of allergic rhinitis (Cauwenberge et al.,2000) by the following symptoms: itching in the nose, sneezing, watery rhinorrhoea and nasal obstruction. Headache, impaired smell, and conjunctivitis may occur as other symptoms.

Allergic rhinitis is the manifestation of allergy, IgE-mediated and associated with inflammatory cell infiltration of the nasal mucosa. An inflammation develops in the mucosa and it contributes to the formation of nasal symptoms and the development of nasal nonspecific hyperreactivity. Nasal mucosa responds to incentives in four ways. Congestion is based on the vasodilatation and increased vascular permeability. Itching and sneezing cause stimulation of sensory nerves. Secretion from the nose is the result of stimulation of the glands and increased vascular permeability.

2.1 Pathophysiology

The inflammatory responses of upper respiratory tract are similar in nature to those in the lower airways. The main difference is that the deterioration in the nasal passage area lies in the changes in vascular tone (the predominant influence of vasodilatation and vascular filling capacity), whereas in the bronchi it leads to a significant contraction of smooth muscles.

The human upper respiratory tract (as opposed to experiments on rodents) does not respond to increasing vascular permeability of irritants. Neurological responses include central mechanisms (cholinergic) and local (axonic) neurogenic reflexes (Bascom et al, 1999). The emergence of rhinitis symptoms can generally be provoked by both allergens and irritants.

2.2 Etiopathogenesis

Inhaled allergens of external environment interact with specific IgE bound to mast cell receptor of nasal mucosa. After binding to allergen-specific IgE there are preformed mediators and newly developed mast cells released and after the release of cytokines it leads to the development of nasal inflammation. This inflammatory process is associated with endothelial cell activation and accumulation of eosinophils from the circulation into tissues.

In the epithelium of the nasal mucosa there are located not only mast cells and eosinophils, but also T lymphocytes, and basophils. Also epithelial cells are activated in case of allergic diseases and the mediators released from them contribute to the spread of symptoms of allergic rhinitis.

We distinguish the early phase, in which itching, sneezing, runny nose and nasal congestion dominate. The development of symptoms is associated with elevated levels of histamine, tryptase, devoid glandins, leukotrienes and kinins. These findings are a manifestation of mast cell degranulation.

The early phase is followed by a late phase, which reflects the activation of basophils. There is a late accumulation of eosinophils, activation of T lymphocytes and a rise of adhesive molecules on the surface of vascular epithelium. In addition to cellular processes and their regulations neural influence are applied. In addition to autonomic control of glandular secretion and nasal vascular tone, also non-adrenergic and non-cholinergic control in the nose is present.

Activation of sensory nerves and local release of mediators causes vasodilatation and enhance microvascular permeability through stimulation of local and axonic reflexes and modifications ganglion neurotransmission (Horwath,1999).

The late phase of chronic allergic rhinitis is clinically characterized by predominance of nasal blockade, impaired sense of smell and constant nasal hyperreactivity.

2.3 The distribution of allergic rhinitis

According to the new International consensus (Cauwenberge et al.,2000), allergic rhinitis can be divided into perennial, seasonal and professional.

Chronic rhinitis resulting in causal connection with the work may be associated not only with the immunopathological mechanism of formation - allergic rhinitis, but also with non-immunological pathogenesis. In that case we speak about a non-allergic rhinitis.

3. Occupational rhinitis

Definition of occupational rhinitis is a medico-legal term. Occupational allergic rhinitis is an allergic rhinitis, which has been objectively proved thar the cause or the major (predominant) cause of the disease is pollutant, or that the patient was exposed in their working environment. Professional diagnosis of rhinitis cannot be based only on anamnestic data and routine laboratory tests, but it must be properly objectified. Early diagnosis is extremely important from the prognostic point of view, because the allergic rhinitis can be the initial phase of more serious disease such as asthma. (Vignola,1998)

In the Czech Republic it was not classified as an occupational diseases until the Government Regulation No. 290/1995 Coll. establishing a list of occupational diseases, and which came into force on 1 January 1996. In Chapter III paragraph 10, there are listed allergic diseases of upper respiratory tract, if they occur at workplace, for which there is some evidence of exposure to dust or gaseous substances with allergenic effects. By definition, the professionalism of Chapter III/10 should be considered especially when diagnosing allergic rhinitis.

As occupational characteristics are considered either allergens occurring commonly in the environment, but in the workplace is their amount increased (flour in bakeries, grain dust in farming), or allergens, which are specific for certain industrial work environment (acid anhydrides in the production of plastics, platinum salts in galvanic works etc).

As in the case of occupational asthma when the professional formation of allergic rhinitis applied as high-molecular substances (animal and vegetable proteins, grain dust, insect antigens, latex, proteolytic enzymes) and low molecular weight compounds (diisocyanates, anhydrides of acids, substances contained in the rosin, antibiotics etc.)

3.1 Etiopathogenesis of occupational rhinitis

Repeated contact with professional allergen leads to IgE-dependent activation of mast cells in the nasal mucosa These cells produce mediators that are collected in their granules (histamine, tryptase). These mediators in conjunction with others (leukotrienes, prostaglandins, platelet activating factor, cytokines and others) cause vasodilatation and increased vascular permeability with edema, resulting in obscure in nasal passages. Increased secretion of glands produces mucous rhinorrhoea.

Stimulation of afferent nerve mediators can cause itchy nose, sneezing and in case of the local axonal reflex can also release neuropeptides that cause further mast cell degranulation. A characteristic feature of allergic inflammation is the local accumulation of inflammatory cells, including basophils and neutrophils, T lymphocytes and eosinophils, which was also involved in the cascade of immunopathological processes. (Mamessier et al.,2007, Braunstahl et al., 2000)

There is accumulating evidence that the workplace environment can induce or trigger a wide spectrum of rhinitis conditions involving immunological and nonimmunological mechanisms. (Castano et al, 2006) These various conditions should be referred to as a work-related rhinitis and should be further distinguished according to the clinical features, etiopathogenic mechanisms and strength of evidence supporting the casual relationship.

According to the revised nomenclature for allergy recently recommended by the European Academy of Allergy and Clinical Immunology (Johansson et al.,2001) and the classification of work-related asthma proposed by panels of experts, different types of work-related rhinitis may be delineated as summarized in Figure 1. (Moscato et al., 2008)

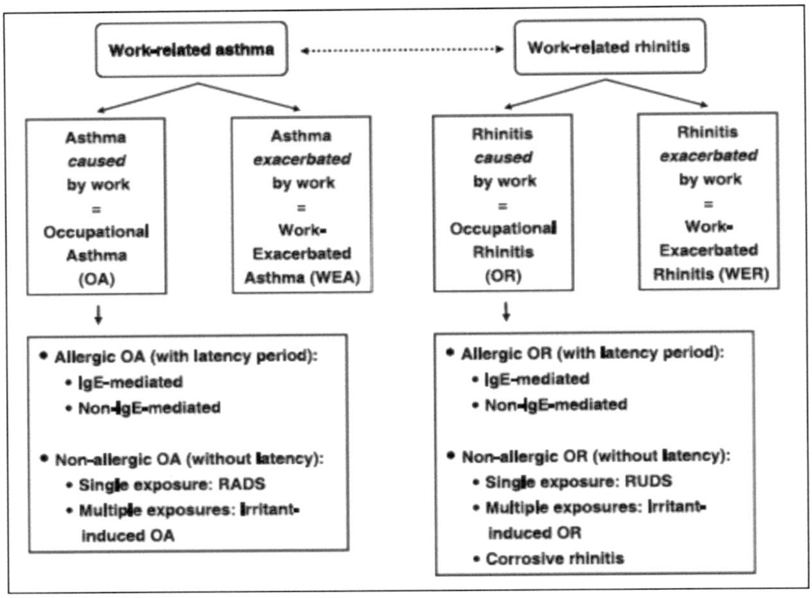

Fig. 1. Parallel classification of occupational rhinitis and asthma. RADS, reactive airways dysfunction syndrome; RUDS, reactive upper airways dysfunction symndrome

3.2 The clinical picture of occupational disease

Acute allergic rhinitis is defined as an inflammatory disease of the nasal mucosa, which occurs in response to airborne allergen occurring in the workplace.

The main symptoms are itching and irritation in the nose, sneezing and watery secretion, often associated with congestion of the nasal mucosa. It can be accompanied by itching in the throat, eyes and ears, which are often present symptoms of asthma.

Because this is a type I immune response, symptoms appear within minutes after the start of exposure and usually disappear within a short time after its completion. During the work week it usually causes deeper trouble. The improvement or disappearance of symptoms occur on weekends and holidays. (Storaas et al.,2005)

Depending on the amount of exposure and individual sensitivity, with some patients there may occur a late-phase allergic reaction within 6-12 hours that results in nasal hyperreactivity. This can be either specific (a specific allergen sensitization) or nonspecific (increased sensitivity to irritants that trigger an allergic reaction). As a by a professional unrecognized and untreated disease can rhinitis (after months or years) lead to chronicity.

Then the clinical picture is dominated by a sense of blocked nose and thick mucus. Sneezing and itching are infrequent or absent. They are observed in chronic conjunctive changes, swelling of eyelids, increased lacrimation. (Slavin, 2003)

3.3 Complex diagnostic procedure

A consensus diagnostic algorithm has been elaborated - see Fig 2 (Moscato et al, 2008) – by taking into account the following practical constraints:

a. the validity of tests used for diagnosing remains largely uncertain and

b. the level of reliability may vary according to the purpose of the diagnostic evaluation and its expected socio-economic impact.

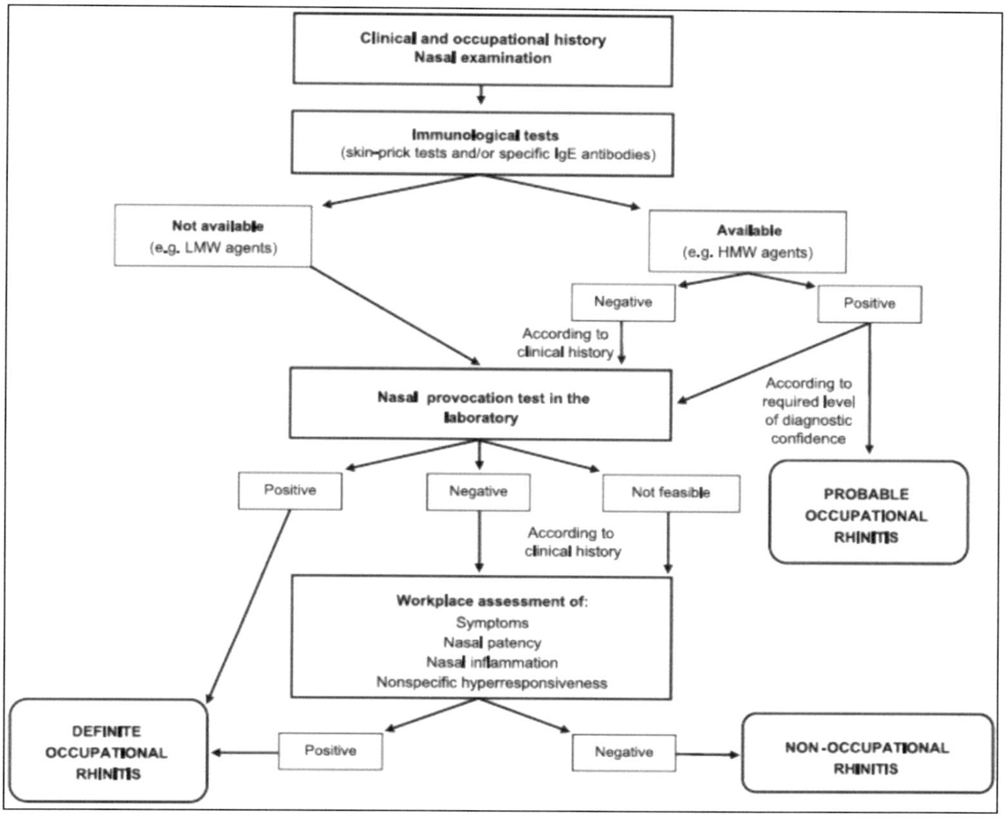

Fig. 2. Diagnostic algorithm

Complex diagnosis procedure for suspected occupational allergic rhinitis must focus on several steps:

1. **History**: (presence of clinical symptoms linked to the workplace): i.e. clinical symptoms, the onset of the first difficulties related to working environment, the total length of exposure to the noxa in the workplace, the current presence of breathing problems, other allergic manifestations with or without a link to the work environment, the incidence of allergic disease in the family.
2. **ENT examination**: it includes a front and rear rhinoscopy, nasal pathology exclusion type of nasal septum deviation, nasal polyps, foci, and the state of the nasal mucosa. A finding of pale, swollen mucous membrane is evident with the allergic rhinitis outside the period of manifest clinical signs.
3. **Allergy tests**: it includes intradermal skin or pointed-tip (SPT) tests, determination of serum total IgE, determination of allergen-specific IgE in serum by ELISA.
4. **Bacteriological examination** of swabs and nasal and throat: cytological analysis in allergic rhinitis is considered a pointer to increase the number of eosinophils.
5. **X-ray** paranasal sinuses and chest.
6. **Blood tests**: blood count with leukogramem, erythrocyte sedimentation rate.
7. **Rhinomanometrie**: measures the resistance of the nasal passages using quantitative measurement of nasal flow and pressure. Usually, front rhinomanometrie is used. A

finding of pale, swollen mucous membrane is evident with the allergic rhinitis outside the period of manifest clinical signs.

8. **Nasal provocation tests:** these tests are still considered the gold standard for confirming the diagnosis of occupational rhinitis allergica. Nasal provocation tests can be performed either under controlled conditions in a laboratory or under natural conditions at work. (Airaksinen et al., 2007). These are methods that can be used to deliver occupational agents and to measure nasal response during nasal provocation tests.

3.4 Assessment of occupational rhinitis allergica

Next to the typical history, the clinical picture and a specific immune response are crucial to assess occupational rhinitis allergica. Nasal provocation tests with suspected inhalation of workplace noxa are the best possibility for objectification.. Nasal provocation tests have confirmed a causal relationship between the induction of symptoms and exposure to inhaled allergens in the workplace.

The most important aspect of the nasal provocation test is a comparison of objective and subjective parameters of patient's discomfort before and after nasal provocation. (Arandelovic et al.,2004)

There are provided objective evaluations of the decrease in nasal flow values (significant for the allergic reaction is a decrease of - 40% or more compared to the native value) and of the rise of resistance value (significant for the allergic reaction is a rise of +60% or more compared to the native value)

Subjective difficulties are assessed according to a symptom score (see Table 1). Clinical symptoms assess as positive when reaching a total sum of at least 4 points or more.

Symptoms:	**Intensity:**	**Scoring**
Nasal Secretion	*Without (Nothing)*	0
	Low (Medium)	1
	Lot of (Significant)	2
Sneezing	*0-2*	0
	3-5	1
	>5	2
Eyes Watering		1
Itching Palate		1
Itching Ears		1
Conjuntivitis		2
Chemosis (swelling of the conjuctiva)		2
Urticaria		2
Cough		2
Dyspnoea		2

Table 1. Nasal symptom score

3.4.1 The procedure for nasal provocation tests

First the patient must be informed about the nature of examinations - about examination procedure and duties assigned to it in the test result.

During testing, we follow the basic contraindications and take into account other important factors:

a. Contraindications:
- Acute inflammatory diseases of paranasal sinuses
- Nasal acute allergic-type reactions quickly manifest in other organs
- Patients with a higher degree of sensitivity - based on skin tests or IgE
- Pregnancy
- Ongoing vaccination against influenza

b. Other:
- any signs of nasal obstruction
- anatomical deformities (septal deviation, nasal polyps)
- last alcohol consumption at least 24 hours ago
- consumption of hot beverages (including coffee and tea) and food
- smoking
- elimination of nasal medication, if the patient's condition allows it

c. Recommendations for withdrawal therapy before the test:
- Nasal corticosteroids and nasal drops (Avamys etc.) - at least 3 days prior to the examination
- Corticosteroids (Prednisone, Beclomet, Pulmicort, etc.) - at least 3 days before testing
- Antihistamines (Zyrtec, Clarinin etc.) - at least 3 days prior to the examination
- Sodium cromoglycate, ketotifen (Zaditen) - at least 2 days before testing
- Xantin derivatives (Syntophylin, Euphylin) - 1-2 days prior to the examination
- Inhaled anticholinergics (Atrovent, Berodual) - at least 8-12 hours before testing
- Inhaled beta2 agonists (Berotec, Ventolin) - at least 6-8 hours before testing

Tests can be performed earlier than 6 weeks after abatement of symptoms of upper respiratory tract inflammation, at least 4 weeks after application of anti-influenza vaccine.

4. Nasal provocation tests include

1. **Native patient examination**

Firstly, the native rhinomanometric curve is recorded. According to the European Commission recommendations for standardization in rhinomanometry, only nasal active front rhinomanometry is used and a reference value is measured at a pressure of 150 Pa. It is based on the principle of transnasal pressure and nasal resistance, which is then calculated from the nasal flow and transnasal pressure. The relationship between pressure and flow is a complex function of changing the turbulent air flow and the relationship between pressure and flow. (Guideline, 2008) the beginning of this test, eartips of olive-sized amount are inserted into the patient´s nose, which correspond to anatomical dimensions of the nostrils, so that the exhaled air is not escaping out of olives. An olive with pressure sensor is inserted into the nostril of examined nasal cavity and a nasal flow is then recorded from the second nasal cavity. Then the nostrils are changed.

At Occupational Medicine Clinic at St..Anne in Brno ZAN 100 Handy device is used for the rhinomanometry examination. (See Picture 1.)

2. **Application of control saline**

Nasal mucosa is exposed to the physiological solution, which excludes non-specific nasal hyperreactivity. The rhinomanometry curve is recorded.

3. **Custom nasal provocation**

In occupational medicine, there are a wide range of potential etiological agents. First we use nonspecific methacholine nasal provocation test. Positive test tells us that there is a reaction of the nasal mucosa and we can proceed to further investigations of the causal nox itself.

4. **Nasal provocative test perform the following alternatives**:

   a. Simulated reexposive test with a suspicious noxa from the workplace:
      We test only those substances that the patient was actually exposed to in the workplace. The patient is situated in a closed cabin, where he/she is manipulating with the material for 30 minutes at the most, like in the workplace.

   b. Reexposive test directly in the workplace:
      We test only in that environment, in which the patient was exposed. The test is performed during normal working hours.

After the end of the provocation, we record another rhinomanometry curve and evaluate nasal symptom score. The patient must be monitored for at least 24 hours to record also delayed responses.

5. **Rating of nasal provocation tests:**

The test is positive when the nasal resistance increases by 60% or more, and the nasal flow decreases by 40% or more, compared with values after application of control solution. (See Picture 2.)

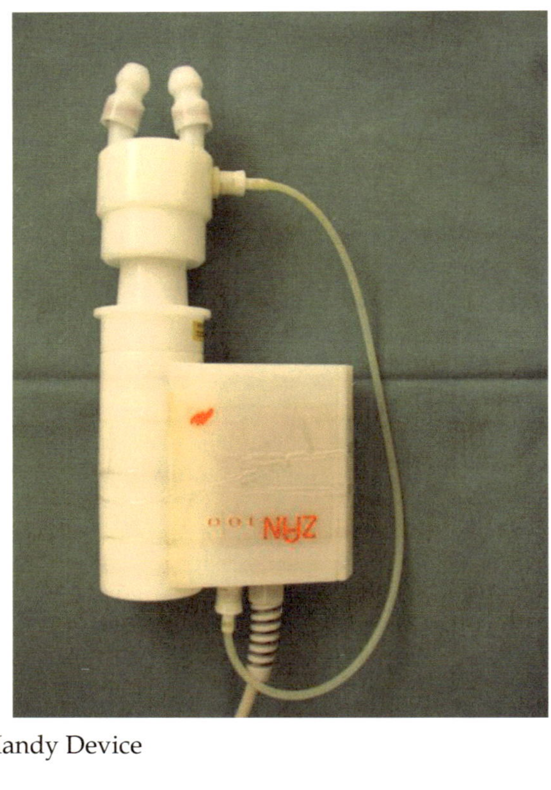

Picture 1. ZAN 100 Handy Device

3.5 Differential diagnosis

It is necessary to distinguish the differential diagnosis of allergic rhinitis from other occupational allergic of different etiology, particularly seasonal allergic rhinitis, perennial rhinitis, infectious rhinitis, and others (idiopathic, irritation, hormonal, drug-induced, alimentary, psychogenic etc.)

It is also necessary to take in account other pathological processes in the nasal cavity, paranasal sinuses and secondary processes (polyps, mechanical changes, tumours, granulomas, cerebrospinal fluid). (Horwath et al, 1999)

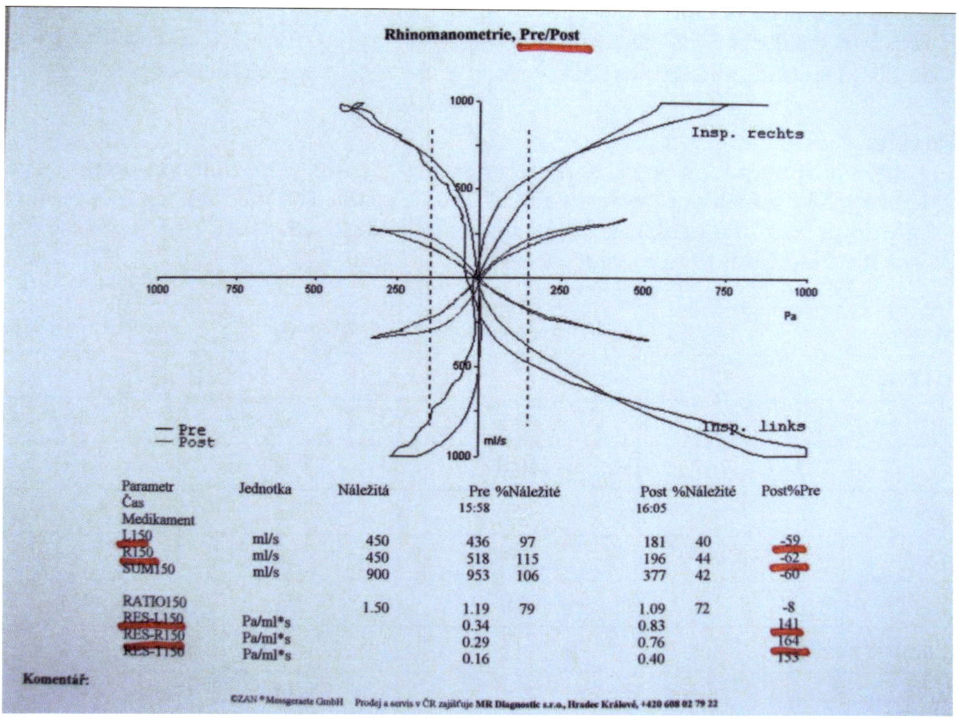

Picture 2. Rating of Nasal Provocation Test

3.6 Treatment of occupational allergic rhinitis

The basic essential step is the permanent removal of patient contact with the allergen professional. Drug treatment is identical to the unprofessional treatment of allergic rhinitis - it means antihistamines, local eventually systemic corticosteroids. As the mast cell stabilizer disodium cromoglycate is used, you can also use anticholinergics, which absorb watery rhinorrhea but have no effect on nasal obscuration.

3.7 Special precautions

In terms of technical measures, it should be ensured that the permissible exposure limits at workplaces are not. There should be preferred safe technological processes and they should be preceded by emergency conditions. In case of high-risk procedures, the protection respirators should be ensured.

Furthermore, patients with allergic rhinitis should not be working in the environment with a presence of known professional allergens and involvement of atopic in such operation should be carefully considered.

4. Cases of occupational rhinitis allergica in southern Moravia

4.1 Examined group and methods

There were analyzed all the cases of occupational rhinitis, which have been recognized and reported to the Occupational Medicine Clinic Hospital St. Anne in Brno and the Faculty of Medicine at the Masaryk University in Brno in the period from 1.1.2004 to 31.12.2006.
The statistical analysis was performed using Microsoft Office Excel and Statistica for Windows. Considering the lack of data normality, we used nonparametric tests.

4.2 Results

During the reporting period 86 cases of occupational rhinitis were diagnosed and reported. Of this group, 59 (68.6%) were women and 27 (31.4%) men. The median age (median) of the whole group at the time of notification of occupational disease was 39.5 years, age range was wide, it varied from 19 to 63 years. (See Table 2, 3 and 4)

Parameter	**Women (n=59)**	**Men (n=27)**	**Total (n=86)**
Age (Years)			
Mean	40,4	35,2	38,7
SD	10,8	9,96	10,8
Median	42	32	39,5
Min.	19	23	19
Max.	63	63	63
Exposure (Years)			
Mean	8,8	10,46	9,32
SD	7,24	8,06	7,5
Median	7	8	7
Min.	0,83	2	0,83
Max.	30	27	30

n = the amount of patients, SD = standard deviation, min. = lowest value, max. = highest value

Table 2. Basic Group Data

Mean duration of exposure to etiological noxa (median) was 7 years, duration of exposure varied from 0.83 to 30 years. (See Table 5).
We also investigated the time elapsed since the first manifestation of symptoms of rhinitis to recognition of occupational disease, the median was 1 year (see Table 3).
There was no statistically significant difference among women and men (Mann-Whitney´s U test, $p > 0.05$) in any of the parameters mentioned above.

Parameter	Rhinitis (n=40)	Rhinitis and Astma (n=46)	Total (n=86)
Age (Years)			
Mean	36,6	40,6	38,7
SD	10,2	10,8	10,8
Median	37	41,5	39,5
Min.	19	22	19
Max.	57	63	63
Exposure (Years)			
Mean	8,1	10,4	9,32
SD	6,4	8,1	7,5
Median	5,5	8	7
Min.	0,83	1	0,83
Max.	23	30	30
The Duration of Symptoms to the Notification of Occupational Disease (Years)			
Mean	1,17	1,68	1,44
SD	0,69	1,17	1,01
Median	1	1,75	1
Min.	0,33	0,33	0,33
Max.	3	7	7

n = the amount of patients, SD = standard deviation, min. = lowest value, max. = highest value

Table 3. Next Group Data

Professions, in which the affected were employed are summarized in Table 6. The work in bakeries, textile industry and livestock production prevailed. Rye or wheat flour and textile fibres (cotton, wool, synthetics are usually applied as professional etiological agents), others included different feed mixtures, wood dust, straw, preservatives, varnishes and adhesives.

Age (Years)	Women (n)	Men (n)	Total (n)	%
15-19	1	0	1	1,2
20-24	4	1	5	5,8
25-29	9	8	17	19,8
30-34	4	8	12	13,9
35-39	6	2	8	9,3
40-44	12	4	16	18,6
45-49	10	0	10	11,6
50-54	9	3	12	13,9
55-59	4	0	4	4,7
60-64	0	1	1	1,2
Total	**59**	**27**	**86**	**100**

n = the amount of patients

Table 4. Distribution by age at the time of notification of occupational disease

Exposure (Years)	Amount of Patients	%
do 2,9	13	15,1
3,0-5,9	23	26,7
6,0-8,9	14	16,4
9,0-11,9	11	12,9
12,0-14,9	5	5,8
15,0-17,9	5	5,8
18,0-20,9	3	3,5
21,0-23,9	7	8,1
24,0-26,9	3	3,5
27,0-29,9	1	1,1
30,0 and more	1	1,1
Total	**86**	**100**

Table 5. Distribution by the length of exposure to etiological noxa

Profession	Number of occupational diseases
Baker	29
Worker in a bakery	9
Milkmaid	8
Seamstress	6
Dressmaker	5
Confectioner	5
Repairman	3
Nurse	3
Cabinetmaker	2
Printer	2
Painter	2
Cook	2
Electrician	2
Worker in Production of Compound Feed	2
Workers in Pasta Plant	1
Worker in Chemical Industry	1
Developer	1
Worker at Service Lines	1
Worker at mill	1
Worker in army	1
Total	86

Table 6. Distribution according to profession

At the time of reporting rhinitis allergica as an occupational disease, 46 of 86 probands - 54% of the sample - had currently suffered with bronchial asthma.
The basic time parameters in a group of patients with rhinitis were compared to a group of patients also affected by bronchial asthma. When comparing the median length of exposure and the median time of the first manifestations of nasal symptoms in the recognition of occupational disease, we can see that in the group, where there was reported only rhinitis, the exposure of noxa symptoms and their length of shorter than with those with asthma. (See Table 3) However, the differences observed were not statistically significant (Mann-Whitney´s U test, p> 0.05).
We were also interested in the number of smokers in the examined group. 18.6 % of probands of the sample smoked cigarettes at the time of recognition of occupational disease, 72.1 % patients were non-smokers and the rest of probands (9.3%) were former smokers.
We compared the value of symptom scores at the time of recognition of occupational diseases with the value acquired the year after the recognition of occupational disease. Symptom score was evaluated by adding the points according to Table 1.
Table 7 shows a statistically significant (Wilcoxon paired test, p-value p<0,001) decrease of symptom score at the time of recognition of occupational disease compared with symptom score one year after rhinitis has been recognized as an occupational disease.

Parameter	**Rhinitis (n=40)**	**Rhinitis and Asthma (n=46)**	**Total (n=86)**
Symptom score at the time of recognition of occupational disease			
Mean	12,87	12,67	12,76
SD	1,27	1,44	1,37
Median	12	13	12,5
Min.	11	10	10
Max.	16	16	16
Symptom score - one year after the recognition of occupational disease			
Mean	4,71	4,75	4,73
SD	0,8	0,92	0,87
Median	5	5	5
Min.	2	3	2
Max.	6	7	7

n = the amount of patients, SD = standard deviation, min. = lowest value, max. = highest value

Table 7. Nasal Symptom score

When comparing individual items of the nasal symptom score, we came to the conclusion that even there was a statistically significant (Wilcoxon paired test, p-value p<0,001) decrease of each parts of symptom score. For details see Figure 3.

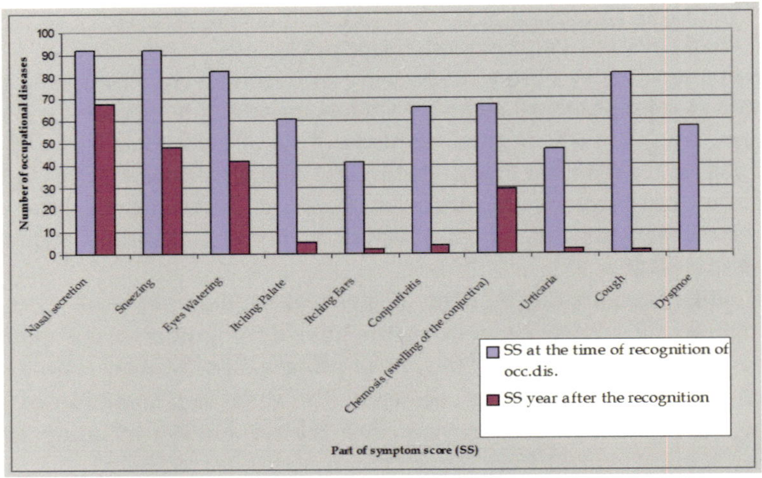

Fig. 3. Parts of symptom score

4.3 Discussions

Occupational rhinitis participated in the occupational diseases reported in southern Moravia between 2004 and 2006 in 7.2% of all the cases.

Compared with a period of years 1996 - 1999 (Brhel et al, 2000), there are no major changes. In both periods, there were more women in the group and the most common age of both groups are from 40 to 44 years. The overall average age is now slightly higher (38.7 versus 34.7 years).

Length of exposure necessary for developing the disease is now also slightly higher (median 7 versus 5), but not statistically significant (Mann-Whitney´s U test, p> 0.05).

The number of recognized diseases of occupational rhinitis has been gradually decreasing, not only at the Department of Occupational Diseases, St. Anne´s Hospital and Masaryk University Brno, but also in the whole country, as shown in Figure 4.

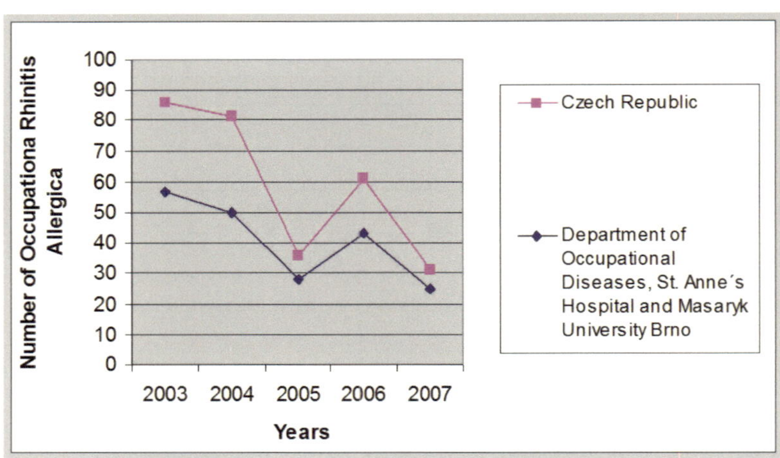

Fig. 4. Number of Occupational Rhinitis

If we look at the etiological noxa and individual professions of occupational rhinitis now and in the past, there have been minor changes - there are the same professions, such as workers in bakeries, textile industry and livestock production.
When comparing the number of smokers, the data show that the number of smokers has decreased and we can consider it good news.

5. Conclusion

Allergic rhinitis occurs all over the world. We are spending many hours a day in the work environment, so it is necessary to monitor all inhaled allergens.
Nasal provocation tests assess the clinical relevance of sensitization verified skin or serological tests. Mostly we use tests in the test room at Departments of Occupational Medicine under controlled conditions - tests are performed only with substances that occur in the workplace. In some cases, also nasal provocation tests must be performed directly at the workplace.
Allergic rhinitis makes the quality of life significantly worse and it is often associated with other comorbidities. When we investigate occupational allergic rhinitis, we should always confirm the causal link between allergic rhinitis and working environment, so we must find etiological agents (noxa).
A careful history, occupational health knowledge, willingness to consider the causal link and following the recommended use of investigative procedures will enable early detection of occupational rhinitis.
After the recognition of occupational disease it is necessary to avoid the patient´s contact with the causal noxa exposure. This avoids the potential for occupational development of asthma bronchiole and other related diseases that accompany chronic allergic rhinitis.

6. References

Airaksinen L. et al.: Use of nasal provocation test in the diagnostics of occupational rhinitis. Rhinology, 2007, 45, pp. 40–46.

Arandelovic M., Stankovic, I.: Allergic rhinitis-possible occupational disease-criteria suggestion. Acta Fac. Med. NAISS., 2004, 21, 2, pp. 65–71.

Bascom R., Shusterman D. Occupational and environmental exposures and the upper respiratory tract. In: Naclerio R. M., Durham S. R., Mygind N. (eds.). Rhinitis mechanisms and management. New York-Basel-Hongkong: Marcel Dekker Inc., 1999: p. 65- 99.

Braunstahl, GJ et al: Nasal provocation results in bronchial inflammation in allergic rhinitis patients. Am.J respir Crit Care Med 2000; 161: A, p. 325.

Brhel P.,Vomelová K., Říhová A.: Profesionální rinitida na jižní Moravě, Pracov. Lék., 52, 2000, 3, pp. 116-119

Castano R, Theriault G, Gautrin D., The definition of rhinitis and occupational rhinitis needs to be revisited, Acta Otolaryngol 2006: 126: pp.1118-1119

Cauwenberge van P., Bachert C., Passalacqua G., et al.: Consensus statement on the treatment of allergic rhinitis. Allergy, 55, 2000: pp 116-134

Guideline: Management of allergic rhinitis and its impact on asthma. Geneva (Switzerland): World Health Organization (WHO); 2008.

Horwath P. H.: Mucosal Inflammation and Allergic Rhinitis. In: Rhinitis Mechanism and Management (Naclerio R. M., Durham S. R., Mygind N., eds.), Marcel Dekker Inc., New York-Basel-Hongkong, 1999: pp 109-133

Johansson SG, Hourihane JO, Bousquet J et al., A revised nomenclature for allergy. An EAACI position statement freom ESSCI nomenclaturetask force, Allergy 2001:56: pp 813-824

Mamessier E., Milhe F., Guillot C. et al.: T-cell activation in occupational asthma and rhinitis, Allergy, Oxford 2007. Vol. 62, 2, pp. 162-169

Moscato et al, Occupational Rhinitis, Allergy 2008:63: pp 969-980

Slavin R. G.: Occupational Rhinitis. Annals of Allergy, Asthma & Immunology, 90,2003, 5, pp. 2-6

Storaas T. et al.:Occupational rhinitis: diagnostic criteria, relation to lower airway symptoms and IgE sensitization in bakery workers. Acta Oto-Laryngologica, 2005, 125, pp. 1211–1217

Vignola A. M: Relationship between rhinitis and asthma. Allergy, 53, 1998: pp. 833-839

10

Nasal Provocation Test in the Diagnosis of Allergic Rhinitis

Graça Loureiro, Beatriz Tavares, Daniel Machado and Celso Pereira
Immunoallergy Department, Coimbra University Hospital
Portugal

1. Introduction

The specific provocation tests, since its introduction by Blackley in 1853, have been widely used in the investigation of pathophysiological mechanisms, immunological and therapeutic aspects of allergic disease, as they mimic the response to allergen exposure, under controlled conditions. However, it has not been broadly used in the diagnosis of allergic disease in clinical practice, because of the lack of standardization of the methodology and the need of other complementary diagnostic tests for monitoring specific provocation tests. Nevertheless, the importance of such test is enormous in many circumstances, since it is the only method that can establish the exact etiology of allergic disease. Although the usefulness of these tests has not been questioned, the need to standardize the methodology for monitoring the response has been stressed. In this review, these aspects will be discussed.

2. Allergic rhinitis

Rhinitis is generally subdivided into two groups: allergic and non-allergic. It has been estimated that allergic rhinitis has a high prevalence in the general population (5 to 20%), and non-allergic rhinitis alone is thought to affect more than 200 million people worldwide. So, this is a very common but under diagnosed disease. The correct diagnosis has an enormous impact in public health, since it would involve several health and economic benefits (Bousquet & ARIA Workshop Group, 2001).

Allergic rhinitis is an IgE mediated inflammatory chronic disease affecting nasal mucosa, characterized by the presence of itching, rhinorrea, sneezing and congestion (Bousquet & ARIA Workshop Group, 2001). The diagnosis of allergic rhinitis is based mostly in clinical evidence. In fact, a positive correlation between the clinical history and the allergen sensitization is usually enough to support the diagnosis of allergic rhinitis and its aetiology. However, in some circumstances (table 1), additional approaches are required to reach a correct diagnosis in allergic rhinitis patients, namely nasal provocation test (NPT). Indeed, the specific NPT is the method of choice for the reproducibility of the allergic reaction, and it is indicated when discrepancies arise in the assessment of a patient's medical history and the results of skin and/or serological tests, as reviewed by several authors (Litvyakova LI & Baraniuk JN. 2001; Loureiro, 2001; Dordal et al, 2011; Mellilo, 1997; Naclerio & Norman, 1998).

Clinical practice	• Multissensitized patients • Local allergic rhinitis • Occupational allergic rhinitis • Correlation between allergy and other morbidities
Investigational research	• Mechanisms of allergic reaction • Mechanisms of immunotherapy • Efficacy of new treatments

Table 1. Indications for NPT: clarifying the pathogenesis and diagnostic evidence, in particular situations of allergic rhinitis

2.1 Multissensitized patients

Atopic patients are frequently sensitized to multiple allergens. In some circumstances, clinical history is not clearly related to allergen specific IgE. A NPT could be performed to differentiate the relevant allergenic aetiology in multissensitized patients, since these patients need specific therapeutic approaches.

2.2 Local allergic rhinitis

Patients with allergic rhinitis have allergen-specific IgE demonstrable both systemically as well as local IgE produced in the nasal mucosa. On the other hand, the concept of non allergic rhinitis is supported by negative skin tests. However, in a subset of patients who have positive NPT to allergens despite having a negative skin prick test, it has been hypothesized that these patients have localized allergic rhinitis. Huggins made the first description of local allergic rhinitis (Huggins & Brostoff J, 1975). Recently, several studies have strengthened the existence of this allergic disorder and the immunological mechanisms involved in the immediate and late responses to NPT have been described (Kim & Jang, 2010; López S et al, 2010; Rondón et al, 2007, 2009, 2010a, 2010b). A type 2 helper T cell inflammatory pattern in nasal secretions in response to allergen exposure was demonstrated. Accordingly, local production of IgE and mast cell / eosinophil activation with its inflammatory mediators was also founded in these patients. These findings support the hypothesis of a localized inflammatory response and the concept of local allergic rhinitis. As discussed, local allergic rhinitis involves nasal production of specific IgE in the absence of atopy. Evidence of this entity is supported by suggestive clinical symptoms and a positive NPT. So it is a useful tool for detecting patients with local allergic rhinitis in previously diagnosed idiopathic / non-allergic rhinitis patients, as defended by several authors and evidenced by our group (Loureiro et al, 2011). In our experience, the specific NPT reproduced the clinical manifestations in some patients, supporting the concept of local allergic rhinitis in a subset of patients with perennial rhinitis. We studied 15 patients with an average age of 22.2±14.8 years (77.7% were female) with typical clinical symptoms of perennial rhinitis, negative skin prick test to common aeroallergens and negative specific IgE. The period of symptoms evolution was 5.37±3.9 years. A *Dermatophagoides* specific NPT (BialAristegui, Bilbao, Spain) was performed with clinical monitoring. Total nasal symptom scores were assessed using a validated questionnaire and a positive NPT was considered if a score of 5 or greater was recorded (Linder, 1988). The NPT was considered positive in 8 patients. Several studies proved that house dust mites could have a pro-inflammatory activity independent of IgE (Fujisawa et al, 2008; Gregory et al, 2009; Hammad et al, 2009; Wong et al, 2006). This fact could explain the positive result in NPT, in our study however, all patients were negative to a non-specific NPT. Despite the few number of patients included, our data highlight the need for the most complete diagnostic approach. The correct differential diagnosis with non-allergic rhinitis is crucial for therapeutic purposes, since some of these misdiagnosed patients may benefit of specific immunotherapy. Indeed, in our findings, all the patients with the diagnosis of local allergic rhinitis were submitted to specific immunotherapy, with clinical improvement (data not published).

Because the concept of local allergic rhinitis is based in positive NPT, some authors emphasize the need to standardize this procedure to better understand its usefulness in the diagnostic approach of this new entity. It has still controversial aspects to be defined, as discussed by some authors (Alvares & Khan, 2011; Khan 2009). In a review of the studies that evaluated patients with negative skin tests using NPT, these authors argued that several aspects could explain the different data in the literature. For instance, the prevalence ranges from 0% to 100% of skin test negative individuals. This wide range in prevalence could be explained by the differences in methodology (allergen manufacturers, concentrations, and numbers of allergens tested) and, perhaps most importantly, criteria for a positive nasal challenge. In another review of the literature, the concept of entopy was also considered controversial (Forester & Calabria, 2010). In spite of this, they recognize that there are a large number of non-allergic rhinitis patients for whom current treatment regimens are suboptimal, considering the need to better understand the subjacent immunological mechanisms to achieve an optimal diagnosis and treatment in this subset of patients.

2.3 Occupational allergic rhinitis

The occupational exposure to immunogenic substances, such as chemicals and biologic products is enormous in the workplace, since it is the place were people spend more time. Despite an increasing estimated prevalence of 5 to 15%, occupational allergic diseases, namely occupational rhinitis it is still underestimated. Several factors are pointed, including the worker reluctance to complain and the failure to diagnose. More than 400 substances have been implicated as cause of occupational respiratory allergy. It is recognized that exposure to these substances can result in increased nasal hyperreactivity and can predispose to occupational rhinitis. It presents a major impact in quality of life, as well in professional performance. Further the legal impact, a correct etiologic identification in occupational allergic rhinitis as an enormous impact in the natural history of this disease. Indeed it is assumed that occupational rhinitis coexists and it may precede occupational asthma. Despite this, occupational asthma has been better evaluated than occupational rhinitis, both in epidemiological and physiopathological approaches.

The real incidence and prevalence of occupational disease is not known. Occupational disease has been recognized by physicians and epidemiologists. However, there are a few publications about occupational rhinitis. NPT is an fundamental diagnostic approach of occupational Allergic Rhinitis (Loureiro, 2008).

New allergens (high molecular weight as well as low molecular weight agents) are continuously being described in occupational asthma and/or rhinitis. Standardized extracts for skin testing are not available. A complementary diagnostic approach in occupational rhinitis, to better recognise and early diagnose this disease, includes specific NPT with clinical and functional monitoring. In fact, NPT is the ideal methodology to confirm or refute the diagnosis of occupational allergic rhinitis because it confirms the clinical symptoms and its causality. For instance, using NPT our group could reached the correct etiologic diagnosis of the first case of fungal lipase allergy in a patient not sensitized to amylase working in the pharmaceutical industry (Loureiro, 2009). It has well known that occupational allergy to lipase has been reported in the detergent industry (Brant et al, 2004, 2006; Lindstedt et al, 2005; van Kampen et al, 2000). While the main allergenic enzyme in the pharmaceutical industry is amylase, there have been reports of lipase sensitization, albeit without clinical relevance (Park et al, 2002; Zentner et al, 1997). The NPT was the supporting approach methodology to obtain this diagnosis confirmation, in our patient. Several cases of occupational allergic rhinitis are described in the literature, based directly on positive NPT, both in confirming the diagnosis and the etiological identification. The NPT reproduces the nasal symptoms and can be performed on the workplace, or under controlled conditions in hospital environment (Gosepath et al, 2005; Hytonen & Sala 1996; Hytonen et al, 1997; Litvyakova & Baraniuk, 2001; Loureiro, 2008). In a relevant study, 507 NPT were performed in 165 patients and the authors concluded that NPT is an essential, easy and safe tool in the diagnosis of allergic occupational rhinitis (Airaksinen et al, 2007). Recently, there has been a growing scientific interest in work-related rhinitis, because the relationship to asthma has been evaluated (Vandenplas, 2010). Considerations of the epidemiology of work-related rhinitis (both occupational rhinitis and work-exacerbated rhinitis) and its medico-legal implications have stressed the need to better identify this entity. Recent consensus have been presented to better define, classify and diagnosis occupational rhinitis, emphasizing the importance of NPT (EAACI Task Force on Occupational Rhinitis, 2008; Moscato et al, 2011; Dordal et al, 2011).

2.4 Investigational research

The applicability of NPT on investigational research is widely described in the literature, namely in the study of several aspects of allergic disease, namely the mechanisms of allergic reaction, the mechanisms of immunotherapy, the efficacy of new treatments and also in the study of the link between allergy and other morbidities, namely ENT diseases.

In a prospective controlled study, the possible role of nasal allergy in chronic disease of the maxillary sinuses was evaluated using NPT combined with radiography and ultrasonography (Pelikan, 2009). It was concluded that nasal allergy might be involved in some patients with chronic sinusitis. In these patients the NPT was a useful diagnostic tool and allowed to achieve a better diagnostic of co-morbidity and, consequently, therapeutic measures.

Otitis media with effusion (OME) is a very prevalent disease, particularly in children. The OME pathogenesis is considered multifactorial, and it has been related to viral upper respiratory tract infection and eustachian tube disfunction. Allergy has been implicated in OME pathogenesis by several authors, but it is a matter still controversial. It has been assumed that there is insufficient evidence of therapeutic efficacy or a causal relationship between allergy and OME. For instance, 123 children with OME (and 141 controls) were submitted to NPT. The prevalence of the allergic rhinitis in children with OME did not differ significantly when compared to control subjects, and the abnormalities in Eustachian tube function were the same in both groups (Yeo et al, 2007). A recent review of literature pointed to a strong possibility of allergy as a risk factor for OME. Thus patients with allergic rhinitis should be evaluated for OME and patients with OME should be considered for an allergy evaluation. Allergy should be treated aggressively in these patients, because OME has important and severe sequelae (Lack et al, 2011; Skoner et al, 2009). Our group studied 34 children with diagnosis of adenoids hypertrophy with or without OME, with 7.60±1.76

years. They were submitted to skin prick test with common aeroallergens battery. 24 were sensitized to *Dermatophagoides pteronyssinus*. The link between allergy and OME was evaluated in each patient with *Dermatophagoides pteronyssinus* specific NPT (BialAristegui, Bilbao, Spain). The NPT was monitored using symptom scores and it was considered positive if a total score ≥ 5. The NPT was positive in 20.8% of the sensitized children. The therapeutic management of these patients included immunotherapy with clinical improvement, supporting the link between allergy and OME in a subset of patients.

Concerning investigational research in the yield of the allergic disease, NPT has been widely used to better understand the underlying mechanisms. Pereira C, 2009 showed that the cell response starts at an early stage, in parallel with the immediate allergic response. The IgE mediated response induces immunolymphatic involvement of the adjacent structures. This amplifies the allergic response to locoregional lymphoid organs, while leukocyte recirculation involves the primary lymphoid organs (thymus and bone marrow). These central organs are responsible for the systemic immune response induced by a focused allergen challenge, in this case, a nasal challenge.

3. Nasal provocation test

The NPT is an "*in vivo*" diagnostic method that mimics the allergen natural exposure. The allergic reaction is triggered by allergenic exposure, and symptoms are recorded. Although not standardized, it is an extremely helpful method as it has several important indications in the diagnosis of allergic rhinitis (table 1), as described above. Indeed, specific allergen challenge tests are still the gold standard for allergic diseases diagnosis, being an important tool to assess the treatment outcomes. Moreover, they have been essential in research, namely in the progressive understanding of the pathophysiology, immunology and pharmacotherapy of allergic diseases.

The first allergen challenge was performed in 1873, by Blackley, who elicited a nasal response after an application of fresh pollen to the membrane of his own nostrils (Blackley, 1873). After this first NPT, several consensus and guidelines have been published trying to achieve a better diagnostic approach of allergic disease and its knowledge (Dordal et al, 2011; Druce & Schumacher, 1990; Gosepath et al, 2005; Litvyakova & Baraniuk, 2001, 2002; Lund et al, 1994; Malm et al, 2000; Mellilo et al, 1997; Schumacher, 1992).

3.1 Methodology

The anterior section of the inferior turbinate allows direct and visible application of the allergen extract, with consequent allergic reaction development (Dordal et al, 2011; Litvyakova & Baraniuk, 2001; Melilo et al, 1997; Naclerio & Norman, 1998). Despite the availability of the published international consensus guidelines, several difficulties are described in the assessment of the technique standardization, namely the type of allergen extracts to be used (lyophilized, aqueous or paper disc), the dose of allergen (which defaults to increase the doses) and the technique of administration of allergen (drops, micropipette to extract volumes, paper disks impregnated with solutions, nebulized extracts). The NPT should only be performed after a pharmacological washout period, namely H1-antihistamines, benzodiazepines, corticosteroids and mastocyte stabilizers. It should be performed at least 4 weeks after an undercurrent infectious disease and avoidance of exercise. Room conditions of temperature and humidity must be fulfilled. Aqueous solution and lyophilized powder are the most common commercial allergen extract presentations. In most studies it is administered unilaterally by various methods: spray (without propellant gas), instillation (pipette, dropper, syringe) or application of small pieces of cotton or paper discs with impregnated allergen. The use of different concentrations is recommended, therefore the dose-response could be evaluated and hence the real sensitivity to that allergen can be assessed. The starting dose for the NPT must be calculated from the minimum concentration used for skin prick tests that induces a wheal diameter of 3mm. Alternatively the initial concentration recommended could be 1 / 100 of the concentration that induced a positive skin prick test. After establishing the initial concentration, it should be scheduled a progressive increment of doses. All NPT should be initiated with the previous administration of saline, to evaluate a possible irritant effect. The interval between administrations of the allergen at different concentrations should be performed in 15 to 60 minutes. The terminus of the procedure occurs when there are symptoms of rhinitis or signs of mucosal inflammation. The application of the allergen must occur at the level of the previous section of the inferior turbinate, which is easily accessible, while the patient is asked a nasal expiration. The duration of expiration is not established, but the objective is to minimize bronchial inhalation. Several reviews in the literature analyse a variety of techniques and approaches, dosing and concentration of allergen extracts, delivery systems, and also the outcome-evaluation method (Dordal et al, 2011; Litvyakova & Baraniuk, 2001,2002; Tantilipikorn et al, 2010). In our experience we used commercial extracts prepared in an aqueous solution administered as a spray, directly to the anterior section of the inferior turbinate. The starting dose for the NPT was the concentration that induced a wheal diameter of 3mm in each patient.

3.2 Monitoring

The response to NPT is clinical and laboratory assessable. Several parameters could be used to evaluate the immediate and late allergic response, namely the symptoms score, the evaluation of nasal congestion (nasal Peak Inspiratory Flow Rate (nPIFR), rhinomanometry, acoustic rhinometry) and inflammatory cells / mediators analysis in nasal secretions, as reviewed in the published consensus. None of the methods that evaluate the response to NPT is standardized. In many publications the assessment of nasal response is based exclusively on symptom scores. Some authors suggested objective measurements together with symptom scoring. Thus, the response to NPT should be determined by the combination of symptom scores and / or rhinomanometry (Dordal et al, 2011; Litvyakova & Baraniuk, 2001).

3.2.1 Clinical symptom scores

Despite symptom scores is a qualitative and subjective method, it is the most used to evaluate the response to NPT, both in clinical practice and investigational research, since it mimics a spontaneous allergic response. To assess the nasal response to NPT, it could be used a score based on a visual analog scale (Bachert, 1997) or scales of semi-quantitative and subjective clinical assessments (Lebel et al, 1988; Linder, 1988). Usually our group uses the symptom scoring scaling according to Litvyakova & Baraniuk, 2001. Simple rating scales from 0 to 3 are used, for each nasal or non-nasal symptom, with defined criteria such as 0 = no symptoms, 1 = mild symptoms (symptoms that are present but not particularly bothersome), 2 = moderate symptoms (symptoms that are bothersome but do not interfere with daily activities), and 3 = severe symptoms (symptoms that are bothersome and interfere with daily activities or disturb sleep). Even though the known individual variability and the variability between patients, several authors have been tried to standardized the symptom score. In all reports, symptom scores are compared with objective parameters, supporting the relevance of the use of the symptom score in the monitoring of NPT. For instance, 155 patients with allergic rhinitis to *Dermatophagoides* were submitted to NPT to evaluate the optimal cut-off values of symptom changes after NPT for predicting perennial allergic rhinitis, as well as the nPIFR evaluation (Chusakul et al, 2010). In another study, the symptom score change and acoustic rhinometry values were combined, before and after NPT in 208 patients with allergic rhinitis and in 222 controls (Kim & Jang, 2011).

3.2.2 Methods to evaluate nasal congestion: Nasal Peak Inspiratory flow rate, rhinomanometry and acoustic rhinometry

The assessment of nasal congestion could be evaluated by subjective parameters (symptom score) and by an objective and quantitative method. Several techniques are available for assessing changes in nasal airflow resistance, patency, and nasal cavity geometry. Such techniques provide objective measurement of nasal congestion, namely nPIFR, rhinomanometry and acoustic rhinometry. These methods provide an objective and quantitative measurement whose value is based on the comparison of results over procedures (diagnostic or therapeutic) in each individual. In spite of this, standardized methodologies assessing functional abnormalities are not sufficiently developed (Nathan et al, 2005). Comparison of results between different patients is not yet standardized. Recently, several studies have been tried to standardize these methods as they can be useful in clinical practice and applied as a diagnostic tool in allergic rhinitis (Chusakul et al, 2010; Kim & Jang, 2011).

Nasal Peak Inspiratory Flow Rate. This technique assesses the nasal airflow. It is easy to perform and inexpensive, but it is difficult to reproduce because is partially dependent on lung capacity (Wihl & Malm, 1988). Some studies demonstrated that nPIFR values correlate with airway resistance, but this is impracticable in case of intense rhinorrea (Holmstrom et al, 1990; Jones et al, 1991).

Rhinomanometry. This standardized technique measures the resistance to the airflow in nasal cavities (Schumacher, 1989). Increases in resistance in one or both nasal cavities have been considered as an objective parameter in positive responses to NPT (Clement, 1984; Kirerleri et al, 2006). The technique depends on patient cooperation and it cannot be used in cases of septum perforation, intense rhinorrhea or nasal obstruction (Nathan et al, 2005).

Acoustic rhinometry. This is a sound-based technique used to evaluate the nasal geometry, which measures nasal cavity area and volume. It has been validated by comparison to measurements with computed tomography and magnetic resonance imaging. It is used to diagnose and evaluate therapeutic responses in conditions such as rhinitis and to measure nasal dimensions during NPT (Keck et al, 2006; Kim et al, 2008; Uzzaman et al, 2006). Acoustic rhinometry is easy to perform and reproducible, but there are no reference values (Corey et al, 1998). It requires little cooperation from the patient, so it could be a useful method for children, and it is not affected by the presence of rhinorrhea or intense nasal obstruction. However, it cannot be applied in cases of septal perforation. Some interpretation caution should be made, when assessing changes in NPT. The nasal cavity volume between 2 cm and 6 cm is the most important parameter, because it corresponds to

the head of the turbinate, while the nasal cavity volume between 6 cm and 10 cm provides information about the sinuses and ostia. The intrinsic bias of the nasal cycle should not be overlooked, consequently, the cross-sectional areas and volumes of both nasal cavities should be measured after NPT (Gotlib et al, 2005).
When comparing both techniques, acoustic rhinometry does not seem to be a better diagnostic method than active rhinomanometry in the monitoring of NPT (Keck et al, 2006).

3.2.3 Laboratorial measurements: Inflammatory allergic mediators and cells

The analysis of nasal cytology is essential to distinguish non-inflammatory from inflammatory nasal diseases. Additionally, the pattern of inflammatory mediators reflects the underlying immunological response. So the analysis of these inflammatory allergic mediators and cells are useful in the assessment of the response to NPT, namely in the diagnosis of allergic disease and in the evaluation of the treatment efficacy. Indeed, the NPT has been used to characterize and to clarify the immunological mechanisms involved in allergic reaction, and reciprocally, known inflammatory allergic mediators and cells have also been used to diagnose allergic rhinitis (for example local allergic rhinitis, as mentioned above) and to monitor the response to NPT. Allergic rhinitis is an allergen-induced IgE-mediated inflammatory disease of the nasal mucosa. Several inflammatory mediators (histamine, tryptase, ECP, leucotrienes, cytokines and chemokines) are involved and the cellular infiltrate is characterized of mast cells, basophils, eosinophils and T cells. The usefulness of nasal cytology depends on several factors, namely obtaining adequate specimens, appropriate samples staining, and the materials interpretation.

3.2.3.1 Methods to collect nasal samples

Various techniques have been used for obtaining, processing, evaluating, and interpreting nasal specimens. The different methods for collecting samples are nasal lavage, nasal swab, nasal brushing, nasal curettage, nasal biopsy and collection of nasal secretions, allowing the assay of cells and inflammatory mediators. Several comparative studies show the usefulness of these non-standardized different methods. Each technique has advantages and disadvantages, so the selection of each method must be carefully decided. Description of the different techniques was reviewed elsewhere, in detail. (Dordal et al, 2011; Howarth et al, 2005).
Nasal lavage. Naclerio first described this technique (Naclerio et al; 1983). This is a frequently used method to collect and to identify cells and inflammatory mediators. It has been used in research studies. In addition to nasal lavage, the collection of nasal secretions could be analyzed to look for both cellular and inflammatory mediators.
Nasal brushing and Nasal biopsy should be performed on the inferior turbinate, to obtain cellular samples. Nasal brushing is usually performed at the middle third of the inferior turbinate, with easy sampling of the superficial of nasal mucosa. Nasal biopsy is usually performed on the lower part of the inferior turbinate, requires anaesthesia, and reaches deeper tissues. However it cannot be systematically repeated because it is traumatic.

3.2.3.2 Difficulties in assessment of inflammatory response

These techniques helped to attain the actual knowledge about the characteristics of allergic disease. However, its usefulness in the evaluation of the response to NPT is restricted to research trials, in order to better understand immunological allergic mechanisms and effects of new therapies. In clinical practice, the assessment of these inflammatory parameters is not enough to evaluate the response to NPT.

In our Immunoallergy Department, we performed a study to evaluate the concentrations of the chemokines, eotaxin and RANTES, in nasal lavage and analyze the applicability of the determination of chemokines in nasal secretions as a parameter of immune response to specific nasal provocation test (Loureiro et al, 2003). We included 17 patients with allergic rhinitis to *Parietaria judaica* (64% male; 36.3±11.2 years old). All the patients were submitted to NPT with *Parietaria judaica* commercial extract (Leti, Madrid, Spain) outside the pollen season. Nasal lavages were performed, before, 30 minutes and 6 hours after NPT, for quantification of inflammatory mediators. NPT response was monitored through symptom score. The NPT was positive in all patients, reproducing the clinical reactivity to the allergen, with a peak in the symptom scores at the first minute with subsequent decreasing till the sixth hour. Eotaxin was not measurable in any of the nasal lavage specimens collected. The chemokine RANTES levels were 4.2±2.1pg/ ml before NPT and 3.96±0.98 pg/ml and 3.90±0.99 pg/ml in the specimens collected at 30 minutes and 6 hours after NPT respectively. These results did not correlate with symptoms progression during NPT. This could be interpreted as a discrepancy between the time of sampling and the dynamics of inflammatory mediators in response to NPT.

In the same group of patients, during the same procedure, we also analysed the tryptase and ECP levels, in nasal lavage, as immunological markers of immediate and late response in allergic reaction, respectively (Loureiro et al, 2004). Tryptase was detected in only three patients. Nasal brushings were also performed to harvest cells. Cellular phenotyping (CD3, CD4, CD8 and CD 125) was assayed by flow citometry, before and 6 hours after NPT, to recognize the cellular dynamics during NPT. Our findings showed an increase in CD3 and CD8 cells in all patients. In a subset of patients submitted to immunotherapy we observed a CD4 cells increase and a CD125 cells decrease, after NPT, while the other patients not submitted to immunotherapy does not showed any dynamic alterations in these cells (figure 1). The differences observed in each group could be explained by different therapeutic approaches in each group. However the dynamic cellular changes after NPT were not as expected. These findings could be explained by premature sampling before cellular trafficking occurred. Another possible explanation is the insufficiency of these sampling methods to harvest the sufficient cellular infiltrate.

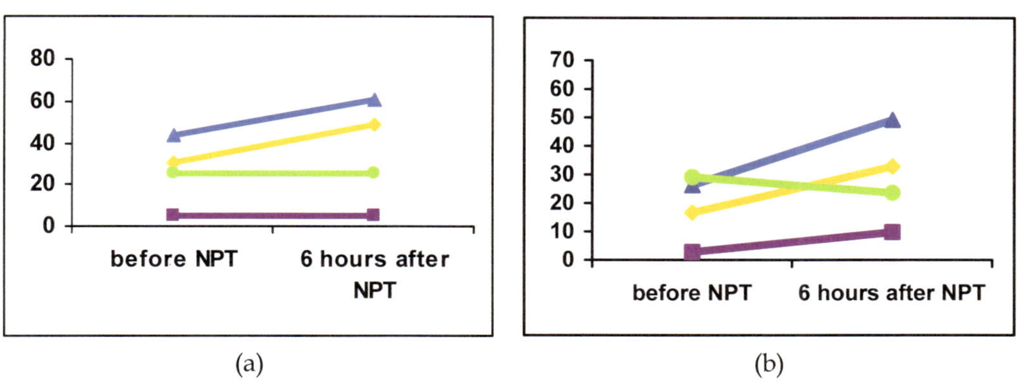

Fig. 1. Nasal cell typing before and after nasal provocation test (NPT) (% of cells): A - in a group of patients submitted to immunotherapy for one year; B - in a group of patients not submitted to immunotherapy (Legend: ▲ - CD3; ■ - CD4; ♦ -CD8; ● - CD125)

In another study conducted by our group, 21 allergic patients were submitted to *Dermatophagoides pteronyssinus* specific NPT (BialAristegui, Bilbao, Spain). Secretions, namely tears and nasal secretions, were collected after NPT and inflammatory mediators, such as interleukins and chemokines were measured (data not published). These inflammatory mediators were measurable only in 21% of the tear samples and in 71.5% of the nasal secretion samples. According to these findings, nasal secretions recovery could be acceptable to be considered as an objective tool in the evaluation of inflammatory mediators. However we could not find out a pattern of mediator release since the inflammatory mediators were inconsistently detected in the different samples.

Although the analysis of immunological parameters has been described as an objective approach to monitor the response to NPT, in our experience, these laboratorial measurements are difficult to perform because of the scheduling of sampling. Additionally, the cost-effectiveness of these procedures does not allow its implementation in the clinical practice. It should be reserved to investigational research.

3.2.4 Assessment on nasal Nitric Oxide

Determination of nasal Nitric Oxide (nNO) provides an indirect measure of the inflammation of the nasal mucosa. A decrease in nNO levels with NPT coincided with maximal symptom intensity, in five patients with pollen-induced allergic rhinitis (Kharitonov et al, 1997). Although nNO promises as a diagnostic non-invasive management tool, its value in nasal pathology is still not clear, mainly due to the lack of standardization of the test. Different methods of measurement have been used in published studies and the results reported are not comparable (Dordal et al, 2011).

3.3 Criteria for positive NPT

Besides diverse combined criteria have been discussed in the literature none of them are standardized criteria to define NPT positivity. This is summarized in the Table 2.

4. NPT as a diagnostic approach in respiratory allergy

The first allergen provocation test was performed in 1873, by Blackley, who elicited a nasal response after an application of fresh pollen to the membrane of his own nostrils (Blackley, 1873). Currently, the indications of NPT are widely known. In this manuscript, the applicability of NPT as a diagnostic tool of allergic rhinitis was discussed. But the usefulness of NPT is not restricted to the diagnostic approach of allergic rhinitis. Supported by the concept of *"one airway, one disease"*, several studies have pointed out that the NPT is a good alternative to Bronchial Provocation Test (BPT), even in the absence of nasal symptoms. In spite of BPT being a standardized diagnostic tool, it is not frequently used in clinical practice because of its technically and methodologically requirement. Indeed, NPT is safer and better tolerated

Reference	Assessment of nasal response	Description of positivity criteria
Hytonen et al, 1997	Symptom score	$\Delta \geq 4$, considering Δ = (obstruction score + rhinorrhea score) after NPT - (obstruction score + rhinorrhea score)
Lebel B et al, 1988	Symptom score	Lebel Symptom Score Scale: Positive if ≥ 5 (maximum possible score 11 points)

Reference	Assessment of nasal response	Description of positivity criteria
Linder A, 1988	Symptom score	Linder Symptom Score Scale: Positive if ≥ 5 (maximum possible score 13 points)
Terrien et al, 1999	nPIFR assessment	Fall in nPIFR ≥ 40%
Cimarra & Robledo, 2001	Rhinomanometry	Airflow resistance increases by 100%
Valero & Picado, 2000	Acoustic rhinometry	MCA and nasal cavity volume vary by 25-30%
Álvarez Eire et al, 2006	Combined symptom score and nPIFR	At least two of the following criteria: five sneezing, runny nose, nasal congestion documented by a decrease ≥ 20% of nPIFR
Gosepath et al, 2005	Combined symptom score and rhinomanometry	A 40% reduction in airflow at 150 Pa in active anterior rhinomanometry, regardless of the symptom score, or a 20% reduction of in airflow at 150 Pa with a symptom score of more than 2
Rondón C et al, 2007	Combined symptom score and acoustic rhinometry	a 30% increase in the symptom score using a visual analog scale and a 30% reduction in nasal cavity volume by acoustic rhinometry
Kim & Jang, 2011	Combined symptom score and acoustic rhinometry	1) symptom score change: more than 2 points in the case of nasal obstruction and more than 1 point for the case of rhinorrea or itching; 2) more than 24.5% change of total nasal volume and 3) more than 20% change of the minimal cross-sectional area.
Wihl, 1986	Combined nasal secretions amount and nPIFR	0.5 mL (0.5 g) of nasal secretion with 5 or more sneezes and a >20% reduction in nPIFR
Pirila & Nuutinen, 1998	Combined nasal secretions amount, rhinomanometry and acoustic rhinometry	30 minutes after NPT: 100 mg of nasal secretion with a 15% decrease in MCA and 50% increase in nasal airflow resistance; 60 minutes after NPT: 210 mg of nasal secretion with a 30% decrease in MCA and 100% increase in nasal airflow resistance
Ganslmayer et al, 1999	Combined acoustic rhinometry and nPIFR	29% decrease in MCA and 26% decrease in nPIFR

Table 2. Some criteria do define NPT positivity, adapted from Dordal et al, 2011.

method in asthmatic patients than BPT (Hervás et al, 2011; Marcucci *et al*, 2007; Oddera *et al*, 1998). So, NPT has been used to the diagnosis of asthma, as reviewed by Olive Pérez, 1997. Thus, based on the *united airways disease* concept, the NPT could be considered as a model of specific provocation test that is easy and quick to perform, in the demonstration of the immediate and late phase response of type I hypersensitivity reaction. It is well known that the nose is an integral part of the upper airway, and anatomically related to several airway structures, such as ears and paranasal sinuses, and as well the eyes. There is an epidemiological relationship between rhinitis and asthma. Rhinitis and asthma are often associated, rhinitis typically precedes the development of asthma and can contribute to insufficient asthma control (Compalati et al, 2010). On the other hand, in cross-sectional and longitudinal studies, the vast majority of patients with asthma have rhinitis, and rhinitis is a major independent risk factor for asthma (Togias, 2003). Treating allergic rhinitis would probably ameliorate other associated upper airway diseases such as acute rhinosinusitis, nasal polyposis, adenoidal hypertrophy, and OME (Marple, 2010). In addition to improve allergic rhinitis outcome, the treatment of subjacent inflammatory disorder reduces asthma-associated health care consuming. A close interaction between the nose and contiguous or distant organs was described and it has been progressively clarified, supporting this epidemiological and clinical relation (Baroody, 2011). The upper and lower airways are not anatomically and functionally distinct areas (Slavin, 2008). It is currently established that the impaired function of the upper airways causing nasal obstruction, retention of secretions, and disturbed conditioning of the inspired air plays an important role in the development of lower airway symptoms (Virchow, 2005). There are important relationships between both the nose and the paranasal sinuses and asthma. Apart from the intrinsic physiological interaction, extensive evidence exists to sustain the concept that the respiratory system functions as an integrated unit (Krouse, 2008), where rhinitis and asthma are manifestations of one syndrome, the chronic allergic respiratory syndrome, in both parts of the respiratory tract (Togias, 2003). It has been described that parallel immunopathological processes involve the upper airway generally occur in conjunction with lower airway diseases, and diffuse inflammation often affects mucosal surfaces of the middle ear, nose, sinuses, and tracheobronchial tree simultaneously (Krouse, 2008). Recent studies show that the deposition of allergen into the lower respiratory tract leads to increased inflammation of the upper respiratory tract, even if the patients are only suffering from allergic rhinitis (Virchow, 2005). Additionally, studies indicate that treatment of the upper respiratory tract inflammation reduces the manifestation of allergen-associated symptoms in the lower respiratory tract, and also have preventive effects if started early on the disease evolution (Bousquet & ARIA Workshop Group, 2001). Both asthma and allergic rhinitis have now been recognized as inflammatory diseases with similar manifestations in the mucous membranes of the upper (nose and paranasal sinuses) and lower respiratory tract (Virchow, 2005). There is increasing evidence that even in patients with rhinitis who do not have asthma, sub-clinical changes in the lower airways and inflammatory mediators can be detected (Compalati et al, 2010). These and other findings support that allergic diseases have a systemic component (Virchow, 2005). The interactive mechanisms of allergic rhinitis and associated conditions highlights the relevance of a bidirectional "unified airway" respiratory inflammation model. Currently, it is accepted that IgE mediated allergic reactions are not confined to the area where the trigger occurred, inducing a secondary systemic immune response (Braunstahl, 2005, 2006; Togias, 2004). The systemic inflammation is produced after local allergic reactions (Togias, 2003). The link between local exposure to allergen and distant response has been clarified. Although some authors defend that this systemic response could result from allergen entering in the systemic circulation from the local of exposure (Hens et al, 2007) this could activate circulating basophils, inducing an anaphylactic reaction, which is a rare condition (Togias, 2004). Both systemic cell circulation and the nervous system activation are two major ways through which local allergic reactions propagate. Mast cell mediators locally released, increase the expression of adhesion molecules on postcapillary venules. This can lead to homing of circulating leukocytes, which may infiltrate distant tissues. This cell recirculation and focalization makes the IgE mediated allergic disease a dynamic and systemic process. Pereira C showed that this cell response starts at an early stage, in parallel with the immediate allergic response (Pereira, 2009). The IgE mediated response induces immunolymphatic involvement of the adjacent structures. This amplifies the allergic response to loco-regional lymphoid organs, while circulating leukocytes recirculation compromises the primary lymphoid organs (thymus and bone marrow). These central organs are responsible for the systemic immune response induced by a localized allergen challenge, in this case, a nasal challenge (Pereira, 2009). The nervous system activation could be involved by, any or both pathways, namely neurogenic inflammation and neuronal reflexes. Neurogenic inflammation is characterized by specific neuromediators closely related to neuro-immune-endocrine system, and it is both a stimulus to and a consequence of allergic inflammation. The naso-nasal and the naso-ocular reflexes are some examples of the role of the nervous system in the propagation of the allergic disease. They seem to be predominantly mediated by parasympathetic and cholinergic pathways, respectively (Baroody et al, 1994, 2008). Histamine release during the acute response to allergen and substance P seem to have an important role in these neural mechanisms (Baroody et al, 1994, 2008; Fujishima et al 1997; Micera et al, 2008; O'Meara et al, 2005; Sheahan et al, 2005). Multiple evidences support a close interaction and influence of the nose on contiguous and distant organs via neural reflex and systemic inflammatory processes (Baroody, 2011). In summary, a local triggered allergenic inflammation is systematically extended, with the early connection of the immune central organs. Independently of the involved pathway, immediate symptoms are clinically manifested.

Besides the limitations of NPT, this is a feasible and easily method to be performed, since the nasal cavities provide easy access to specific provocation. The concept of "*One airway, one disease*" allows assuming the similarity of response to the provocation of both the upper and lower airways, so the nasal allergic reaction could be accepted as predictor of bronchial response. Supported by the concept of the bidirectional "unified airway" respiratory inflammation, a local provocation test is useful in the diagnosis of allergic respiratory disease. Concerning these aspects, the NPT is the method of choice for the reproducibility of the allergic reaction (Litvyakova & Baraniuk, 2001; Loureiro, 2001; Mellilo, 1997; Naclerio & Norman, 1998). Thus the NPT may be considered a model of respiratory provocation test, easy to perform, in the demonstration of the immediate and late phase of type I hypersensitivity reaction.

5. Characterization of NPT score symptom response

According to all the mentioned above, the clinical symptom score is widely used in clinical practice, alone or associated to objective measurements of nasal obstruction, namely nPIFR,

rhinomanometry and acoustic rhinometry. The other methods, such as immunological measurements, should be reserved to research procedures related to the investigation of inflammatory network. However, due to the lack of standardization of parameters in the monitoring of NPT response, its reproducibility remains to be defined. The main problem includes the great variability of the responses in each patient and between patients. Although this is an important limitation, concerning NPT response interpretation, the symptom score has been used in the description of positive criteria to NPT response.
As pointed out above, many authors use the symptom score as a method of monitoring and criteria for positivity in response to the NPT. According to the great variability in each patient and between patients, it has been assumed the absence of pattern of response to the NPT. The attempt to standardize this methodology was characterized by the symptom score quantification, through the use of symptoms scaling. One of the most important limitations of this symptoms scaling, is the overemphasis on nasal obstruction, since firstly not all patients value the perception of this symptom, and secondly, when it is present, it can result from concomitant obstructive and inflammatory causes. Besides there is no clinical pattern of response to NPT, our data showed a response profile, which can not be accepted as standard, but it can be useful in monitoring the NPT, namely in the evaluation of the dynamics of the response to NPT, as described bellow.

5.1 Clinical symptom score pattern

In our experience, the symptom score has supported the positivity of NPT. We analysed that the most frequent and intense symptoms occurred within the first 30 minutes after NPT, agreeing to immediate phase of allergic reaction. From all the studies conducted by our group, we did not observe a clinical score symptom pattern. However, we describe a clinical symptom score profile, which was frequent and was characterized by the presence of nasal and extra-nasal symptoms within the first 30 minutes, with a peak at 5 minutes.

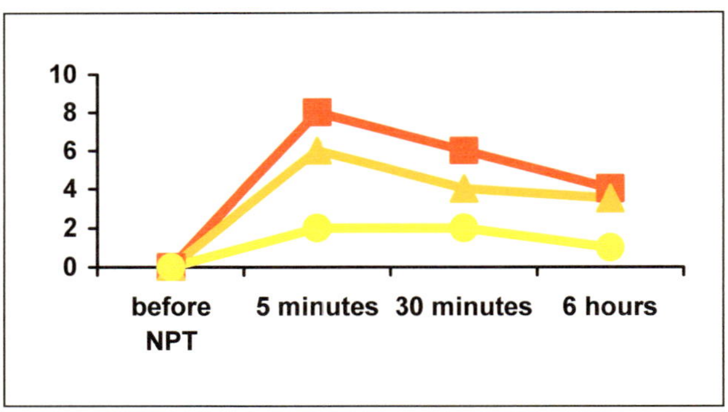

Fig. 2. Score symptoms after *Parietaria judaica* specific nasal provocation test (NPT) (legend: ■ total score; ▲ nasal score; ● non-nasal score).

Indeed, in a group of patients allergic to *Parietaria judaica*, as described above, specific NPT was performed and a symptom score was recorded. The figure 2 presents the total, nasal and non-nasal symptom scores. The higher total score of symptoms was recorded at the fifth minute with progressively decreasing symptoms till 30 minutes and then till 6 hours. Each nasal symptom followed this pattern. The non-nasal symptoms showed a different pattern, having a lower score, with similar values at both the fifth and the 30th minutes, followed by a decline till 6 hours. Looking at the score of each nasal symptom (Figure 3), except for nasal obstruction, all of them followed the response pattern of total symptoms score, with a peak of symptoms at the fifth minute. Sneezing was the predominant symptom at the fifth minute, while nasal obstruction was the predominant symptom at the 30th minute and the sixth hour.

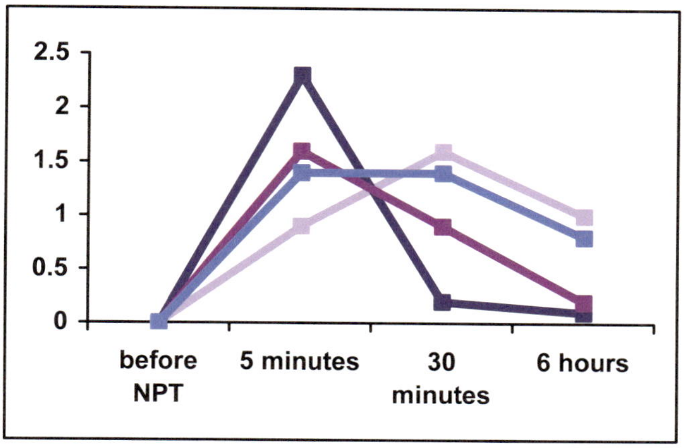

Fig. 3. Nasal symptom score after specific *Parietaria judaica* nasal provocation test (NPT): evolution of each nasal symptom (Legend: ■ nasal congestion; ■ pruritus; ■ sneezing; ■ rhinorrea).

In another study mentioned above, the *Dermatophagoides pteronyssinus* specific NPT were performed in 34 children with OME. Those who had positive NPT, showed a response dynamics characterized by a rapid increase of symptoms score till a peak at the 5th minute (monitored till 1 hour), as shown in figure 4. Looking at the score of each nasal symptom (Figure 5), except for nasal pruritus, all followed the response pattern of total symptoms score, with the peak of symptoms at the fifth minute.

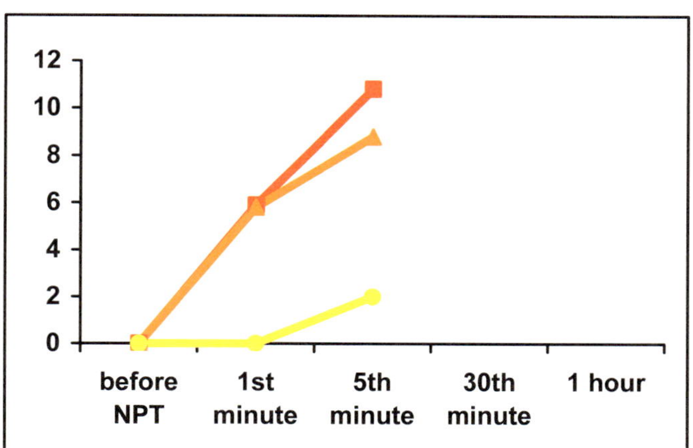

Fig. 4. Score symptoms after *Dermatophagoides pteronyssinus* specific nasal provocation test (NPT); (Legend: ■ total score; ▲ nasal score; ● non-nasal score).

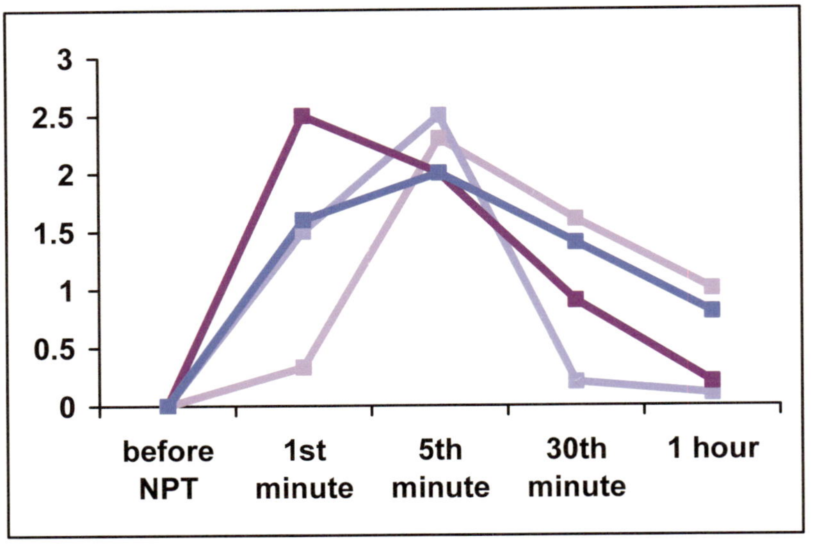

Fig. 5. Nasal symptom score after specific *Dermatophagoides pteronyssinus* nasal provocation test (NPT): evolution of each nasal symptom (Legend: nasal congestion; pruritus; sneezing; rhinorrea).

Beyond the description of symptoms score obtained during NPT, it is also important to compare them with the usual symptoms described by the patient. This looks particularly relevant in the diagnosis of local allergic rhinitis.

In our study related to local allergic rhinitis diagnosis, we included 15 patients with typical clinical symptoms of perennial rhinitis, negative skin prick test to common aeroallergens and negative specific IgE, as mentioned above (Loureiro G et al, 2011). The patients had an average age of 22.2±14.8 years, 77.7% were female. A *Dermatophagoides pteronyssinus* specific NPT was performed with clinical monitoring. Total nasal symptom scores were assessed using a validated questionnaire and a positive challenge was considered if a score of five or greater was recorded. NPT supported the diagnosis of local allergic rhinitis in a group of patients previously diagnosed with "non-allergic rhinitis". They presented a period of symptoms evolution of 5.37±3.9 years. The symptom scores reported during natural exposure and after NPT are shown in figure 6. During natural exposure, the nasal total score was 6.2±2.05. Nasal congestion was always reported and it had the highest recorded value (2.8±0.35). The highest nasal recorded value during NPT was 6.4±2.19. Nasal congestion and pruritus were always reported and this second symptom had the higher recorded value (2.4±0.5). None of the 15 patients had conjunctivitis or asthma. Furthermore, in the 8 patients that had positive NPT, extra-nasal symptoms were recorded, namely conjunctival symptoms, oropharyngeal pruritus, cough and dyspnea, although with lower values.

Concerning the occurrence of non-nasal symptoms, the major non-nasal symptoms observed were those localized in the conjunctiva, followed by oropharyngeal pruritus. Dyspnea and cough were recognized rarely. Non-nasal symptoms were documented in 20 up to 100% of the positive NPT performed, considering the different studies conducted in our Immunoallergy Department.

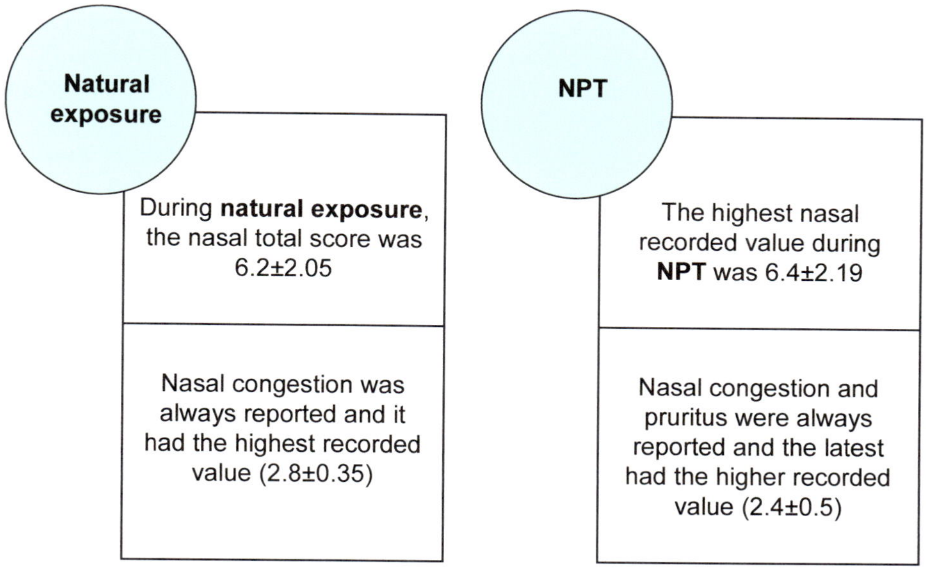

Fig. 6. Symptom scores reported during natural exposure and after nasal provocation test (NPT).

5.2 Comparison of *Dermatophagoides pteronyssinus* nasal provocation test *versus* conjunctiva provocation test

Our group and others authors have been using clinical scores to evaluate NPT response. According to our findings described previously, in respect to the symptoms scores pattern in response to NPT, we conducted a study to characterize the clinical response to NPT comparing to conjunctiva provocation test (CPT). As CPT is easy to perform and systemic reactions are uncommon, some authors have studied the concordance between NPT and CPT in the diagnosis of allergic rhinitis (Andersen et al, 1996; Leonardi et al, 1993; Malmberg et al, 1978; Petersson et al, 1986; Riechelmann et al, 2003) and asthma (Mosbech et al, 1987) using clinical score symptoms and/or objective methods. However, we are not aware of any publication describing the clinical pattern of NPT and CPT responses, neither about its comparison.

Our aim was to compare the dynamics of clinical responses induced by NPT and CPT, using a clinical score system.

5.2.1 Material and methods

5.2.1.1 Subjects

We studied two groups of voluntary adult patients, referred to our outpatient Immunoallergy Department, with *Dermatophagoides pteronyssinus* (*Dp*) allergic rhinitis/rhinoconjunctivitis with or without associated bronchial asthma, according to ARIA (Bousquet & ARIA Workshop Group, 2001) and GINA guidelines, respectively. All patients were clinically stable at the time of the study. Patients with past or ongoing immunotherapy for *Dermatophagoides*, an exacerbation of allergic disease or a respiratory tract infection in the last month, a nasal surgery in the last 3 months or nasal pathology such as polyps or a deviated nasal septum, were excluded. H1-antihistamines and costicosteroids, either nasal or oral, were withheld for 2 weeks and 4 weeks prior to the challenge test, respectively. All patients underwent the challenge between January and February of 2009, a period of low natural exposure to mites in Portugal. A *Dp* NPT was performed in 21 patients and the conjunctival provocation test (CPT) was performed in the other 21 patients. The local ethics committee approved the study and all the participants gave written informed consent before entry. A respiratory function test (pletismography using *Master screen Body Jaeger®*) was performed by all the participants, before specific provocation tests, with all presenting a baseline $FEV_1 \geq 80\%$ and $FEV_1/FVC \geq 80$. After provocation, all patients were asked for the presence of dyspnoea, thoracic oppression, wheezing or cough.

5.2.1.2 Specific nasal and conjuctival provocation tests

A skin prick test aqueous extract of *Dp* with a 5 mg/ml concentration (23 µg/ml of *Der p* 1, BialAristegui, Bilbao, Spain), with 1/1, 1/10, 1/100 and 1/1000 dilutions were performed; negative and positive controls were performed in all patients, according to standardized procedures (Dreborg & Frew A, 1993). The concentration used to specific provocation was the minimum that induced a prick test wheal at least equal to that induced by histamine, which curiously was the 1/10 dilution in all patients. Specific NPT with *Dp* extract were performed in the morning and after an adaptation to room temperature for 30 minutes, in both groups. NPT was performed with unilateral nasal application of 2 consecutives puffs (total volume of 160 µl) of the *Dp* extract to the inferior nasal turbinate of the less congested nostril, using a nasal applicator spraying and patients were asked to perform apnoea during the allergen spraying. CPT consisted in unilateral ocular application of 1 drop (50 µl) of the *Dp* extract in the inferior and external quadrant of the bulbar conjunctiva. Nasal and eye symptoms were recorded at the 1st and 5th minutes after specific provocation tests, using a clinical score system to assess the response (Linder A, 1988).

5.2.1.3 Clinical score scaling

Clinical responses were evaluated using a nasal clinical score (NCS) and an ocular clinical score (OCS), at the 1st and the 5th minutes. An adaptation of the previously used NCS (Linder A, 1988) and OCS (Mortemousque, 2007) were applied. A total clinical score (TCS), representing the sum of NCS (range: 0-15) and OCS (range: 0-13) was also used, ranging from 0 to 28 points. Rhinorrhea, sneezing, itchy nose, itchy ear/throat, nasal obstruction, watery eyes, redness of eyes and burning of eyes were rated on a scale from 0 to 3 points (0, none; 1, mild; 2, moderate; 3, severe). Itchy eyes were scored from 0 to 4 points (0, none; 1, mild; 2, moderate; 3, severe; 4, very severe). A positive response to NPT was considered when NCS ≥ 3 (Linder A, 1988) and to CPT when OCS ≥ 5 (Mortemousque, 2007). Clinical evaluation was interrupted after the 5th minute to collect humours for further investigation to determine inflammatory markers within a research investigation of immunologic mechanisms in allergic disease (Pereira, 2011, *in press*).

5.2.1.4 Statistical analysis

Statistical analysis were performed using SPSS® Statistics 17.0 software. Comparisons between NPT and CPT were studied using Chi-Square test. Intra-groups differences between the 1st and the 5th minutes after provocation were analyzed using a Mann-Whitney U-test. A statistical significant difference was assumed with $p < 0.05$.

5.2.2 Results

Demographical and clinical data are presented in Table 3. Table 4 shows the number of patients that presented nasal and ocular responses at the 5th minute, induced by NPT and CPT, as well as the number of positive challenges at the 1st and the 5th minutes. A progressive increase in clinical score was observed in both provocations. The NPT progressive response was linear while for the CPT it was exponential, as shown in figures 7. CPT response was stronger than NPT at the 5th minute, achieving borderline significance (p=0.05). Clinical score results for NPT and CPT are shown in Table 5.

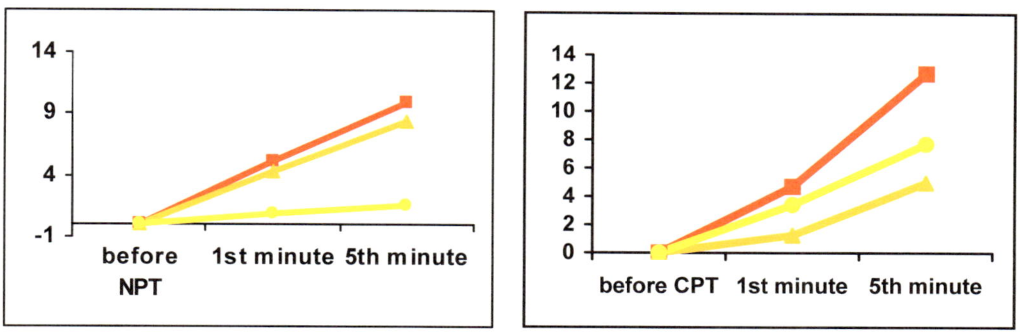

(a) (b)

Fig. 7. Dynamics of symptoms score in response to: A – NPT (Linear progression); B – CPT (Exponential progression) Legend: ■ - Total Symptom score; ▲ - Nasal symptom score; ● - Non-nasal symptom score)

The most frequent symptoms were nasal obstruction, itchy ear/throat and itchy nose, for NPT, and ocular hyperaemia and burning eyes, for CPT in all patients. In NPT, nasal obstruction was observed in 100% of the group. CPT induced ocular hyperaemia and burning eyes in all patients. There were neither bronchial symptoms nor systemic reactions in any of the provocation tests.

The highest scores were reached by nasal obstruction and rhinorrhea in NPT and by ocular hyperaemia in CPT. The average intensity of each sign/symptom at the 5th minute is shown in figure 8.

	NPT	CPT
n	21	21
Average age (years)	28.0 ± 9.0	28.1 ± 5.7
Gender ♀ (%)	57.1	66.7
Rhinitis (n)	20	16
Rhinoconjunctivitis (n)	1	5
Associated asthma (%)	42.8	90.5
Cutaneous reactivity to Dp (mm)	6.5 ± 2.1	8.6 ± 3.6
Specific IgE to Dp (KU/L)	29 ± 24.9	36.3 ± 37.2
Disease evolution (years)	13 ± 10	12.3 ± 8.5

Table 3. Demographical and clinical data of patients submitted to NPT and CPT (Legend: NPT – nasal provocation test; CPT – conjunctiva provocation test)

	NPT	CPT	*p*
Nasal response at 5th min Ocular response at 5th min	21 (100%) 10 (47.6%)	20 (95.2%) 21 (100%)	ns 0.0001
Number of positive challenges: 1st min 5th min	 15 21	 6 21	0.005

Table 4. Frequency of nasal and ocular symptoms at the 5th minute and NPT and CPT outcomes at the 1st and the 5th minutes (Legend: NPT - nasal provocation test; CPT - conjunctiva provocation test; ns - not significant).

Comparing NPT and CPT, in the first one the response was faster at the 1st minute (p=0.005) while for CPT it was stronger at the 5th minute (p=0.05).
Although the inoculation of allergen was unilateral, NPT induced bilateral nasal symptoms in 100% and bilateral ocular symptoms in 47.6%. On the other hand, CPT induced unilateral ocular symptoms in 100% and bilateral nasal symptoms in 95.2%. There were neither bronchial symptoms nor systemic reactions.

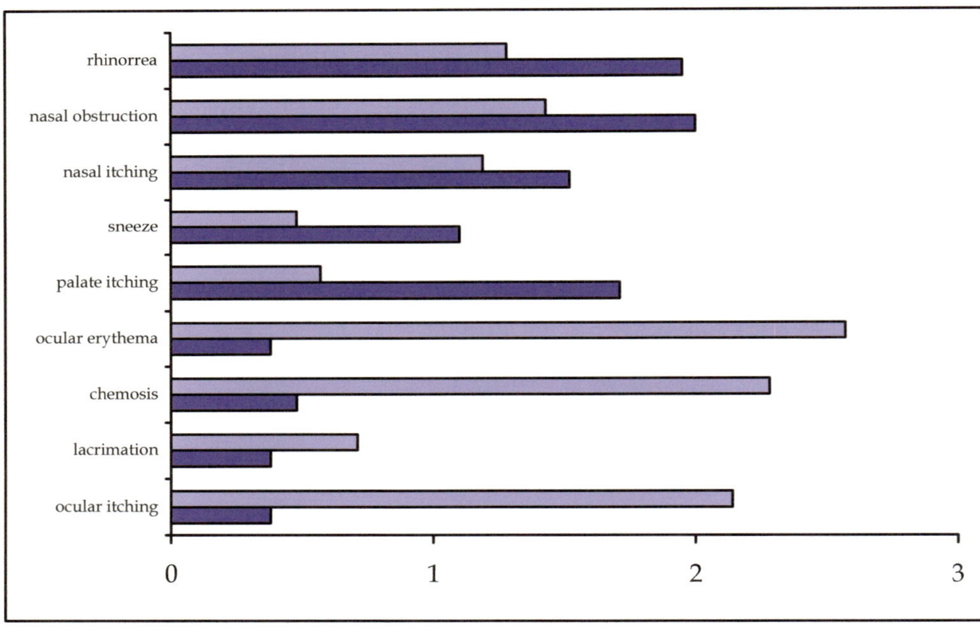

Fig. 8. The average intensity of each sign/symptom at the 5th minute; (Legend: ■ - Nasal provocation test; ■ - Conjunctiva provocation test)

5.2.3 Discussion

Although the importance of the objective monitoring of specific provocation tests is unquestionable, its applicability in clinical practice is not always possible. Usually it is limited to the evaluation of only one symptom, such as nasal patency by nasal peak flow, acoustic rhinometry and/or rhinomanometry (Nathan et al, 2005); however it is not always the most perceived symptom by patients. Clinical scoring systems, even though more subjective, reflect

	NPT	CPT	p
Total			
1st min	5.2 ± 3.8	4.7 ± 3.6	ns
5th min	9.9 ± 4.4	12.7 ± 4.4	ns (0.05)
5th - 1st	4.6 ± 4.57	8.0 ± 3.87	0.011
Nasal (NCS)			
1st min	4.28 ± 2.6	1.24 ± 2.1	<0.0001
5th min	8.29 ± 2.9	4.95 ± 2.8	0.001
Ocular (OCS)			
1st min	0.95 ± 1.8	3.4 ± 3	<0.0001
5th min	1.57 ± 2.3	7.7 ± 3	<0.0001

Table 5. Clinical score results for NPT and CPT (Legend: NPT – nasal provocation test; CPT – conjunctiva provocation test; ns – not significant).

all symptoms, are easy and costless to apply in clinical practice. The validity and reproducibility of CPT based on clinical score systems were demonstrated in several studies (Abelson et al, 1990; Moller et al, 1984; Mortemousque, 2007; Rimas et al, 1992).

According to our findings, we can describe a dynamic response profile to specific provocation. In our study, NPT response at the 1st minute was faster than CPT (p=0.005), with 15/21 patients presenting a positive NPT *versus* 6/21 patients with positive CPT. We speculate that this can eventually be explained by the existence of particular characteristics in nasal and ocular mucosa, resulting in differences related to the contact with the allergen and/or the time response of type I hypersensitivity. The NPT progressive response was linear whereas CPT one was exponential, till the 5th minute of response.

On the other hand, CPT response was stronger at the 5th minute when comparing to NPT, achieving borderline significance (p=0.05). This corroborates other results related to the evaluation of patient discomfort of NPT *versus* CPT using a visual-analogue scale, with a higher discomfort being appointed to CPT (Riechelmann et al, 2003). Apparently, these results are different from the study of Malmberg et al, 1978, in which the conjunctiva of 55% of the patients that underwent both NPT and CPT, using sequentially diluted allergen solutions, was less sensitive to allergen challenge than nasal mucosa. However, the intensity of the positive CPT response was not described in this study. Our patients submitted to CPT had higher specific IgE values, but it is unlikely that this could explain the higher intensity symptoms score. The absence of a direct correlation between the degree of allergen sensitization and the severity of clinical symptoms is well known.

As expected by direct allergen exposure, the higher intensity of nasal response was induced by NPT, while CPT was responsible for the higher intensity of ocular response.

At the 5th minute, procedures to collect secretions were performed, and consequently the clinical evaluation of the response to specific provocation tests was disrupted. However, patients were clinically monitored till 4th hour. Interestingly, after the 5th minute, the intensity of the conjunctival response rapidly decreased while a similar intensity of nasal response persisted for a longer period. This data is not shown because the procedures for collection of secretions could alter the dynamic of response.

Even though the allergen was unilaterally inoculated, NPT induced bilateral nasal symptoms in 100% and bilateral ocular symptoms in 47.6%. On the other hand, CPT induced unilateral ocular symptoms in 100% and bilateral nasal symptoms in 95.2%. This is in accordance with previous studies and can be explained by different mechanisms mentioned above (Section 4. NPT as a diagnostic approach in respiratory allergy). An additional explanation for the higher number of patients with nasal symptoms induced by CPT, when comparing with the number of patients in whom NPT induced ocular symptoms, is the direct contact of the inoculated allergen with the nasal mucosa, through its passage via naso-lacrimal duct.

This study describes, for the first time to our knowledge, the clinical patterns of NPT and CPT responses, using a clinical score system. NPT is faster than CPT and has a linear progression, while CPT has an exponential progression and has a stronger response. The induction of both nasal and ocular responses by NPT or CPT, corroborates the systemically response triggered by local allergen application. Although both methodologies can elicit extra-local symptoms, these are safe procedures. Finally, these data support the applicability of CPT in the diagnosis of allergic rhinitis, even in the absence of ocular signs/symptoms, surpassing some NPT limitations (such as nasal polyps or deviated nasal septum) and decreasing specific challenge risk.

6. Conclusion

The specific provocation tests have been widely used in the investigation of pathophysiological mechanisms, immunological and therapeutic aspects of allergic disease, since they mimic the response to allergen exposure, under controlled conditions. It is well known that NPT has limitations, but it has been helpful to a better clarification of the underlying mechanisms of allergic reaction, and also to recognize the systemic framework of allergic disease. The usefulness of NPT is focused in the diagnosis of allergic rhinitis itself, but it has also a relevant role in the diagnosis of allergic respiratory disease. The upper and lower airways do not exist as anatomically and functionally distinct areas. There are important relationships between both the nose and the paranasal sinuses, and asthma. These epidemiological, clinical and immunopathologic concordance between allergic rhinitis and asthma supports the concept of bidirectional "unified airway" respiratory inflammation model. Multiple evidence supports a close interaction and influence of the nose on contiguous and distant organs via neural reflex and systemic inflammatory processes.

In clinical practice, NPT plays a central role in the diagnosis of allergic rhinitis in some circumstances, as described. This is the only method that could establish the correct aetiology of the allergic disease, namely local allergic rhinitis and occupational rhinitis. The specific therapeutic implications emphasize the attempt to reach the most complete diagnostic approach.

The monitoring of the response to NPT is not standardized, but several parameters have been used, for example symptom scores. Our data suggest that the clinical symptom pattern to NPT develops has a dynamic response which is characterized by a linear progression of symptoms intensity till a 5th minute peak. The prevalence of non-nasal symptoms had a great variability in the studies performed by our group. Those symptoms had a lower score comparing to nasal symptoms. In our opinion, the symptom score is a valuable method to monitor the NPT response.

7. Acknowledgements

We would like to acknowledge Dr Borja Bartolomé, Bial Aristegui, I&D Department, Bilbao, Spain; Dr António Martinho & Dr Artur Paiva, PhD, Histocompatibility Center, Coimbra, Portugal.

8. References

Abelson, MB.; Chambers, WA. & Smith, LM. (1990). Conjunctival allergen challenge. A clinical approach to studying allergic conjunctivitis. *Arch Ophthalmol,* Vol.108, No.1, (January 1990), pp. 84-88, ISSN 0003-9950

Anderson, DF.; McGill, JI. & Roche, WR. (1996). Improving the safety of conjunctival provocation test. *J Allergy Clin Immunol,* Vol.98, No.5 Pt 1, (November 1996), pp. 1000, ISSN 0091-6749

Alvares, ML. & Khan, DA. (2011) Allergic rhinitis with negative skin tests. *Curr Allergy Asthma Rep,* Vol.11, No.(2), (April 2011), pp. 107-114, ISSN 1529-7322

Eire, MA.; Pineda, F.; Losada, SV.; de la Cuesta, CG. & Villalva, MM. (2006). Occupational rhinitis and asthma due to cedroarana wood dust allergy. *J Investig Allergol Clin Immunol,* Vol.16, No.6, (November 2011), pp. 385-387, ISSN 1018-9068

Airaksinen, L.; Tuomi, T.; Vanhanen, M,; Voutilainen, R. & Toskala, E. (2007). Use of nasal provocation test in the diagnostics of occupational rhinitis. *Rhinology,* Vol.45, No.1, (March 2007), pp. 40-46, ISSN 0300-0729

Bachert, C. (1997). Nasal provocation test: critical evaluation. In: *New trends in Allergy IV,* J. Ring; H.D. Behrendt & D. Vieluf (Ed.), pp. 277-280, Springer-Verlag, ISBN 978-3540611202, Berlin, Germany

Baroody, FM.; Ford, S.; Lichtenstein, LM.; Kagey-Sobotka, A. & Naclerio, RM. (1994). Physiologic responses and histamine release after nasal antigen challenge: effect of atropine. *Am J Respir Crit Care Med,* Vol.149, No.6, (June 1994), pp. 1457-1465, ISSN 1073-449X

Baroody, FM.; Foster, KA.; Markaryan, A.; deTineo, M. & Naclerio, RM. (2008). Nasal Ocular reflexes and eye symptoms in patients with allergic rhinitis. *Ann Allergy Asthma Immunol,* Vol.100, No.3, (March 2008), pp. 194-199, ISSN 1081-1206

Baroody, FM. (2011). How nasal function influences the eyes, ears, sinuses and lungs. *Proc Am Thorac Soc,* Vol.8, No.1, (March 2011), pp. 53-61, ISSN 1546-3222

Bousquet, J.; Van Cauwenberge, P.; Khaltaev, N.; Aria Workshop Group & World Health Organization. (2001). Allergic rhinitis and its impact on asthma. *J Allergy Clin Immunol,* Vol.108, No.5 Suppl, (November 2001), pp. S147-S334, ISSN 0091-6749

Blackley, C. (1873). *Experimental researches on the causes and nature of catarrhus aestivus* (first edition), Balliere Tindal & Cox, ISBN 1-871395-00-3, London

Brant, A.; Hole, A.; Cannon, J.; Helm, J.; Swales, C.; Welch, J.; Taylor, NA. & Cullinan, P. (2004). Occupational asthma caused by cellulase and lipase in the detergent industry. *Occup Environ Med,* Vol.61, No.9, (September 2004), pp. 793-795, ISSN 1351-0711

Brant, A.; Zekveld, C.; Welch, J.; Jones, M.; Taylor, NA. & Cullinan, P. (2006). The prognosis of occupational asthma due to detergent enzymes: clinical, immunological and employment outcomes. *Clin Exp Allergy,* Vol.36, No.4, (April 2006), pp. 483-488, ISSN 0954-7894

Braunstahl, GJ. (2005). The unified immune system: Respiratory tract–nasobronchial interaction mechanisms in allergic airway disease. *J Allergy Clin Immunol*, Vol.115, No.1, (January 2005), pp. 142-148, ISSN 0091-6749

Braunstahl, GJ. & Hellings, PW. (2006). Nasobronchial interaction mechanisms in allergic airways disease. *Curr Opin Otolaryngol Head Neck Surg*, Vol.14, No.3, (June 2006), pp. 176–182, ISSN 1068-9508

Chusakul, S.; Phannaso, C.; Sangsarsri, S.; Aeumjaturapat, S. & Snidvongs, K. (2010). House-dust mite nasal provocation: a diagnostic tool in perennial rhinitis. *Am J Rhinol Allergy*, Vol.24, No.2, (March 2010), pp. 133-136, ISSN 1945-8924

Cimarra, M & Robledo, T. (2001). Aplicacion en provocacion nasal especifica, In: *Manual de rinomanometria*, A. Valero; J.M. Fabra; F. Márquez; C. Orus; C. Picado; J. Sastre; J.I. Sierra, (Ed.), pp. 55-63, MRA Medica, Barcelona

Clement, PAR. (1984). Committee report on standardization of rhinomanometry. *Rhinology*, Vol.22, No.3, (September 1984), pp. 151-155, ISSN 0300-0729

Compalati, E.; Ridolo, E.; Passalacqua, G.; Braido, F.; Villa, E. & Canonica, GW. (2010). The link between allergic rhinitis and asthma: the united airways disease. *Expert Rev Clin Immunol*, Vol.6, No.3, (May 2010), pp. 413-423, ISSN 1744-666X

Corey, JP.; Gungor, A.; Nelson, R.; Liu, X. & Fredberg, J. (1998). Normative standards for nasal cross-sectional areas by race as measured by acoustic rhinometry. *Otolaryngol Head Neck Surg*, Vol.119, No.4, (October 1998), pp. 389-393, ISSN 1097-6817

Dordal, MT.; Lluch-Bernal, M.; Sánchez, MC.; Rondón, C.; Navarro, A.; Montoro, J.; Matheu, V.; Ibáñez, MD.; Fernández-Parra, B.; Dávila, I.; Conde, J.; Antón, E.; Colás, C.; Valero, A. & SEAIC Rhinoconjunctivitis Committee. (2011). Allergen-specific nasal provocation testing: Review by the Rhinoconjunctivitis Committee of the Spanish Society of Allergy and Clinical Immunology. *J Investig Allergol Clin Immunol*, Vol.21, No.1, (January 2011), pp. 1-12, ISSN 1018-9068

Dreborg, S. & Frew, A. (1993). EAACI Position paper: allergen standardization and skin tests. *Allergy*, Vol.48, No.Suppl 14, (February 1993), pp. 1-82, ISSN 0105-4538

Druce, HM. & Schumacher, MJ. (1990). Nasal provocation challenge. The Committee on Upper Airway Allergy. *J Allergy Clin Immunol*, Vol.86, No.2, (August 1990), pp. 261-264, ISSN 0091-6749

EAACI Task Force on Occupational Rhinitis; Moscato, G.; Vandenplas, O.; Gerth Van Wijk, R.; Malo, JL.; Quirce, S.; Walusiak, J.; Castano, R.; De Groot, H.; Folletti, I.; Gautrin, D.; Yacoub, MR.; Perfetti, L. & Siracusa, A. (2008). Occupational rhinitis. *Allergy*, Vol.63, No.8, (August 2008), pp. 969-980, ISSN 0105-4538

Forester, JP & Calabria, CW. (2010). Local production of IgE in the respiratory mucosa and the concept of entopy: does allergy exist in nonallergic rhinitis? *Ann Allergy Asthma Immunol*, Vol.105, No.4, (October 2010), pp. 249-255, ISSN 1081-1206

Fujisawa, T.; Katsumata, H. & Kato, Y. (2008). House dust mite extract induces interleukin-9 expression in human eosinophils. *Allergol Intern*, Vol.57, No.2, (June 2008), pp. 141–146, ISSN 1323-8930

Fujishima, H.; Takeyama, M.; Takeuchi, T.; Saito, I. & Tsubota, K. (1997). Elevated levels of substance P in tears of patients with allergic conjunctivitis and vernal keratoconjunctivitis. *Clin Exp Allergy*, Vol.27, No.4, (April 1997), pp. 372–378, ISSN 0954-7894

Ganslmayer, M.; Spertini, F.; Rahm, F.; Terrien, MH.; Mosimann, B. & Leimgruber, A. (1999). Evaluation of acoustic rhinometry in a nasal provocation test with allergen. *Allergy*, Vol.54, No.9, (September 1999), pp. 974-979, ISSN 0105-4538

Gosepath, J.; Amedee, RG. & Mann, WJ. (2005). Nasal provocation testing as an international standard for evaluation of allergic and non-allergic rhinitis. *Laryngoscope*, Vol.115, No.3, (March 2005), pp. 512-516, ISSN 0023-852X

Gotlib, T.; Samoliński, B. & Grzanka, A. (2005). Bilateral nasal allergen provocation monitored with acoustic rhinometry. Assessment of both nasal passages and the side reacting with greater congestion: relation to the nasal cycle. *Clin Exp Allergy*, Vol.35, No.3; (March 2005), pp. 313-318, ISSN 0954-7894

Gregory, LG.; Causton, B.; Murdoch, JR.; Mathie, SA.; O'Donnell, V.; Thomas, CP.; Priest, FM.; Quint, DJ. & Lloyd, CM. (2009). Inhaled house dust mite induces pulmonary T helper 2 cytokine production. *Clin Exp Allergy*, Vol.39, No.10, (October 2009), pp. 1597–1610, ISSN 0954-7894

Hammad, H.; Chieppa, M.; Perros, F.; Willart, MA.; Germain, RN. & Lambrecht, BN. (2009). House dust mite allergen induces asthma via Toll-like receptor 4 triggering of airway structural cells. *Nat Med*, Vol.15, No.4, (April 2009), pp. 410–416, ISSN 1078-8956

Hens, G.; Bobic, S.; Reekmans, K.; Ceuppens, JL. & Hellings, PW. (2007). Rapid systemic uptake of allergens through the respiratory mucosa. *J Allergy Clin Immunol*, Vol.120, No. 2, (August 2007), pp. 472-474, ISSN 0091-6749

Hervás, D.; Rodriguez, R. & Garde, J. (2011). Role of aeroallergen nasal challenge in asthmatic children. *Allergol Immunopathol*, Vol.39, No.1, (January 2011), pp. 17-22, ISSN 0301-0546

Holmström, M.; Scadding, GK.; Lund, VJ. & Darby, YC. (1990). Assessment of nasal obstruction. A comparison between rhinomanometry and nasal inspiratory peak flow. *Rhinology*, Vol.28, No.3, (September 1990), pp. 191-196, ISSN 0300-0729

Howarth, PH.; Persson, CG.; Meltzer, EO.; Jacobson, MR.; Durham, SR. & Silkoff, PE. (2005). Objective monitoring of nasal airway inflammation in rhinitis. *J Allergy Clin Immunol*, Vol.115, No.3 Suppl 1), (March 2005), pp. S414-S441, ISSN 0091-6749

Huggins, KG. & Brostoff, J. (1975). Local Production of specific IgE antibodies in allergic rhinitis patients with negative skin tests. *Lancet*, Vol.2, No.7926, (July 1975), pp. 148–150, ISSN 0099-5355

Hytonen, M. & Sala, E. (1996). Nasal provocation test in the diagnostics of occupational allergic rhinitis. *Rhinology*, Vol.34, No.2, (June 1996), pp. 86-90, ISSN 0300-0729

Hytönen, M.; Leino, T.; Sala, E.; Kanerva, L.; Tupasela, O. & Malmberg, H. (1997). Nasal provocation test in the diagnosis of hairdressers' occupational rhinitis. *Acta Otolaryngol.*, Vol.117, No.S529, (May 1997)pp. 133-136 , ISSN 0001-6489

Jones, AS.; Viani, L.; Phillips, D. & Charters, P. (1991). The objective assessment of nasal patency. *Clin Otolaryngol Allied Sci*, Vol.16,No.2, (April 1991), pp. 206-211, ISSN 0307-7772

Keck, T.; Wiesmiller, K.; Lindemann, J. & Rozsasi, A.. (2006). Acoustic Rhinometry in nasal provocation test in perennial allergic rhinitis. *Eur Arch Otorhinolaryngol*, Vol.263, No.10, (October 2006), pp. 910–916, ISSN 0937-4477

Khan, DA. (2009). Allergic rhinitis with negative tests: does it exist? *Allergy Asthma Proc*, Vol.30, No.5, (September 2009), pp. 465-469, ISSN 1088-5412

Kharitonov, SA.; Rajakulasingam, K.; O'Connor, B.; Durham, SR. & Barnes PJ. (1997). Nasal nitric oxide is increased in patients with asthma and allergic rhinitis and may be modulated by nasal glucocorticoids. *J Allergy Clin Immunol,* Vol.99, No.1 Pt 1, (January 1997), pp. 58-64, ISSN 0091-6749

Kim, YH.; Yang, TY.; Lee, DY.; Ko, KJ.; Shin, SH. & Jang, TY. (2008). Evaluation of acoustic rhinometry in a nasal provocation test with allergic rhinitis. *Otolaryngol Head Neck Surg,* Vol.139, No.1 , (July 2008), pp. 120–123, ISSN 0194-5998

Kim, YH & Jang, TY. (2010). Clinical characteristics and therapeutic outcomes of patients with localized mucosal allergy. *Am J Rhinol Allergy,* Vol.24, No.4, (July 2010), pp. 89–92, ISSN 1945-8924

Kim, YH. & Jang TY. (2011). Proposed diagnostic standard using visual analogue scale and acoustic rhinometry in nasal provocation test in allergic patients. Auris Nasus Larynx, Vol.38, No.3, (June 2011), pp. 340-346, ISSN 0385-8146

Kirerleri, E.; Guler, N.; Tamay, Z. & Ones, U. (2006). Evaluation of the nasal provocation tests for its necessity in the diagnosis of nasal allergy to house dust mite. *Asian Pac J Allergy Immunol,* Vol.24, No.2-3, (June 2006), pp. 117-121, ISSN 0125-877X

Krouse, JH. (2008). The unified airway-concptual framework. *Otolaryngol Clin North Am,* Vol.41, No.2, (April 2008), pp. 257-266, ISSN 0030-6665

Lack, G.; Caulfield, H. & Penagos, M. (2011). The link between otitis media with effusion and allergy: a potential role for intranasal corticosteroids. *Pediatr Allergy Immunol,* Vol.22, No.3, (May 2011), pp. 258-266, ISSN 0905-6157

Lebel, B.; Bousquet, J.; Morel, A. Chanal, I.; Godard, P. & Michel FB. (1988). Correlation between symptoms and the threshold for release of mediators in nasal secretions during nasal challenge with grass-pollen grains. *J Allergy Clin Immunol,* Vol.82, No.5 Pt 1, (November 1988), pp. 869-877, ISSN 0091-6749

Leonardi, A.; Battista, MC.; Gismondi, M.; Fregona, IA. & Secchi, AG.. (1993). Antigen sensitivity evaluated by tear-specific and serum-specific IgE, skin tests, and conjunctival and nasal provocation tests in patients with ocular allergic disease. *Eye,* Vol.7, No.Pt 3, (May 1993), pp. 461-464, ISSN 0950-222X

Linder, A. (1988). Symptom scores as measures of the severity of rhinitis. *Clin Allergy,* Vol.18, No.1 (January 1988), pp 29-37, ISSN 0009-9090

Lindstedt, M.; Schiött, A,; Johnsen, CR.; Roggen, E.; Johansson-Lindbom, B.; & Borrebaeck, CA. (2005). Individual with occupational allergy to detergent enzymes display a differential transcriptional regulation and cellular immune response. *Clin Exp Allergy,* Vol.35, No.2 (February 2005), pp.199-206, ISSN 0954-7894

Litvyakova, LI & Baraniuk, JN. (2001). Nasal provocation testing: a review. *Ann Allergy Asthma Immunol,* Vol. 86, No. 4 (April 2001), pp. 355-65, ISSN 1081-1206

Litvyakova, LI & Baraniuk, JN. (2002). Human nasal allergen provocation for determination of true allergic rhinitis: methods for clinicians. *Curr Allergy Asthma Rep,* Vol. 2, No.3 (May 2002), pp. 194-202, ISSN 1529-7322

Lopez, S.; Rondón, C.; Torres, MJ.; Campo, P.; Canto, G.; fernadez, R.; Garcia, R.; Martínez-Cañavate, A.; & Blanca, M. (2010). Immediate and dual response to nasal challenge with Dermatophagoides pteronyssinus in local allergic rhinitis. *Clin Exp Allergy,* Vol. 40, No. 7 (July 2010), 1007–1014, ISSN 0954-7894

Loureiro, G. (2001). Provocação nasal específica no controlo da imunoterapia. *Rev Port Imunoalergol,* 9, 123-5

Loureiro, G.; Loureiro, C.; Garção, F.; Alves, V.; Santos Rosa, M.; Chieira, C. (2003). Avaliação da resposta imunológica à prova de provocação nasal específica: estudo de quimiocinas em secreções nasais. *Rev Port Imunoalergologia*, 11, 380-90

Loureiro, G.; Loureiro, C.; Alves, V.; Garção, F.; Santos Rosa, M.; Chieira, C. (2004). Padrão de resposta à prova de provocação nasal específica em doentes alérgicos submetidos a imunoterapia específica. *Rev Port Imunoalergologia*, 12, 224-38

Loureiro, G. (2008). Rinite ocupacional: Dificuldades no diagnóstico e enquadramento epidemiológico. *Rev Port Imunoalergologia*, 16 (1), 7-27

Loureiro, G.; Tavares, B.; Pereira, C.; Lundberg, M.; & Chieira, C. (2009). Occupational Allergy to Fungal Lipase in the Pharmaceutical Industry. *J Investig Allergol Clin Immunol, Vol.* 19, No. 3 (March 2009), pp. 242-244, ISSN 1018-9068

Loureiro, G et al. (2011). Specific Nasal provocation test as a diagnostic tool in local allergic rhinitis. (abstract) Allergy, 66 (Suppl 94) 1371, ISSN 0105-4538

Lund, VJ.; & International Rhinitis Management Working Group (1994). International Consensus Report on the diagnosis and management of rhinitis. *Allergy*, Vol. 49, Suppl 19, 1-34, ISSN 0105-4538

Malm, L.; Gerth van Wijk, R.; & Bachert, C. (2000). Guidelines for nasal provocations with aspects on nasal patency, airflow, and airflow resistance. International Committee on Objective Assessment of the Nasal Airways, International Rhinologic Society. *Rhinology*, Vol. 38, No. 1 (March 2000), pp. 1-6, ISSN 0300-0729

Malmberg, CH.; Holopainen, EE.; & Stenius-Aarniala, BS. (1978). Relationship between nasal and conjunctival tests in patients with allergic rhinitis. *Clin Allergy, Vol.* 8, No. 4 (July 1978), pp. 397-402, ISSN 0105-4538

Marcucci, F.; Passalacqua, G.; Canonica, GW.; Frati, F.; Salvatori, S.; Di Cara, G.; Petrini, I.; Bernini, M.; Novembre, E.; Bernardini, R.; Incorvaia, C.; & Sensi, LG. (2007). Lower airway inflammation before and after house dust mite nasal challenge: an age and allergen exposure-related phenomenon. *Respir Med,* Vol. 101, No. 7 (July 2007), pp.1600-1608, ISSN 0954-6111

Marple, BF. (2010). Allergic rhinitis and inflammatory airway disease: interactions within the unified airspace. *Am J Rhinol Allergy*, Vol. 24, No. 4 (July-August 2010), pp. 249-254, ISSN 1945-8924

Mellilo, G.; Bonini, S.; Cocco, G.; Davies, RJ.; de Monchy, JGR.; Frelund, L.; & pelican, Z. (1997). Provocation tests with allergens. *Allergy*, Vol. 52, Suppl 35, (june 1997), pp. 5-35, ISSN 0105-4538

Micera, A.; Lambiase, A.; & Bonini, S. (2008). The role of neuromediators in ocular allergy. *Curr Opin Allergy Clin Immunol*, Vol 8, No. 5 (October 2008), pp. 466–471, ISSN 1528-4050

Möller, C.; Björksten, B.; Nilsson, G.; & Dreborg, S. (1984). The precision of the conjunctival provocation test. *Allergy*, Vol. 39, No. 1 (January 1984), pp. 37-41, ISSN 0105-4538

Mortemousque, B. (2007). Les tests de provocation conjonctivaux. *J Fr Ophtalmol*, Vol. 30, No. 3 (March 2007), pp. 300-305, ISSN 0181-5512

Mosbech, H.; Dirksen, A.; Madsen, F.; Stahl Skov, P.; & Weeke, B.(1987). House dust mite asthma. Correlation between allergen sensitivity in various organs. *Allergy*, Vol. 42, No. 6 (August 1987), pp. 456-463, ISSN 0105-4538

Moscato, G.; Rolla, G.; & Siracusa, A. (2011). Occupational rhinitis: consensus on diagnosiss and medicolegal implications. *Curr Opin Otolaryngol Head Neck Surg,* Vol. 19, No. 1 (February 2011), pp. 36-42, ISSN 1068-9508

Naclerio, RM.; Meier, HL.; Kagey-Sobotka, A.; Adkinson, NF. Jr; Meyers, DA.; Norman, PS.; & Lichtenstein, LM. (1983). Mediator release after nasal airway challenge with allergen. *Am Rev Respir Dis* , Vol. 128, No. 4 (xxx), pp. 597-602, ISSN 0003-0805

Naclerio, RM & Norman, PS. (1998). In vivo methods for the study of allergic rhinitis. In: *Allergy Principles & Practice*, Middleton E, Reed C et al. Eds. St Louis, CV Mosby, 5th edition, 440-453, ISBN 0815100728

Nathan, RA.; Eccles, R.; Howarth, PH.; Steinsvåg, SK.; & Togias, A. (2005). Objective monitoring of nasal patency and nasal physiology in rhinitis. *J Allergy Clin Immunol,* Vol. 115, No. 3, Suppl (March 2005), pp. 442-459, ISSN 0091-6749

O'Meara, TJ.; Sercombe, JK.; Morgan, G.; Reddel, HK.; Xuan, W.; & Tovey, ER. (2005). Reduction of rhinitis symptoms by nasal filters during natural exposure to ragweed andgrass pollen. *Allergy,* Vol. 60, No. 4 (April 2005), pp. 529–532, ISSN 0105-4538

Oddera, S.; Silvestri, M.; Penna, R.; Galeazzi, G.; Crimi, E.; & Rossi, GA.. (1998). Airway eosinophilic inflammation and bronchial hyperresponsiveness after allergen inhlation challenge in asthma. *Lung,* Vol. 176, No. 4 (July 1998), pp. 237-47, ISSN 0341-2040

Olive Pérez, A. (1997). Rhinitis and asthma: nasal provocation test in the diagnosis of asthma. *J Investig Allergol Clin Immunol,* Vol. 7, No. 5 (May 1997), pp. 397-399, ISSN 1018-9068

Park, HS.; Kim, HY.; suh, YJ.; Lee, SJ.; Lee, SK.; Kim, SS.; & Nahm, DH. (2002). Alpha amylase is a major allergenic component in occupational asthma patients caused by porcine pancreatic extract. *J Asthma,* Vol. 39. No. 6 (June 2002), pp. 511-516, ISSN 0277-0903

Pelikan, Z. (2009). Diagnostic value of nasal allergen challenge combined with radiography and ultrasonography in chronic maxillary sinus disease. *Arch Otolaryngol Head Neck Surg,* Vol. 135, No. 12 (December 2009), pp. 1246-55, ISSN 0886-4470

Pereira, C. (2009). *In Thesis,* Dinâmica da inflamação alérgica e da imunoterapia específica. Contribuição para o seu estudo *in vivo.* Dissertação de Doutoramento. Faculdade de Medicina da Universidade de Coimbra. Universidade de Coimbra, 1-546

Pereira, C et al. (2011) T cell receptor excision circles (TREC) and recent thymic migrant cells in specific immunotherapy and respiratory allergy to *Dermatophagoides pteronyssinus. Eur Ann Allergy Clin Immunol. In press*

Petersson, G.; Djueborg, S.; & Ingestad, R. (1986). Clinical history, skin prick test ans RAST in the diagnosis of birch and timothy pollinosis. *Allergy,* Vol 41, No. 6 (August 1986), pp.398-407, ISSN 0105-4538

Pirila, T & Nuutinen, J. (1998). Acoustic rhinometry, rhinomanometry and the amount of nasal secretion in the clinical monitoring of the nasal provocation test. *Clin Exp Allergy,* vol. 28, No. 4 (April 1998), pp. 468-477, ISSN 0954-7894

Riechelmann, H.; Epple, B.; & Gropper, G. (2003). Comparison of conjuctival and nasal provocation test in allergic rhinitis to house dust mite. *Int Arch Allergy Immunol,* Vol. 130, No. 1 (January 2003), pp. 51-59, ISSN 1018-2438

Rimas, M.; Gustafsson, PM.; Kjellman, NIM.; & Bjöorkstéen, B. (1992). Conjunctival provocation test: high clinical reproducibility but little local temperature change. *Allergy*, Vol. 47, No. 4 (August 1992), pp. 324-326, ISSN 0105-4538

Rondón, C., Romero, J.; López, s.; Antúnez, C.; Martin-Casañez, E.; Torres, MJ.; Mayorga, C.; Pena, R.; & Blana, M. (2007). Local IgE production and positive nasal provocation test in patients with persistent nonallergic rhinitis. *J Allergy Clin Immunol*, Vol. 119, No. 4 (April 2007), pp. 899-905, ISSN 0091-6794

Rondón, C.; Férnandez, J.; López, S.; Campo, P.; Doña, I.; torres, MJ.; Mayorga, C.; & Blanca, M.(2009). Nasal inflammatory mediators and specific IgE production after nasal Challenge with grass pollen in local allergic rhinitis. *J Allergy Clin Immunol*, Vol. 124, No. 5 (November 2009), pp. 1005-1011, ISSN 0091-6794

Rondón, C. ; Canto, G. ; & Blanca, M. (2010a). Local allergic rhinitis: a new entity, characterization and further studies. *Curr Opin Allergy Immunol*, Vol 10, No. 1 (February 2010), pp. 1-7, ISSN 1528-4050

Rondón, C.; fernadez, J.; Canto, G.; & Blanca, M. (2010b). Local allergic rhinitis: concept, clinical manifestations and diagnostic approach. *J Investig Allergol Clin Immunol*, Vol. 20, No. 5 (May 2010), pp. 364-371, ISSN 1018-9068

Schumacher, MJ. (1989). Rhinomanometry. *J Allergy Clin Immunol* 1989, 83, 711-8, ISSN 0091-6794

Schumacher, MJ. (1992). Nasal provocation test. *Rhinology*, 14, 242-6, ISSN 0300-0729

Sheahan, P.; walsh, RM.; Walsh, MA.; & Costello, RW. (2005). Induction of nasal hyper responsiveness by allergen challenge in allergic rhinitis: the role of afferent and efferent nerves. *Clin Exp Allergy*, Vol. 35, No. 1 (January 2005), pp. 45-51, ISSN 0954-7894

Skoner, AR.; Skoner, KR.; & Skoner, DP. (2009). Allergic rhinitis, histamine and otitis media. *Allergy Asthma Proc*, Vol. 30, No. 5 (September-October 2009), pp. 470-481, ISSN 1088-5412

Slavin, RG. (2008). The upper and lower airways: the epidemiological and pathophysiological connection. *Allergy Asthma Proc*, Vol. 29, No. 6 (November-December 2008), pp. 553-556, ISSN 1088-5412

Tantilipikorn, P.; Vichyanond, P.; & Lacroix, JS. (2010). Nasal Provocation test: how to maximize its clinical use? *Asian Pac J Allergy Immunol*, Vol. 28, No. 4 (December 2010), pp. 225-231, ISSN 0125-877X

Terrien, M-H.; Rahm, F.; Fellrath, JM.; & Spertini, F. (1999). Comparison of effects of terfenadine with fexofenadine on nasal provocation tests with allergen. *J Allergy Clin Immunol*, Vol. 103, No. 6 (June 1999), pp. 1025-30, ISSN 0091-6794

Togias, A. (2003). Rhinitis and asthma: evidence for respiratory system integration. *J Allergy Clin Immunol* , Vol. 111, No. 6 (June 2003), pp. 1171-83, ISSN 0091-6794

Togias, A. (2004). Systemic effects of local allergic disease. *J Allergy Clin Immunol*, Vol. 113, No. 1,Supll (January 2004), pp. 8-14, ISSN 0091-6794

Uzzaman, A.; Metclafe, DD.; & Komarow, HD. (2006). Acoustic rhinometry in the practice of allergy. *Ann Allergy Asthma Immunol*, Vol. 97, No. 5, pp. 745-751, ISSN 1081-1206

Valero, AL & Picado, C. (2000). Pruebas de provocación nasal específicas. In: *Manual de rinometría acústica*. Valero AL, Fabra JM, Márquez F, Orús C, Picado C, Sastre J, Sierra JI. Barcelona: MRA Médica, 53-74 van Kampen, V.; Merget, R.; & Baur, X. (2000). Occupational airway sensitizers: an overview on the respective literature. *Am J Ind Med*, Vol. 38, No. 2, pp. 164-218, ISSN 0271-3586

Vandenplas, O. (2010). Asthma and rhinitis in the workplace. *Curr Allergy Asthma Rep*, Vol. 10, No. 5 (September 2010), pp. 373-380, ISSN 1529-7322

Virchow, J. (2005). Asthma, allergic rhinitis, sinusitis. Concept of the "unified respiratory tracts. *HNO*, vol. 53, Suppl 1 (May 2005), pp. 16-20, ISSN 0017-6192

Wihl, JA. (1986). Methodological aspects of nasal allergen challenges based on a three-year tree pollen immunotherapy study. *Allergy* , Vol. 41, No. 5 (May 1986), pp. 357-364, ISSN 0105-4538

Wihl, JA & Malm, L. (1988). Rhinomanometry and nasal peak expiratory and inspiratory flow rate. *Ann Allergy*, Vol. 61, (July 1988), pp. 50-55, ISSN 0003-4738

Wong, CK.; Li, MLY.; Wang, CB.; Ip, WK.; Tian, YP.; & Lam, CWK. (2006). House dust mite allergen Der p 1 elevates the release of inflammatory cytokines and expression of adhesion molecules in co-culture of human eosinophils and bronchial epithelial cells. *Int Immunol*, Vol. 18, No. 8 (August 2006), pp. 1327–1335, ISSN 0953-8178

Yeo, SG.; Park, DC.; Eun, YG.; & Cha, C. (2007). The role of allergic rhinitis in the development of otitis media with effusion: effect on Eustachian tube function. *Am J Otolaryngol*, Vol. 28, No. 3 (May-June 2007), pp. 148-152, ISSN 0196-0709

Zentner, A.; Jeep, S.; Wahl, R.; Kunkel, G.; & Kleine-Tebbe, J. (1997). Multiple IgE-mediated sensitizations to enzymes after occupational exposure: evaluation by skin prick test, RAST, and immunoblot. *Allergy*, Vol. 52, No. 9 (September 1997), pp. 928-934, ISSN 0105-4538

11

Phototherapy for the Treatment of Allergic Rhinitis

Ko-Hsin Hu[1,2,3] and Wen-Tyng Li[3]
[1]*Department of Otorhinolaryngology, Keelung Hospital*
[2]*School of Traditional Chinese Medicine, Chang Gung University*
[3]*Department of Biomedical Engineering, Chung-Yuan Christian University*
Taiwan

1. Introduction

Allergic rhinitis (AR) is one of the most common allergic diseases, affecting 20% of the adult population and up to 40% of children (Salib et al., 2003). It is associated with decreased learning, performance and productivity at work and school, as well as a reduced quality of life. The detrimental effects of AR on quality of life (QOL) include fatigue, irritability, memory deficits, excessive daytime somnolence, and depression. The annual economic impact of AR is calculated to be between $ 6.3 billion and $ 7.9 billion without counting its detrimental effects on QOL (Fineman, 2002). Current therapeutic options such as allergen avoidance, medication and immunotherapy are far from ideal. It is important to develop an effective modality to relieve the symptom except for targeting the complexity of underlying inflammatory mechanism of AR.

Phototherapy is the application of light to a pathological area to promote tissue regeneration, reduce inflammation and relieve pain. Several types of phototherapeutic devices are currently used for medical treatment using selected wavelengths and controlled dosage of irradiation. Significant suppression on the clinical symptoms of AR by the phototherapy treatment of ultraviolet (UV) and visible light was reported (Csoma, et al., 2004, 2006; Koreck, et al., 2005, 2007). Narrow-band red light phototherapy was found to markedly alleviate the clinical symptoms of AR (Neuman & Finkelstein, 1997). In addition to UV and visible light therapy, far infrared ray (FIR) therapy is also reported to have beneficial effects to patients with AR (Hu & Li, 2007). Photochemical effect is elicited using UV and visible light irradiation, whereas thermal effect is induced with FIR irradiation. Although different mechanisms are involved when light sources with different ranges of wavelengths are employed, phototherapy represents a noninvasive, alternative intervention for the treatment of AR.

This chapter is organized as follows. First, pathophysiology and traditional management of AR are briefly reviewed. Second, photobiology and phototherapy related to AR are summarized. Finally, the clinical outcomes of FIR therapy as well as red light acupoint stimulation on patients with AR are described.

2. Pathophysiology of allergic rhinitis

AR is defined as an abnormal inflammation of the membrane lining the nose, which is mediated by immunoglobulin E (IgE). The clinical symptoms of AR include sneezing, itching of the nose, rhinorrhea and nasal congestion. Additionally, airway lining hypersensitivity, a loss of the sense of small and an inability to taste may occur. It has become progressively clear that it is a common comorbid condition with asthma, allergic conjunctivitis, sinusitis, otitis media, nasal polyposis and respiratory infections (Berrettini, et al., 1999; Skoner, 2000). Nasal obstruction can often be seen with pale nasal mucosa, enlarged turbinates, clear nasal secretions, and pharyngeal cobble-stoning upon physical examination (Al Suleimani & Walker, 2007). The diagnosis of AR was based on definite symptoms of nasal itching, rhinorrhea, sneezing, nasal obstruction or mouth breathing, as well as positive reactions to blood tests to antigens, such as house dust mite, cockroach, molds, feathers, grass pollen, weed pollens, sage pollen, and local tree pollens, etc. Criteria for positive skin prick test responses were a wheel of 3 mm or greater diameter with erythema of at least 5 mm. Histamine control skin test was read at 10 minutes, allergen and negative control skin tests were read at 15 minutes. The score for each symptom is usually registered on a four-grade scale- absent, slight, moderate or severe (Linder, 1988) as shown in Table 1.

Scoring of eye itching 0: no eye itching 1: rubbing eyes less than 5 episodes a day 2: rubbing eyes 6-10 episodes a day 3: rubbing eyes more than 10 episodes a day	Scoring of rhinorrhea 0: no nasal blowing 1:nasal blowing less than 5 episodes a day 2: nasal blowing 6-10 episodes a day 3: nasal blowing more than 10 episodes a day
Scoring of nasal itching 0: no nasal itching 1: rubbing nose less than 5 episodes a day 2: rubbing nose 6-10 episodes a day 3: rubbing nose more than 10 episodes a day	Scoring of smell impairment 0: no smell impairment 1: hyposmia with mild smell impairment 2: hyposmia with moderate smell impairment 3: anosmia
Scoring of nasal stuffiness 0: no nasal stuffiness 1: nasal stuffiness without mouth breathing 2: nasal stuffiness with sporadic mouth breathing 3: nasal stuffiness with predominant mouth breathing	Scoring of sneezing 0: no sneezing 1: sneezing less than 5 episodes a day 2: sneezing 6-10 episodes a day 3: sneezing more than 10 episodes a day

Table 1. Scoring of symptoms for AR

Various mediators are associated to the pathophysiology of AR. For example, histamine plays a pivotal role in early allergic responses and also acts as stimulatory signal for cytokine production, expression of cell adhesion molecules and HLA class II antigens. Most of the effects of histamine in allergic disease are mediated through H1 receptors (Akdis & Blaser, 2003). Cysteinyl leukotrienes (CysLTs) increase nasal airway resistance and obstruction, and contribute to rhinorrhea via increased vascular permeability and mucus secretion (Okuda, et al., 1988). Prostaglandins cause congestion and rhinorrhea.

Neuropeptides induce vasodilation, thus causing congestion (Howarth, 1997). Cytokine secretion upregulates the expression of adhesion molecules on the vascular endothelial cells, thereby enhancing the activation and adhesion of inflammatory cells. An increase in interleukin-4 (IL-4), IL-5, and granulocyte-macrophage colony-stimulating factor (GM-CSF) is associated with a mucosal eosinophilia (Quraishi, et al., 2004).

3. Traditional management of allergic rhinitis

Effective allergen avoidance can lead to substantial relief of symptoms. However, patients are still not able to avoid their confirmed allergens such as mites or atmospheric pollens under many circumstances. Medication to manipulate the release of mediators is the next step in the management of AR. Table 2 summarizes the classes of pharmacological therapies for the treatment of AR. The two major classes of medication are oral H1 antihistamines and intranasal corticosteroids. According to the guidelines, oral antihistamines are the first-line therapy which relieve sneezing and rhinorrhea (Bousquet, et al., 2001; van Cauwenberge, et al., 2000; Dykewicz, et al., 1998). Topical administration can further minimize systemic adverse effects of antihistamines. H1 antihistamines are often combined with a decongestant to reach sufficient efficacy for nasal congestion (Quraishi, et al., 2004). The new generation of antihistamines acts as inverse agonists that stabilize the inactive conformation of the receptors and reverses constitutive activity of receptors (Oppenheimer & Casale, 2002). Intranasal corticosteroids are recommended as first-line treatment for moderate and severe AR, which are effective in relieving symptoms such as sneezing, rhinorrhea, itching and congestion (Weiner, et al., 1998). Corticosteroids target the inflammatory mechanisms; therefore the amount of oral corticosteroids for long-term treatment should be carefully adjusted to avoid adverse effects such as osteoporosis and growth inhibition in children (Wilson, et al., 1998).

Decongestants can reduce nasal obstruction and congestion by their vasoconstrictive action on α-adrenergic receptors. The application of intranasal decongestants may cause rhinitis medicamentosa. The adverse effects of oral decongestants include elevated blood pressure, tremor, tachycardia, loss of appetite, sleep disturbance. The long term use of decongestant is not recommended. (Quraishi, et al., 2004). Anticholinergics act as muscarinic receptor blocker which inhibits mucus secretion and subsequent rhinorrhea. Through inhibiting degranulation and neosynthesis of inflammatory mediators, mast cell stabilizers are shown to be effective in reducing symptoms of early inflammatory phase and are useful for preventive purposes (Al Suleimani & Walker, 2007). Leukotrienes inhibitors significantly reduce nasal blockade by inhibiting leukotriene synthesis or serving as antagonists for its receptors. Immunotherapy has the potential to provide a permanent cure for the disease. The proposed mechanisms for immunotherapy include suppression of IgE elevation, decrease in neutrophil and eosionophil activity, reduction in mast cell number, inhibition of T-lymphocyte proliferation (Jayasekera, et al., 2007; Pipet, et al., 2009). However, the technique is burdensome which requiring a lengthy series of injection and it may not be applicable to all patients (Naclerio, et al., 2002). Although most of the drugs are effective in treating certain symptoms of AR, they all have limitations due to their adverse effects. Due to the complex mechanisms involved in the AR, the ideal treatment for this disease has yet to be discovered.

Class	Route of administrati-on	Mechanism of action	Symptom relief	Adverse effects
Antihistami-nes	Intranasal, oral	Antagonists or inverse agonists for histamine at the histamine receptor	Sneezing, rhinorrhea, itching	First-generation: sedation, impaired mental performance, dry mouth, dry eyes, urinary retention
Corticostero-ids	Intranasal, oral	Bind to glucocorticoid receptors, affecting the production of various mediators	Sneezing, rhinorrhea, itching, congestion	Intranasal: nose irritation, bleeding Oral: long-term use may cause growth inhibition in children and osteoporosis
Decongestants	Intranasal, oral	Stimulate α-adrenergic receptors to induce vasoconstriction	Congestion	Intranasal: rhinitis medicamentosa Oral: elevated blood pressure, tremor, tachycardia, loss of appetite, sleep disturbance
Anticholinerg-ics	Intranasal	Muscarinic receptor blockade	Rhinorrhea	Minimal
Mast cell stabilizers	Intranasal	Prevent mast cell degranulation and neosynthesis of inflammatory mediators	Sneezing, rhinorrhea, itching, congestion	Minimal
Leukotriene inhibitors	Oral	Leukotriene synthesis inhibitors, antagonists for the leukotriene receptors	Sneezing, rhinorrhea, congestion	Possibility of neuropsychiatric side effects
Immunothera-py	Subcutaneo-us injection	Suppress IgE elevation, neutrophil and eosionophil activity, mast cell number, T-lymphocyte proliferation	Early or late inflammatory phase responses	Unknown effects from the modification of immune system

Table 2. Current therapeutic agents in use for AR

4. Photobiology

Electromagnetic radiation comprises of radio, microwave, infrared (IR), visible light, UV, X-ray and gamma radiation. The phenomenon of light absorption to produce electronic excitation of atoms and molecules has long been accepted by photochemists and photobiologists. In phototherapy, wavelengths used include UV (100-400 nm), visible light (400-800 nm) and IR (800-10^5 nm).

Photobiological reactions often involve the absorption of a specific wavelength of light by the functioning photoacceptor molecule. Photochemical effect is elicited using UV and visible light irradiation, whereas thermal effect is induced with FIR irradiation. Light in the ultraviolet range is absorbed by the protein part of the molecule and the visible and NIR wavelengths are absorbed by the metals. Further analysis of action spectra, it is suggested that the primary photoacceptor for the red-NIR wavelengths in mammalian cells is cytochrome *c* oxidase in terminal respiratory chain (Karu, et al., 2005, 2008). Flavoproteins such as NADH dehydrogenase in the beginning of the respiratory chain is believed to be the photoacceptor for the violet-to-blue spectral range (Karu, 2003). In addition, light induces a wave-like alternating electric field in a medium that is able to interact with polar structures and produce dipole transitions. These dipole transitions may lead to the primary actions at cellular and biochemical levels (Amat, et al., 2006).

Early hypothesis of the mechanism of primary action upon visible light irradiation can be divided into two categories: (1) singlet oxygen hypothesis based on the singlet oxygen generation from the endogenous molecules possessing the properties of photosensitizers, such as porphyrins and flavoproteins, upon irradiation (Vladimirov, et al., 2004), and (2) the oxidation-reduction hypothesis based on the excitation in chromophores of cytochrome-oxidase complex such as Cu_A, Cu_B or heme $a(a_3)$, thereby enhancing the electron transfer rate (Lubart, et al., 2005). Later, the nitric oxide (NO) hypothesis was proposed suggesting that the activity of cytochrome *c* oxidase can be regulated by NO, here light irradiation can reverse the partial inhibition by NO (Karu, et al., 2005). Superoxide anion hypothesis was also suggested because of increased production of superoxide anion by irradiation, possibly through promoting the mitochondrial respiratory chain (Karu, 2003). The transient local heating hypothesis suggested that the irradiation energy may lead to a local transient increase in the temperature of absorbing chromophores, which may cause structural changes and trigger biochemical activity (Hallen, et al., 1993). The primary reactions upon light irradiation mainly occur in the mitochondria, which may lead to the secondary reactions occurring in the nucleus and cytoplasm. The secondary reactions involves cellular signaling cascade including increased intracellular ATP level, activation of transcription factors such as Nuclear factor-kappa B (NF-κB) and AP-1, activation of NADPH oxidase, change of the cellular redox potential to more oxidized direction (increased ROS production), manipulation of Ca^{2+} concentration, alteration of mitochondrial transmembrane potential (ΔΨm), regulation of inducible nitric oxide synthase (iNOS) activity and intracellular pH, and increased DNA/RNA synthesis (Karu, 2003). Other phenomena such as suppression of inflammatory cytokines, up-regulation of growth factor production, modification of extracellular matrix components, inhibition of apoptosis, stimulation of mast cell degranulation, and up-regulation of heat shock protein are also observed (Lin, et al., 2010).

IR are invisible electromagnetic waves which are subdivided into three categories: near-infrared (NIR) (0.8-1.5 μm), middle-infrared (1.5-5.6 μm) and far-infrared (FIR) (5.6-1000 μm). Different photobiological mechanisms are involved when FIR radiation is employed in phototherapy. The main principles of FIR are radiation, deep penetration and absorption of resonance. At molecular level, FIR exerts rotational and vibrational effects that are biologically beneficial. FIR therapy is often used as alternative physical therapy to decrease joint stiffness, relieve muscle spasms, assist soft tissue injury repair, lead to pain relief, and help to resolve inflammatory infiltrated edema. FIR therapy can improve blood flow and survival of the arteriovenous fistula in hemodialysis patients (Lin, et al., 2007). Furthermore, FIR stimulation on acupoints at Qihai, Kuan yuan and Chung chi decreases both stress and fatigue levels as well as stimulates autonomic nervous system activity in hemodialysis patients (Su, et al., 2009). IR radiation is believed to transfer energy that is perceived as heat by thermoreceptors in the surrounding skin (Inoué & Kabaya, 1989). The abdominal skin temperature steadily increased to a plateau between 38 and 39°C when the top FIR radiator was 20 cm above the rats (Yu, et al., 2006). The expression of HSP70 participates in cytoprotection and may be induced by hyperthermia, infection, UV radiation, NO, etc. However, an *in vitro* study demonstrated that FIR radiation inhibited the proliferation of cancer cells by the low expression level of heat shock protein 70A (Ishibashi, et al., 2008). In addition to the thermal effect, the non-thermal biological effects of FIR therapy led to enhance the extensibility of collagen tissue, stimulate the secretion of transforming growth factor-β1, and increase microcirculation via L-arginine/NO pathway (Toyokawa, et al., 2003; Yu, et al., 2006). Repeated FIR therapy could upregulate the expression of endothelial NO synthase (eNOS) (Akasaki, et al., 2006). FIR therapy was found to exert an anti-inflammatory effect via the induction of heme oxygenase-1 in endothelial cells via stimulating NF-E2-related factor (Nrf2) dependent promoter activity. TNF-α-induced expression of E-selectin, vascular cell adhesion molecule-1 (VCAM-1), and intercellular cell adhesion molecule-1 (ICAM-1) were suppressed (Lin, et al., 2008). A study on the mechanism of action demonstrated that FIR radiation activated p38 and extracellular signal-regulated kinase (ERK), but not Akt or c-Jun N-terminal protein kinases (JNK), and significantly promoted angiogenesis by increasing tube formation and the migration of endothelial cells (Rau, et al., 2010). Based on the above studies, the mechanism of action by FIR therapy can be both thermal and non-thermal effects.

5. Phototherapy in allergic rhinitis

Phototherapy is an effective treatment modality in inflammatory and immue mediated dieases. It has been successfully used in dermatology practice for several decades. The XeCl UV-B laser irradiation and mixed irradiation with UV-A (25%), UV-B (5%) and visible light (70%) (mUV/VIS) resulted in a dose-dependent inhibition of the allergen-induced wheal formation on the skin (Cosma, et al., 2004; Koreck, et al., 2004). Development of new phototherapeutic devices made it possible to treat the inflammatory disease of the nasal mucosa. Intranasal UV-B phototherapy with medium-dose 308 nm XeCl excimer significantly suppressed the nsasl symptoms of patients with severe hay fever (Cosma, et al., 2004). Rhinophototherapy consist of using mUV/VIS resulted in a significant improvement of clinical symptoms for sneezing, rhinorrhea, nasal itching, and total nasal score (Koreck, et al., 2005). The number of eosinophils and the level of eosinophil cationic protein and IL-5 were also reduced. Statiscally significant differences were found in the average results of the

Rhinoconjunctivitis Quality of Life Questionnaire (Cingi, et al., 2009). Another prospective, randomized, single-blind study showed that total nasal scores decreased in both mUV/VIS and low-intensity visible light (mUV/VIS without UV) treated groups (Cingi, et al., 2010). But the decrease was highly significant in the mUV/VIS treated group when compared with the low-intensity visible light treated group. However, the impact of endonasal phototherapy on the number of Langerhans cells in the nasal mucosa was limited (Brehmer & Schön, 2010). DNA damage was significantly higher in nasal cytology samples collected immediately after the last treatment (Koreck, et al., 2007). The DNA damage induced by intranasal UV phototherapy was efficiently repaired two months after ending therapy. One of the possible mechanisms that explain the immunosuppressive effect of mUV/VIS is the induction of apoptosis of T cells and eosinophils after UV damage, thus, leading to the inhibition of synthesis and release of pro-inflammatory mediators (Kemény & Koreck, 2007). The side effect of phototherapy is dryness of nasal mucosa, which can be overcome with emollients. Another disadvantage of UV-B treatment is the risk of carcinogenesis. Therefore, it is important to develop phototherapeutic devices using wavelengths other than UV (Morita, et al., 2008).

Very few papers report the application of the light in the other wavelengths in addition to UV light for the management of AR despite that over 2500 papers have been published regarding low level light therapy as a therapeutic modality to speed up tissue repair as well as related biochemical, cellular, histological and functional effects. NIR irradiation suppressed contact hypersensitivity reaction in rats via systemic immunomodulatory effect (Kandolf-Sekulovic, et al., 2003). A double-blind randomized study showed that 70% improvement of clinical symptoms on AR after intranasal illumination at 660 nm (Neuman & Finkelstein, 1997). Thus, light in red or NIR wavelengths with different mechanism of action from UV and visible light may be an ideal candidate for the intervention of AR after systematic study.

5.1 Far infrared irradiation in allergic rhinitis

FIR therapy, a non-invasive and convenient therapeutic modality, can improve blood flow and inflammatory status through both its thermal and non-thermal effects. By applying FIR therapy to the nasal region in the patients with AR, our study demonstrated that FIR therapy could improve significantly for the clinical symptoms of eye itching, nasal itching, nasal stuffiness, rhinorrhea and sneezing during period of therapy (Hu & Li, 2007).

Thirty-one patients with perennial AR enrolled in the study completed the FIR therapy. All patients had daily symptoms despite antihistamines and local steroid spray treatments. Patients with severe deviation of the nasal septum causing bilateral nasal obstruction and suffering from sinusitis were excluded from the study. A FIR emitter was used for FIR therapy in this study. The wavelength of the light generated from the electrified ceramic plates of this emitter was in the range between 5 and 12 μm with a peak at 8.2 μm. The radiator was positioned via facing patient's nasal region at a distance of 30 cm. The therapeutic time was 40 minutes everyday for 7 days. All the FIR therapies were performed in the morning between 9 am and noon. During the course of the study, the patients did not receive any other anti-allergic management. The effects of FIR on the clinical symptoms were analyzed by the paired sample t-test.

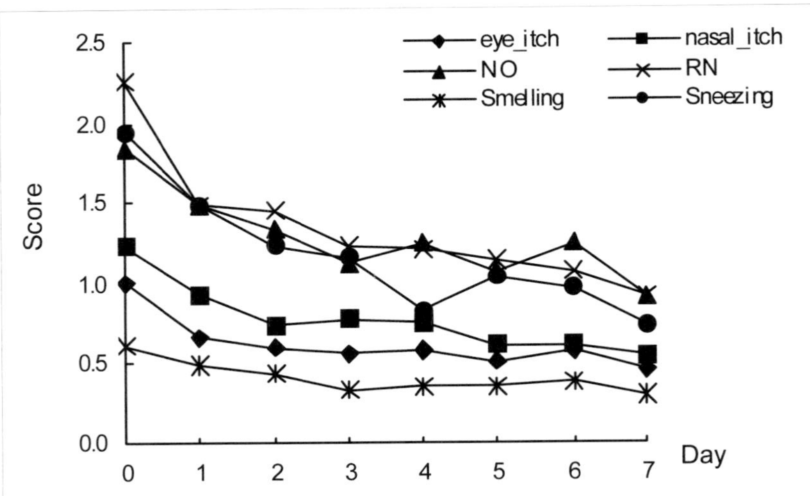

Fig. 1. Mean values of daily scores for six symptoms of AR. The score is given on a scale from 0 = no symptom to 3 = severe symptom. The symptom scores decreased over the period of FIR treatment. Pre-treatment (Day 0); during treatment (Day 1-7).

Mean values of daily registrations for eye itching, nasal itching, nasal stuffiness, rhinorrhea, smell impairment and sneezing after FIR therapy are given in Figure 1. All the symptom scores were reduced by more than 50% by the end of the FIR therapy. The most severe symptom of the pre-treat patients was rhinorrhea, which the mean value of the symptom score was 2.26, followed by sneezing and nasal stuffiness with scores of 1.94 and 1.84, respectively. The least severe symptom of the pre-treat patients was smell impairment with a mean score of 0.61. After the one-week treatment period, significant improvements were observed in all the symptoms of AR patients. The improved clinical symptoms were usually seen 1 day after the start of therapy, and thereafter the improvement was continuous. However, the smell impairment did not reveal significant improvement until after the 7th therapy. This was probably because the pre-treatment score of smell impairment was only 0.61 and not much room for improvement of the score or FIR was not very effective on improving olfactory disorder.

Our study demonstrated the improving effect of FIR therapy on the clinical symptoms of AR. Most of the clinical symptoms improved quickly and significantly. The patients tolerated the treatment well, and no severe adverse effect was observed during FIR treatment.

5.2 Red light acupoint stimulation in allergic rhinitis

Acupuncture involves the stimulation of acupoints that are located at a lines of meridians that correspond to the flow of energy through the body. Traditional treatment for AR by acupuncture may include needling and moxibustion. Modern acupuncture has evolved other methods of stimulating acupoints including the use of an electrical current, by applying pressure to the acupoint (acupressure) or using a low intensity laser or light emitting diodes (LEDs). Evidence suggests that acupuncture is a useful complementary or alternative treatment option for AR in both adults and children (Xue, et al., 2002; Ng, et al., 2004). Points of the ear are sensitive acupuncture treatment sites for a range of clinical conditions. Ear-acupressure is commonly used as a non-invasive alternative stimulation method by using small seeds or metal pellets on ear acupoints. A review based on 92 research papers searched from 21 electronic English and Chinese databases concluded that ear-acupressure was more effective than herbal medicine, as effective as body acupuncture or antihistamine for short-term effect. But it was more effective than anti-histamine for long-term effect. However, the benefit of ear-acupressure for systematic relief of AR is unknown due to the poor quality of included studies (Zhang, et al., 2010).

Allergic symptoms are largely dependent on oxygen radical formation, which were found to be suppressed after red light illumination. Shangyingxiāng Xue is an acupoint at the upper end of nasolabial fold. Acupuncture to Shangyingxiāng Xue helps to relieve symptoms of AR, rhinorrhea with turbid discharge, stuffy nose, and headache. Here, we evaluated the clinical effects of phototherapy using red light to Shangyingxiāng Xue on patients with AR(Hu & Yan, 2009).

Sixty-one AR patients who met the inclusion criteria were enrolled in this study. Patients were divided randomly into the treating group and control group. All patients filled out the informed consent form before treatment and recorded their symptom scores everyday in a diary before and during treatment. Thirty-one patients in the treating group received phototherapy with LEDs consisted of two wavelengths, 660 and 850 nm, to bilateral Shangyingxiāng Xue. Phototherapy was performed once a day for 7 days. The duration of each treatment was 10 minutes. Thirty patients in the control group received antihistamine (Zyrtec, 10 mg) once a day for 7 days. A symptom score of 0 to 3 was assigned for each of the following rhinitis symptoms: eye itching, nasal itching, nasal obstruction, rhinorrhea, smell impairment, sneezing and size of inferior turbinate. The scores of pre- and post-therapy in both groups were collected after the course of treatments and analyzed by using the paired sample t-test.

Thirty-one patients enrolled in the study completed the red light phototherapy. Mean values of daily registrations for eye itching, nasal itching, nasal stuffiness, rhinorrhea, smell impairment and sneezing are given in Figure 2. Most of the symptoms were quickly and significantly improved. The most severe symptom of the pre-treat patients was rhinorrhea, which the mean value of the symptom score was 2.0, followed by sneezing and nasal stuffiness with scores of 1.84 and 1.55, respectively. The least severe symptom of the pre-treat patients was smell impairment with a mean score of 0.71. After the one-week treatment period, significant improvements were observed in all the symptoms of AR patients. The improved clinical symptoms were usually seen 1 to 2 days after the start of therapy, and thereafter the improvement was continuous. However, the smell impairment did not reveal significant improvement until after the third treatment. This was probably because the pre-treatment score was lower than the others that there was not much room for improvement or phtotherapy to acupoint was not so effective on improving olfactory disorder.

Comparing the clinical effects of phototherapy and antihistamine control groups with repeated measures analysis, no difference was observed except the size of inferior turbinate. To sum up, phototherapy to Shangyingxiāng Xue could relieve the symptoms. Its low cost and low side effect suggest that phototherapy to Shangyingxiāng Xue is an attractive alternative to conventional treatment for AR patients.

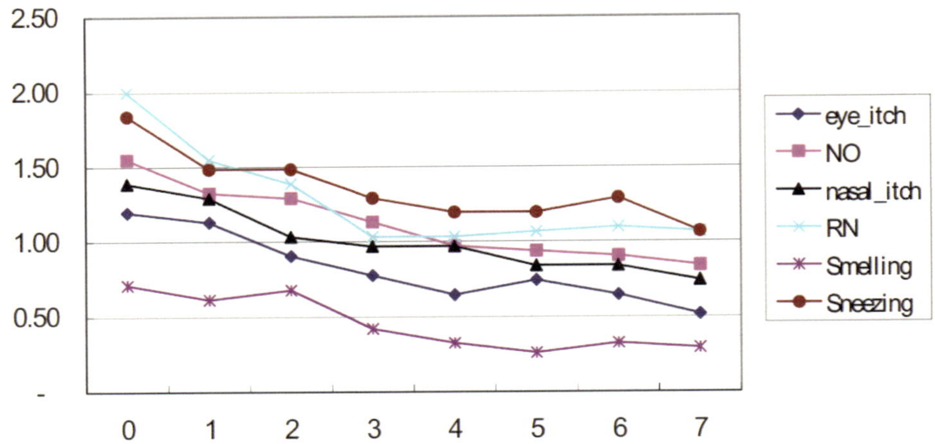

Fig. 2. Mean values of daily scores for symptoms of experimental group by using red light phototherapy. The symptom scores decreased over the period of red light treatment. Pre-treatment (Day 0); during treatment (Day 1-7).

6. Conclusion

Although new medication and topical applications are used with good results in the management of AR, there are cases in which complete resolution of symptoms cannot be obtained. Moreover, the use of drugs is not suitable for pregnant and breast-feeding women. Phototherapy is a safe and promising therapeutic modality for AR. Accumulating evidence supports that phototherapy suppresses the effector phase and results in significant improvement of clinical symptoms of AR. By applying FIR therapy to the nasal region in the patients with AR, our study demonstrated that FIR therapy could improve the clinical symptoms of eye itching, nasal itching, nasal stuffiness, rhinorrhea and sneezing significantly during period of therapy. Employing phototherapy to bilateral Shangyingxiāng Xue (an acupoint at the upper end of nasolabial fold) at 660 and 850 nm, symptom scores of AR had all significantly decreased in the treating group. In addition to UV and visible light, phototherapy with FIR and red light irradiation can improve the symptoms of AR and may serve as a novel modality in the treatment of AR.

7. Acknowledgment

During the writing of this article, supports of the authors were provided by grant from Keelung Hospital (No. 9815); the Department of Health, Executive Yuan, Taiwan(No. 97012), and NSC 99-2221-E-033-027, NSC 99-2627-E-033-001 from National Science Council of Taiwan. No conflict of interest is declared.

8. References

Akasaki, Y., Miyata, M., Eto, H., Shirasawa, T., Hamada, N., Ikeda, Y., Biro, S., Otsuji, Y. & Tei, C. (2006). Repeated Thermal Therapy Up-Regulates Endothelial Nitric Oxide

Synthase and Augments Angiogenesis in a Mouse Model of Hindlimb Ischemia. *Circulation Journal,* Vol.70, No.4, pp. 463-470

Akdis, C.A. & Blaser, L. (2003). Histamine in the Immune Regulation of Allergic Inflammation. *The Journal of Allergy and Clinical Immunology,* Vol.112, No.1, pp. 15-22

Al Suleimani, Y.M. & Walker, M.J. (2007). Allergic rhinitis and its pharmacology. *Pharmacology and Therapeutics,* Vol.114, No.3, pp. 233–260

Amat, A., Rigau, J., Waynant, R.W., Ilev, I.K. & Anders, J.J. (2006). The Electric Field Induced by Light can Explain Cellular Responses to Electromagnetic Energy: A Hypothesis of Mechanism. *Journal of Photochemistry and Photobiology B : Biology,* Vol.82, No.2, pp. 152-160

Berrettini, S., Carabelli, A., Sellari-Franceschini, S., Bruschini, L., Abruzzese, A., Quartieri, F., Sconosciuto, F. (1999). Perennial Allergic Rhinitis and Chronic Sinusitis: Correlation with Rhinologic Risk Factors. *Allergy,* Vol.54, No.3, pp. 242-248

Bousquet, J., van Cauwenberge, P. & Khaltaev, N. (2001). Allergic Rhinitis and Its Impact on Asthma. *The Journal of Allergy and Clinical Immunology,* Vol.108, Suppl.5, pp. S147-S334

Brehmer, D. & Schön, M.P. (2011). Endonasal Phototherapy Significantly Alleviates Symptoms of Allergic Rhinitis, But Has A Limited Impact on the Nasal Mucosa Immune Cells. *European Archives of Oto-Rhino-Laryngology,* Vol.268, No.3, pp. 393-399

Cingi, C., Cakli, H., Yaz, A., Songu, M. & Bal, C. (2010). Phototherapy for Allergic Rhinitis: A Prospective, Randomized, Single-Blind, Placebo-Controlled Study. *Therapeutic Advances in Respiratory Disease,* Vol.4, No.4, pp. 209-213

Cingi, C., Yaz, A., Cakli, H., Ozudogru, E., Kecik, C. & Bal, C. (2009). The Effects of Phototherapy on Quality of Life in Allergic Rhinitis Cases. *European Archives of Otorhinolaryngology,* Vol.266, No.12, pp. 1903-1908

Csoma Z., Koreck, A., Ignacz, F., Bor, Z., Szabo, G., Bodai, L., Dobozy, A. & Kemény, L. (2006). PUVA Treatment of the Nasal Cavity Improves the Clinical Symptoms of Allergic Rhinitis and Inhibits the Immediate-type Hypersensitivity Reaction in the Skin. *Journal of Photochemistry and Photobiology B : Biology,* Vol.83, No.1, pp.21-26

Csoma, Z., Ignacz, F., Bor, Z., Szabo, G., Bodai, L., Dobozy, A. & Kemény, L. (2004). Intranasal Irradiation with the Xenon Chloride Ultraviolet B Laser Improves Allergic Rhinitis. *Journal of Photochemistry and Photobiology B : Biology,* Vol.75, No.3, pp.137-144

Dykewicz, M.S., Fineman, S., Skoner, D.P., Nicklas, R., Lee, R., Blessing-Moore, J., Li, J.T., Bernstein, I.L., Berger, W., Spector, S. & Schuller, D. (1998). Diagnosis and Management of Rhinitis: Complete Guidelines of the Joint Task Force on Practice Parameters in Allergy, Asthma and Immunology. *Annals of Allergy, Asthma and Immunology,* Vol.81, No.5, pp. 478-518

Fineman, S.M. (2002). The Burden of Allergic Rhinitis : beyond Dollars and Cents. *Annals of Allergy, Asthma and Immunology,* Vol. 88, No.4, pp. S2-S7

Hallen, S., Oliveberg, M. & Brzezinski, P. (1993). Light-induced Structural Changes in Cytochrome c Oxidase. Measurements of Electrogenic Events and Absorbance Changes. *FEBS Letters,* Vol.318, No.2, pp. 134-138

Howarth P.H. (1997). Mediators of Nasal Blockage in Allergic Rhinitis. *Allergy,* Vol.52, Suppl.40, pp.12 -18

Hu, K.-H. & Li, W.-T. (2007). Clinical Effects of Far-Infrared Therapy in Patients with Allergic Rhinitis, *Proceedings of the 29th Annual International Conference of the IEEE EMBS,* pp.1479-1482, Lyon, France, August 23-26, 2007.

Hu, K.-H. & Yan, D.-N. (2009). Clinical Effects of Phototherapy to Shangyingxiāng Xue on 31 Patients with Allergic Rhinitis, *Journal of Changchun University of Traditional Chinese Medicine,* Vol.25, No.4, pp 266-267

Inoué, S. & Kabaya, M. (1989). Biological Activities Caused by Far-Infrared Radiation. *International Journal of Biometeorology,* Vol.33, No.3, pp. 15-150

Ishibashi, J., Yamashita, K., Ishikawa, T., Hosokawa, H., Sumida, K., Nagayama, M. & Kitamura, S. (2008). The Effects Inhibiting the Proliferation of Cancer Cells by Far-Infrared Radiation (FIR) Are Controlled by the Basal Expression Level of Heat Shock Protein (HSP) 70A. *Medical Oncology,* Vol.25, No.2, pp. 229-237

Jayasekera, N.P., Toma, T.P., Williams, A. & Rajakulasingam, K. (2007). Mechanisms of Immunotherapy in Allergic Rhinitis. *Biomedicine and Pharmacotherapy,* Vol.61, No.1, pp. 29-33

Kandolf-Sekulovic, L., Kataranovski, M. & Pavlovic, M.D. (2003). Immunomodulatory Effects of Low-Intensity Near-Infrared Laser Irradiation on Contact Hypersensitivity Reaction. *Photodermatology, Photoimmunology and Photomedicine,* Vol.19, No.4, p.203-212

Karu, T.I. (2003). Low Power Laser Therapy, In: *Biomedical Photonics Handbook,* T. Vo-Dinh, (Ed.), 48-1-25, CRC Press, ISBN 978-084-9311-16-1, Boca Raton, FL, USA

Karu, T.I., Pyatibrat, L.V. & Afanasyeva, N.I. (2005). Cellular Effects of Low Power Laser Therapy can Be Mediated by Nitric Oxide. *Lasers in Surgery and Medicine,* Vol.36, No.4, pp. 307-314

Karu, T.I., Pyatibrat, L.V., Kolyakov, S.F. & Afanasyeva, N.I. (2005). Absorption Measurements of a Cell Monolayer Relevant to Phototherapy: Reduction of Cytochrome c Oxidase under Near IR Radiation. *Journal of Photochemistry and Photobiology B : Biology,* Vol.81, No.2, pp. 98-106

Karu, T.I., Pyatibrat, L.V., Kolyakov, S.F. & Afanasyeva, N.I. (2008). Absorption Measurements of Cell Monolayers Relevant to Mechanisms of Laser Phototherapy: Reduction or Oxidation of Cytochrome c Oxidase under Laser Radiation at 632.8 nm. *Photomedicine and Laser Surgery,* Vol.26, No.6, pp. 593-599

Kemény, L. & Koreck, A. (2007). Ultraviolet Light Phototherapy for Allergic Rhinitis. *Journal of Photochemistry and Photobiology B : Biology,* Vol.87, No.1, pp.58-65

Koreck, A., Csoma, Z., Boros-Gyevi, M., Ignacz, F., Bodai, L., Dobozy, A., Kemeny, L. (2004). Inhibition of Immediate Type Hypersensitivity Reaction by Combined Irradiation with Ultraviolet and Visible Light. *Journal of Photochemistry and Photobiology B : Biology,* Vol.77, No.1-3, pp.93-96

Koreck, A., Szechenyi, A., Morocz, M., Cimpean, A., Bella, Zs., Garaczi, E., Raica, M., Olariu, T.R., Rasko, I. & Kemény, L. (2007). Effects of Intranasal Phototherapy on Nasal Mucosa in Patients with Allergic Rhinitis. *Journal of Photochemistry and Photobiology B : Biology,* Vol.89, No.2-3, pp.163-169

Koreck, A.I., Csoma, Z., Bodai, L., Ignacz, F., Kenderessy, A.S., Kadocsa, E., Szabo, G., Bor, Z., Erdei, A., Szony, B., Homey, B., Dobozy, A. & Kemény, L. (2005).

Rhinophototherapy : A New Therapeutic Tool for the Management of Allergic Rhinitis. *The Journal of Allergy and Clinical Immunology,* Vol.115, No.3, pp. 541-547

Koreck, A.I., Csoma, Z., Bodai, L., Ignacz, F., Kenderessy, A.S., Kadocsa, E., Szabo, G., Bor, Z., Erdei, A., Szony, B., Homey, B., Dobozy, A. & Kemeny, L. (2005). Rhinophototherapy: A New Therapeutic Tool for the Management of Allergic Rhinitis. *The Journal of Allergy and Clinical Immunology,* Vol.115, No.3, pp. 541-547

Lin, C.C., Chang, C.F., Lai, M.Y., Chen, T.W., Lee, P.C., Yang, W.C. (2007). Far-Infrared Therapy: A Novel Treatment to Improve Access Blood Flow and Unassisted Patency of Arteriovenous Fistula in Hemodialysis Patients. Journal of the American Society of Nephrology, Vol.18, No.3, pp. 985-992

Lin, C.C., Liu, X.M., Peyton, K., Wang, H., Yang, W.C., Lin, S.J. & Durante, W. (2008). Far Infrared Therapy Inhibits Vascular Endothelial Inflammation via the Induction of Heme Oxygenase-1. *Arteriosclerosis, Thrombosis, and Vascular Biology,* Vol.28, No.4, pp. 739-745

Lin, F., Josephs, S.F., Alexandrescu, D.T., Ramos, F., Bogin, V., Gammill, V., Dasanu, C.A., De Necochea-Campion, R., Patel, A.N., Carrier, E. & Koos, D.R. (2010). Lasers, Stem Cells, and COPD. *Journal of Translational Medicine,* Vol.8, No.16, pp. 1-10

Linder, A. (1988) Symptom Scores as Measures of the Severity of Rhinitis. *Clinical and Experimental Allergy,* 1988, Vol.18, No.1, pp. 29-37

Lubart, R., Eichler, M., Lavi, R., Friedman, H. & Shainberg, A. (2005). Low-energy Laser Irradiation Promotes Cellular Redox Activity. *Photomedicine and Laser Surgery,* Vol.23, No.1, pp. 3-9

Morita, A., Weiss, M. & Maeda, A. (2008) Recent Developments in Phototherapy: Treatment Methods and Devices. *Recent Patents on Inflammation and Allergy Drug Discovery,* Vol.2, No.2, pp. 105-108

Naclerio, R., Rosenwasser, L. & Ohkubot, K. (2002). Allergic Rhinitis: Current and Future Treatments. *Clinical and Experimental Allergy Reviews,* Vol.2, No.4, pp. 137-147

Neuman, I. & Finkelstein, Y. (1997). Narrow-band Red Light Phototherapy in Perennial Allergic Rhinitis and Nasal Polyposis. *Annals of Allergy, Asthma and Immunology,* Vol.78, No.4, pp.399-406

Ng, D.K., Chow, P.Y., Ming, S.P., Hong, S.H., Lau, S., Tse, D., Kwong, W.K., Wong, M.F., Wong, W.H., Fu, Y.M., Kwok, K.L., Li, H. & Ho, J.C. (2004) A Double-Blind, Randomized, Placebo-Controlled Trial of Acupuncture for The Treatment of Childhood Persistent Allergic Rhinitis. *Pediatrics,* Vol.114, No.5, pp.1242-1247

Okuda, M., Watase, T., Mezawa, A. & Liu, C.M. (1988). The Role of Leukotriene D4 in Allergic Rhinitis. *Annals of Allergy,* Vol.60, No.6, pp.537-540

Oppenheimer, J.J. & Casale, T.B. (2002). Next Generation Antihistamines: Therapeutic Rationale, Accomplishments and Advances. *Expert Opinion on Investigational Drugs,* Vol.11, No.6, pp. 807-8174

Pipet, A., Botturi, K., Pinot, D., Vervloet, D. & Magnan, A. (2009). Allergen-specific immunotherapy in allergic rhinitis and asthma. Mechanisms and proof of efficacy. *Respiratory Medicine,* Vol.103, No.6, pp. 800-812

Quraishi, S.A., Davies, M.J. & Craig, T.J. (2004). Inflammatory Responses in Allergic Rhinitis : Traditional Approaches and Novel Treatment Strategies, *The Journal of the American Osteopathic Association,* Vol.104, Suppl.5, pp.S7-S15

Rau, C.S., Yang, J.C., Jeng, S.F., Chen, Y.C., Lin, C.J., Wu, C.J., Lu, T.H. & Hsieh, C.H. (2011). Far-Infrared Radiation Promotes Angiogenesis in Human Microvascular Endothelial Cells via Extracellular Signal-Regulated Kinase Activation. *Photochemistry and Photobiology,* Vol. 87, No. 2, pp. 441-446

Salib, R.J., Drake-Lee, A. & Howarth, P.H. (2003). Allergic Rhinitis : Past, Present and the Future. *Clinical Otolaryngology,* Vol.28, No.4, pp. 201-303

Skoner, D.P. (2000). Complications of Allergic Rhinitis. *The Journal of Allergy and Clinical Immunology,* Vol.105, No.6, pp. S605-S609

Su, L.H., Wu, K.D., Lee, L.S., Wang, H. & Liu, C.F. (2009). Effects of Far Infrared Acupoint Stimulation on Autonomic Activity and Quality of Life in Hemodialysis Patients. *The American Journal of Chinese Medicine,* Vol.37, No.2, pp. 215–226

Toyokawa, H., Matsui, Y., Uhara, J., Tsuchiya, H., Teshima, S., Nakanishi, H., Kwon, A.H., Azuma, Y., Nagaoka, T., Ogawa, T. & Kamiyama, Y. (2003). Promotive Effects of Far-Infrared Ray on Full-Thickness Skin Wound Healing in Rats. *Experimental Biology and Medicine (Maywood),* Vol.228, No.6, pp. 724-729

van Cauwenberge, P., Bachert, C., Passalacqua, G. Bousquet, J., Canonica, G.W., Durham, S.R., Fokkens, W.J., Howarth, P.H., Lund, V., Malling, H.J., Mygind, N., Passali, D., Scadding, G.K. & Wang, D.Y. (2000). Consensus Statement on the Treatment of Allergic Rhinitis. European Academy of Allergology and Clinical Immunology. *Allergy,* Vol.55, No.2, pp. 116-134

Vladimirov, Y.A., Osipov, A.N. & Klebanov, G.I. (2004). Photobiological Principles of Therapeutic Applications of Laser Radiation. *Biochemistry (Mosc),* Vol.69, No.1, pp. 81-90

Weiner, J. M., Abramson, M.J. & Puy, R.M. (1998). Intranasal Corticosteroids versus Oral H_1 Receptor Antagonists in Allergic Rhinitis, Systemic Review of Randomized Controlled Trials. *British Medical Journal,* Vol.317, No.7173, pp. 1624-1629

Wilson, A.M., Sims, E.J., McFarlane, L.C. & Lipworth, B.J. (1998). Effects of Intranasal Corticosteroids on Adrenal, Bone, and Blood Markers of Systemic Activity in Allergic Rhinitis. *The Journal of Allergy and Clinical Immunology,* Vol.102, No.4, pp. 598-604

Xue, C.C., English, R., Zhang, J.J., Da Costa, C. & Li, C.G. (2002). Effect of Acupuncture in the Treatment of Seasonal Allergic Rhinitis: A Randomized Controlled Clinical Trial. *The American Journal of Chinese Medicine,* Vol.30, No.1, pp. 1-11

Yu, S.Y., Chiu, J.H., Yang, S.D., Hsu, Y.C., Lui, W.Y. & Wu, C.W. (2006). Biological Effect of Far-Infrared Therapy on Increasing Skin Microcirculation in Rats. *Photodermatology, Photoimmunology and Photomedicine,* Vol.22, No.2, pp.78-86

Zhang, C.S., Yang, A.W., Zhang, A.L., Fu, W.B., Thien, F.U., Lewith, G., Xue, C.C. (2010). Ear-acupressure for Allergic Rhinitis: A Systematic Review. *Clinical Otolaryngology,* Vol.35, No.1, pp. 6-12

12

Evaluation of Therapeutic Efficacy of *Nigella sativa* (Black Seed) for Treatment of Allergic Rhinitis

Abdulghani Mohamed Alsamarai,
Mohamed Abdul Satar and Amina Hamed Ahmed Alobaidi
Departments of Medicine and Biochemistry, Tikrit University College of Medicine
Tikrit
Iraq

1. Introduction

Allergy in general is a common problem in the community, when all aspects of allergy are considered, this condition may well represent the largest single medical problem seen in the United States today and probably in the world.[1] Allergic rhinitis is the commonest allergic disease. It alone is the sixth most prevalent chronic disease in the world, outranking heart disease. [2] There were six factors that stimulated us to choose this disease in our study: firstly, Allergic rhinitis is the commonest allergic disease in the world, affect 10-25% of population [3], secondly, Although it is not a life threatening but from an economic point of view, allergic rhinitis is not a minor problem based on figures reported elsewhere[4], thirdly, Till now, there is no curative treatment for allergic rhinitis except specific immunotherapy which have many side effects and not suitable for every patient especially when multiple allergens are implicated, which is commonest than single allergen.[5], fourthly, Serious side effects of pharmacotherapy used in treatment of allergic rhinitis especially steroids which reflected in recent years a trend of increasing use of alternative medicines[6-7],fifthly, Allergic rhinitis was frequently trivialized by patients and doctors (particularly non sufferers),this may be because it is not a fatal disease yet it remains a common cause of morbidity, social embarrassment and impaired performance either at school or in the work place, moreover , it may be complicated by a course of other diseases such as sinusitis, otitis media and asthma. [3-8] and lastly, in a previous studies, it has been proved that Nigella sativa is an effective treatment of asthma. It also showed an improvement in the associated nasal symptoms that accompanied asthma [9,10] Administration of black seed oil significantly reduced the level of allergen induced lung remodeling [11].

Allergic rhinitis is a common disease, accounting for at least 2.5% of all physician visits, 2 million lost school days per year, 6 million lost work days, and 28 million restricted work days per year. At least $ 5.3 billion is spent annually on prescription and over-the-counters medications for allergy[12] . Between 10 and 25% of the population is affected[3] and the prevalence in urban areas is increasing .The prevalence is lowest in children below age 5 , rises to a peak in early adulthood and declines thereafter. The 4 year remission rate reported to be 10% in males and 5% in females.[13]

N.S. is a an annual famous herb, the respect of which in the medical field is taken from a religious origin when the prophet Mohammed ρ advised people to use it in order to treat different diseases. The seeds of N.S are considered as carminative, stimulant, galactoguge, anti tussive, anti flu and anti flatulence e.t.c. (2). Anti allergic effects of N.S. was reported (2). The active ingredient is thymoquinone with its carbonyl polymer. (14) Recently reported study suggest the N. sativa could reduce the presence of the nasal mucosal congestion, nasal itching, runny nose, sneezing attacks, turbinate hypertrophy, and mucosal pallor during the first 2 weeks(15). Furthermore, N. sativa supplementation during specific immunotherapy of AR may be considered a potential adjuvant therapy (16) and it was equal therapeutic activity in relieving the symptoms of seasonal AR to cetirizine, without its side effects (17).

1.1 AIm of the study

To evaluate the therapeutic effect of systemic forms of black seed oil in allergic rhinitis

2. Materials and methods

2.1 Study population

A total of 188 patients with allergic rhinitis symptoms of different severities (mild, moderate and severe) with age ranging from 6-45 years, were included in this study [Table 1]. This double blinded clinical trial was performed during the period between January 2009 to June 2010 in the out- patient clinic of centre of allergy in Tikrit Teaching Hospital (TTH) in Salahuldean governorate, Iraq. The patients were either referred from medical or ENT departments, from the out patients in the same hospital and those who attended the allergy centre to have immunotherapy.

2.2 Diagnosis of asthma and allergic rhinitis

The diagnosis of asthma and classification was performed by specialist physicians based on the National Heart Blood and Lung Institute / World Health Organization (NHLBI/WHO) workshop on the Global Strategy for Asthma (18). Allergic rhinitis diagnosis was performed according to previously reported guidelines (19).

2.3 Skin prick test

The skin prick tests were performed for all patients and control and evaluated in accordance with European Academy of Allergy and Clinical Immunology subcommittee on allergy standardization and skin tests using standards allergen panel (Stallergen, France). The panel for skin test include: dust mite (Dermatophagoides farina, Dermatophagoides peteronyssinus), Aleternaria, Cladosprium, Penicillum mixture, Aspergillus mixture, Grasses mixture, Feather mixture, Dog hair, Horse hair, Cat fur, Fagacae, Oleaceae, Betulaceae, Plantain, Bermuda grass, Chenopodium and Mugworth. All tests were performed in the outpatient Asthma and Allergy Centre, Mosul by a physician using a commercial allergen extracts (Stallergen, France) and a lancet skin prick test device. A wheal diameter of 3 mm or more in excess of the negative control was considered as positive test result.

2.3.1 Allergen extracts for skin prick test

Therapeutic vaccines containing allergen extracts were purchased from Stallergen, France. Both aqueous and glycenerated extracts were used to achieve a concentrate of 1:100 w/v of the mixed extract. In standardized extracts the stock formulation was prepared by tenfold dilution. Separate vial was used for allergen extract to reduce proteolysis degradation. All extracts were stored at 8 ^{0}C . Therapeutic vaccine varied with each individual patient based on specific allergen identified during testing. Moist patients received a variety of aeroallergen combination.

Variable	Active group	Control group	Total Number [%]
Patients total number	115	95	210
Patients completed study	102	86	188
Female/Male	58/44	48/38	106/82
Mild group			
Total number	35	30	65
Patient completed study	31	27	58
Female/Male	18/13	16/11	34/24
Moderate group			
Total number	50	40	90
Patient completed study	44	37	81
Female/Male	25/19	20/17	45/36
Severe group			
Total number	30	25	55
Patient completed study	27	22	49
Female/Male	15/12	12/10	27/22
Gender			
Male			82 [43.6]
Female			106 [56.4]
Age in year			
6 -15			60 [31.9]
16-25			75 [39.8]
26-35			36 [19.1]
36-45			17 [9.0]
Duration in year			
Mild			1-4
Moderate			2-7
Severe			2.5–11
Skin test			
Single			63 [33.5]
Multiple			125 [66.5]
Two			76 [40.4]
Three			40 [21.3]
Four			9 [4.8]
HDM			103 [54.7]
Candida			70 [37.2]
Molds			65 [34.5]
Grass mixture			58 [30.8]
Animal dander			32 [17.0]
Other pollen			43 [22.8]
Associated diseases			
Conjunctivitis	68 [66.6]	43 [50]	111 [59]
Asthma	33 [32.3]	26 [30.2]	59 [31.4]
Sinusitis	15 [14.7]	17 [19.7]	32 [17]
Urticaria	12 [11.7]	5 [5.8]	17 [9]
Otitis media	4 [3.9]	3 [3.4]	7 [3.7]
Polyps	4 [3.9]	2 [2.3]	6 [3.2]

Variable	Active group	Control group	Total Number [%]
Exacerbating factor			
Allergen exposure	89 [87.2]	64 [74.2]	153 [81.4]
URT infection	39 [38.2]	24 [27.9]	63 [33.5]
Temperature change	26 [25.4]	22 [25.5]	48 [25.5]
Smoke & irritants	21 [20.5]	14 [16.2]	35 [18.6]
Hormonal	4 [3.9]	2 [2.3]	6 [3.2]
Severity			
Mild	31 [30.4]	27 [31.4]	58 [30.8]
Moderate	44 [43.1]	37 [43.0]	81 [43.1]
Severe	27 [26.5]	22 [25.6]	49 [26.1]
Pattern			
Seasonal	41 [40.2]	37 [43.0]	78 [41.5]
Mild	11 [26.8]	9 [24.3]	20 [25.6]
Moderate	20 [48.8]	20 [54.1]	40 [51.3]
Severe	10 [24.4]	8 [21.6]	18 [23.1]
Pereniall	61 [59.8]	49 [57.0]	110 [58.5]
Mild	20 [32.8]	18 [36.7]	38 [34.5]
Moderate	24 [34.3]	17 [34.7]	41 [37.3]
Severe	17 [27.9]	14 [28.6]	31 [28.2]
Family atopy			
Mild			
Atopic	11 [35.5]	13 [48.1]	24 [41.3]
Non-atopic	20 [64.5]	14 [51.9]	34 [58.7]
Moderate			
Atopic	21 [47.7]	19 [51.4]	40 [49.3]
Non-atopic	23 [52.3]	18 [48.6]	41 [50.7]
Severe			
Atopic	17 [63]	14 [63.6]	31 [63.2]
Non-atopic	10 [37]	8 [36.4]	18 [36.8]
IgE IU/ml			
Mild	143	168	
Moderate	176	188	
Severe	393	361	

Table 1. Patients characteristics at time of enrolled in the trial.

2.4 Determination of total serum IgE

ELISA was performed to estimate the total serum IgE level as a serological marker for treatment response monitoring.[20] Total serum IgE was determined by enzyme linked immunosorbant assay kit (Biomaghreb). Results were interpreted as allergy not probable if serum IgE was lower than 20 IU/ml, allergy is possible if IgE value is between 20 and 120 IU/ml and allergy is very probable if IgE is more than 120 IU/ml.

2.5 Classification of patients

In classifying the patients, two types of classification were adopted[3,5]

According to severity of symptoms. They were also sub classified into the following: mild group :A total 58 patients (31 active and 27 control); Moderate group: A total 81 patients (44 active and 37 control); and Severe group: A total 49 patients (27 active and 22 control)

According to allergens. The patients were sub classified into the following :

- Seasonal class: A total 78 patients (41 active and 37 control).
- Perennial class: A total 110 patients (61 active and 49 control).

2.6 Family history of allergy

Because allergic diseases are familial diseases, some emphasis was laid on the families of patients to know the percentage of them that had allergic diathesis.

3. Systemic use of the black seed oil

The herb was given in the form of capsules, one capsule three times a day .Each capsule was about 0.6-0.8 gm of oil (which is about half of the dose that used in asthma in a previous study)[9] The control group received same shaped capsules but they contained ordinary food oil. The treatment was given for 6 weeks for both groups . The results were recorded on the patient's questionnaire each visit .The same routine physical examination and laboratory investigations as mentioned earlier were done and recorded in addition to the clinical evaluation which was done according to the following criteria:

3.1 Clinical assessment (symptom score)

During each visit, the patient was examined clinically for vital signs and questioned about the improvement in his day and night symptoms (Rhinorrhoea, nasal obstruction, paroxysm of sneezing, night snoring, daily physical activities, school attendance and affection of life quality). Symptom score was of 4 points scale (0-3) according to the classification of rhinitis symptoms as specified by:

0. No symptoms.
1. Mild symptoms: Symptoms not interfere with sleep, normal daily activities, (sports, leisure), no trouble of some symptoms, sneezing (not more than 3 in each attack or paroxysm), with mild runny nose (of no more than 1hour).[3,5]
2. Moderate symptoms: Are of one or more items of the following: abnormal sleep, impairment of daily activities, (sports, and leisure), problems caused at work, at school with troublesome symptoms: longer attack > 1h. -<8 with uncomfortable stuffy, runny nose, sneering 4-10 sneeze each attack. [3,5]
3. Severe symptoms: The same as moderate but more severe, more nasal blockage and sleep interference with severe distressing stuffy, runny nose for more than 8h. attack with sneeze more than 10 times each paroxysm. [3,5]

3.2 Tolerability to the exacerbating factors

Many precipitating factors such as aeroallergen exposure, cold exposure, infection (sinusitis), drugs ...etc. may precipitate the condition, so the response to the exacerbating factors were assessed in each visit by skin test.

3.3 Other associated allergic diseases

Other allergic diseases such as asthma, conjunctivitis and urticaria were also recorded in each visits.

3.4 Side effects

Side effects that were shown by the patients were recorded for both systemic and nasal uses.

3.5 Statistical analysis

CHI square analytic system (X^2) with Yates correction was used to compare between active and placebo groups. However, Chi Square is calculated only if the expected cell frequencies are equal to or greater than 5. While Fisher Exact Probability Test is used if some cells are less than five. Student t test is used to determine the significance of IgE differences between the groups.

4. Results

For systemic trial, a total of 210 patients were included in the study. Of them 115 patients received the treatment [active group] and 95 patients were the controls. The patients were divided according to their disease severity, and each of the above groups was subdivided into active and control groups. As mentioned earlier, 188 patients completed the course of treatment in this study while 22 patients withdrawn from the study [Table 1].

4.1 Age and sex frequency distribution

The eligible patients for analysis were subdivided into 3 groups as follow:
Mild group: A total of 58 patients were included, of them: 31 patients (18 female and 13 male) were mild active group and 27 patients (16 female and 11 male) were mild control group. Mild group patients accounts for 30.8% of the total .
Moderate group: A total of 81 patients were included , of them : 44 patients (25 female and 19 male) were moderate active group and 37 patients (20 female and 17 male) were moderate control group. Moderate group patients accounts for 43. 1% of the total.
Severe group: A total of 49 patients were included, of them: 27 patients (15 female and 12 male) constitute the severe active group while 22 patients (12 female, and 10 male) constitute the severe control group. Severe group patients accounts for 26.1% of the total. Male patients account for 43.6% and female ones account for 56.4% of total patients. The highest frequency of AR is in the age group of 16 -25 years and then the declines with age.
Frequency distribution of the patients according to the duration of AR : Severe group had the longest duration of the diseases which was from 2.5 years-11 years, while mild group had the shortest duration range which was from 1 years- 4 years.
Classification of the patients according to allergen's type:
One of the important classification of the allergic rhinitis depending on the type of exacerbating allergen into the seasonal and perennial type. Perennial type (110 patient, 58.5%) was more common than seasonal type (78 patient, 41.5%).

4.2 Monthly distribution of the patients

The monthly distribution of the patients indicated that 63.2% of cases were reported in March, April and May.

4.3 Exacerbating factors

The potent exacerbating factor in both groups was allergen exposure which account for 87.2% ,(89 patients) in active group and 74.2% (64 patients) in control group. The upper respiratory tract infection forms 38.2% ,(39 patients) in active group and 27.9% ,(24 patients) in control group. This is followed by temperature and humidity changes with cold exposure which was 25.4%,(26 patients) in active group and 25.5% ,(22 patients) in control group. Then smoke and irritants factor which was about 20.5% ,(21 patients) in active group and 16.2%,(14 patients) in control group .The last exacerbating factor that affect the disease in the studied patients was hormonal factor (i.e. pregnancy) which was 3.9% ,(4 patients) in active group and 2.3% ,(2 patients) in control group.

4.4 Family atopic diathesis

As it is clear from the history of patients as shown in Table 3: atopic family diathesis with positive family history of allergy (in any form of allergy as asthma, eczema, and allergic rhinitis) was found in 41.3% (24 patients) of total mild group (13 control and 11 active) .This increased to 49.3% (40 patients) of total moderate group (19 control and 21active) .While the highest incidence was in severe allergic rhinitis group which was 63.2% (31 patients) (14 control and 17 active) .This means that the disease is generally more severe in patients of atopic diathesis or tendency.

4.5 Associated diseases

Conjunctivitis was the most common associated disease which accounted for 66.6% (68 patients) of total active group and 50% (43 patients) of total control group. Asthma was the second common associated disease. In active group it is accounted for 32.3% (33 patients) and in control group it is 30.2 (26 patients) while sinusitis which comes thirdly, accounted for 14.7% (15 patients) of active group and 19.7% (17 patients) of control group. The lowest associated disease was nasal polyposis which account for 3.9% (4 patients) of total active group and 2.3% (2 patients) of total control group.

4.6 Skin test results

In 33.5% of patients (63 patients) the test was positive to only one allergen and in 66.5% (125 patients) was positive to multiple allergen. Double allergen positive skin test results form 40.4% (76 patients), while triple allergen positive skin test results form 21.3% (40 patients) and lastly quadrant allergen positive skin test results form 4.8% (9 patients) of total 188 patients. For frequency distribution of the skin tests result according to allergens type, the highest incidence was HDM which accounted for 54.7% (103 patients), then Candida albicans 37.2% (70 patients). Animal dander account for 17% (32 patients), forms the lowest frequency.

4.7 IgE serum level

Serum IgE mean was 143 IU/ml in mild active and 168 IU/ml in mild control groups and were lower than those of the moderate groups (active,176 IU/ml; control, 188 IU/ml). This in turn was less than that of severe allergic rhinitis of both active (393 IU/ml) and control (361 IU/ml) groups.

4.8 Effects after 6 weeks systemic treatment

4.8.1 Symptomatic response: [Table 2]

Mild group response: In mild active group,19 patients out of 31,(61.3%), became free from symptoms after a three week of treatment with black seed oil .This percentage is considered highly significant (P=0.000) when it is compared with mild control group of which only 4 patients out of 27 (14.8%) , became free from symptoms. After six weeks of treatment, the results of mild group are as following : 30 patients (96.7%) did not show symptoms .This results is highly significant (P=0.000) when it is compared with mild control group of which only 7 patients (25. 9%) did not show symptoms.

Group		Active group				Control group			
		0W	3W	6W	P value	0W	3W	6W	P value
Mild	Symptomatic	31	12	1		27	23	20	
		(100%)	(38.7%)	(3.2%)		(100%)	(85.1%)	(74.5)	
	Symptom free	0	19	30	0.000	0	4	7	NS
		(0%)	(61.3%)	(96.7%)		(0%)	(14.8%)	(25.9%)	
Moderate	Symptomatic	44	21	9		37	32	29	
		(100%)	(47.7%)	(20.4%)		(100%)	(86.4%)	(78.3%)	
	Improved	0	17	21		0	5	6	
		(0%)	(38.6%)	(47.7%)		(0%)	(13.5%)	(16.20%)	
	Symptom free	0	6	14	0.000	0	0	2	NS
		(0%)	(13.6%)	(31.8%)		(0%)	(0%)	(5.4%)	
Severe	Symptomatic	27	17	11		22	19	17	
		(100%)	(62.9%)	(40.7%)		(100%)	(86.3%)	(77.2%)	
	Improved	0	8	10		0	3	5	
		(0%)	(29.9%)	(37%)		(0%)	(13.6%)	(22.7%)	
	Symptom free	0	2	6	NS	0	0	0	NS
		(0%)	(7.4%)	(22.2%)		(0%)	(0%)	(0%)	

Table 2. Symptomatic response at 6 weeks systemic use

Moderate group response: In moderate group, after 3 weeks of treatment, 17 patients out of 44 (38.6%) demonstrate partial improvement while 6 patients (13.6%) became symptoms free patients. So 23 patients out of 44 (52.2%) demonstrated either partial or total improvement of their signs and symptoms. These results are highly significant (P=0.004) as compared with moderate control group from whom only 5 patients out of 37 (13.5%) got partial improvement at the end of 3 weeks . At the end of 6 weeks treatment in moderate active group; 21 patients (47.7%) show partial improvement and 14 patients (31.8%) were symptoms free. Thus, the total improved patients of moderate active group at the end of 6 weeks (partially and a totally improved) were 35 patients out of 44 , nearly about 79.5% . This is significant with (P=0.02) as compared with moderate control group at 6 weeks treatment of which 6 patients (16.2%) got partial improvement while only 2 patients (5.4%) got no symptoms. Therefore in moderate control group 8 patients (12.5%) improved (partially ,and totally) at the end of the 6 weeks.

Severe group responses: For severe active group, 8 patient out of 27 (29.9%) show partial improvement while 2 patients(7.4%) became free from symptoms after 3 weeks treatment with black seed capsules .This indicate that 10 patients (36.3%) demonstrate treatment benefit (partially or totally). While in severe control group, 3 patients out of 22 (13.6%) got partial improvement after 3 weeks of treatment with ordinary food oil capsules and none became non symptomatic. At the end of 6 weeks of treatment for severe active group: 10 patients (37%) were got partial improvement while 6 (22.2%) got symptoms free. Thus collectively improved patients were 16 patients (59.2%). Clinically, this is considered a good result and is statistically significant (P=0.026) as compared with the results of severe control group were only 5 patients (22.7%) got partial improvement. The differences in clinical improvement between 3 and 6 weeks treatment duration was highly significant (P=0.000) as compared to baseline for both mild and moderate active group. However, it was not significant in case of severe group.

4.9 Serum IgE

The mean serum IgE level in mild active group decreased from 143 IU/ml at the baseline estimation to 91 after a 6 week treatment with N. sativa oil, while in mild control group, it decreased from 168 IU/ml to 131 IU/ml after a 6 week treatment with ordinary food oil. In moderate active group, it decreased from 176 IU/ml at the baseline estimation to 127 IU/ml after 6 weeks of treatment while for moderate control group also there was reduction in the IgE average level from 188 IU/ml to 152 IU/ml. In severe group, the IgE average level of severe active group decreased from 393 IU/ml to 354 IU/ml and the same thing occurred in control group which decreased from 361 IU/ml at the baseline estimation to 335 IU/ml at the end of the 6 week treatment. The reduction in serum IgE means level pre- and post-treatment was significant for both active and control groups, however, there was a significant differences between active and control groups [Table 3].

		Mean IgE IU/ml [SD]		
		Mild	Moderate	Severe
Active	Pretreatment	143 [8.9]	176 [11.3]	393 [18.7]
	Post treatment	91 [7.1]	127 [7.7]	354 [12.3]
	Difference	52	49	39
	P value	0.000	0.000	0.000
Control	Pretreatment	168 [9.6]	188 [10.1]	361 [16.4]
	Post treatment	131 [10.4]	152 [12.5]	335 [17.5]
	Difference	37	36	26
	P value	0.000	0.000	0.000
P value for difference between active & control		0.000	0.000	0.007

Table 3. Effect of systemic treatment with N. sativa on IgE [IU/ ml] serum level.

4.10 Tolerability to the exacerbating factors

Improvement in tolerability of the exacerbating factors in total active group and total control group are shown in Table 6. The response to allergen exposure has improved from 24.5% after 3 weeks (P=0.001) treatment to 37.5% at 6 weeks (P=0.000) treatment in the active group while in control group, the improvement was much less. The allergen exposure tolerability was significant during the treatment course (P=0.000), however, there was no significant difference between 3 and 6 weeks of treatment period. The response to temperature variation has also improved to about 7.8% at the end of 3 weeks (P=0.01) and to about 11.7% at the end of 6 weeks treatment in active group (P=0.001) .This is better than that of control group which was about 2.3 at the end of 3 weeks and increased to 4.6 (4 patients) at the end of 6 weeks . Another environmental factor that showed improvement was exposure to irritant gases which increased from 5.8% at the 3 week (P=0.03) treatment in active group to 9.8% at the end of 6 weeks (P=0.00 3) while in control group, a minor improvement occurred, which was from 2.31 after 3 weeks of treatment to 3.4% after 6 weeks of treatment. [Table 4].

Variable	Active groupNumber [%]	Control groupNumber [%]	P value
Allergen exposure			
3 week	25 [24.5]	3 [3.4]	0.000
6 week	38 [37.2]	5 [5.8]	0.000
P value 0,3 & 6 weeks	0.000	NS	
0 & 3 weeks	0.001	NS	
0 & 6 weeks	0.000	NS	
3 & 6 weeks	NS	NS	
Temperature change			
3 week	8 [7.8]	2 [2.3]	NS
6 week	[11.7]	2 [2.3]	0.02
P value 0,3 & 6 weeks	NS	NS	
0 & 3 weeks	0.01	NS	
0 & 6 weeks	0.001	NS	
3 & 6 weeks	NS	NS	
Irritant exposure			
3 week	6 [5.8]	4 [4.6]	NS
6 week	10 [9.8]	3 [3.4]	NS
P value 0,3 & 6 weeks	NS	NS	
0 & 3 weeks	0.03	NS	
0 & 6 weeks	0.003	NS	
3 & 6 weeks	NS	NS	

Table 4. Tolerability to the exacerbating factors

4.11 Symptomatic response in associated allergic illnesses

The common associated allergic disease allergic rhinitis was allergic conjunctivitis which accounts for 66.6% (68 patients) and this was decreased to 21.5% (22 patients) at the 3 weeks (P=0.000) treatment then became 17.6% (18 patients) at the end of 6 weeks (P=0.000) treatment. While in control group, conjunctivitis affect 50% (43 patients) which showed some improvement after 3 weeks to 44.1% (38 patients) and decreased lastly to 39.5% (34 patients) at the end of 6 weeks treatment . The differences between active and control groups was significant for both 3 and 6 weeks course treatment (P=0.001). Table 5.

Asthma which was presented in 32.3%(33 patients) of active group decreased to 21.5% (22 patients) after 3 weeks and then decreased to 18.6% (19 patients) at end of 6 weeks while in control group, 30.2% (26 patients) have asthma which showed improvement by decreasing in symptomatic patients to 26.7% (23 patients) at 3 weeks treatment, then decreasing to 24.4% (21 patients) at the end of 6 weeks treatment .however, the differences between active and control groups was not significant. Table 5.

The last associated disease was urticaria which showed some improvement : 9.8% (10 patients) were had symptoms at the beginning of the study and decreased to 6.8% (7 patients) at 3 weeks treatment which then decreased to 4.9% (5 patients) at the end of 6 weeks. While in control group, 8.1% (7 patients) have symptomatic urticaria decreased to 6.9% (6 patients) by 3 weeks and remained the same at the end of 6 weeks treatment. The demonstrated differences between active and control groups was not significant. Table 5.

Variable	Active group Number [%]	Control group Number [%]	P value
Conjunctivitis			
0 week	68 [66.6]	43 [50]	0.03
3 week	22 [21.5]	38 [44.1]	0.001
6 week	18 [17.6]	34 [39.5]	0.001
P value 0,3 & 6 weeks	0.000	NS	
0 & 3 weeks	0.000	NS	
0 & 6 weeks	0.000	NS	
3 & 6 weeks	NS	NS	
Asthma			
0 week	33 [32.3]	26 [30.2]	NS
3 week	22 [21.5]	23 [26.7]	NS
6 week	19 [18.6]	21 [24.4]	NS
P value 0,3 & 6 weeks	NS	NS	
0 & 3 weeks	NS	NS	
0 & 6 weeks	0.03	NS	
3 & 6 weeks	NS	NS	
Urticaria			
0 week	10 [9.8]	7 [8.1]	NS
3 week	7 [6.8]	6 [6.9]	NS
6 week	5 [4.9]	6 [6.9]	NS
P value 0,3 & 6 weeks	NS	NS	
0 & 3 weeks	NS	NS	
0 & 6 weeks	NS	NS	
3 & 6 weeks	NS	NS	

Table 5. Symptomatic response in associated allergic illness.

Group	Sub group	Improved patients on 3 and 6 weeks		Withdrawal effect on improved patients	
		3 weeks	6 week	Patients with recurrence of symptoms	Not symptomatic Patients
Mild AR group (58)	Active group 31	19 61.3%	30 96.7%	25 80.6%	5 16.1%
	Control group 27	4 14.8%	7 25.9%	2 7.4%	5 18.5%
	P value			0.000	
Moderate AR group(81)	Active group 44	23 52.2%	35 79.5%	32 72.7%	3 6.8%
	Control group 37	5 13.5%	8 21.6%	3 8.1%	5 13.5%
	P value			0.009	
Severe AR group (49)	Active group 27	10 37.3%	16 59.2%	14 55.5%	2 7.4
	Control group 22	3 13.6%	5 22.7%	2 9%	3 13.6%
	P value			NS	

Table 6. Two weeks systemic oil treatment with drawl effect

4.12 Factors associated with poor response to systemic NS treatment in AR

The following factors seem to be associated with poor response to the systemic herb treatment [Table. 6]: Multiple allergic diseases in the same patients, High IgE serum level, Gender (female), Perennial type more than seasonal one, Atopic diathesis, and Older age group.

4.13 Two weeks systemic oil treatment withdrawal effect

Two weeks systemic oil treatment with drawl effect is shown in Table 9. In mild active group, from 96.7% that improved at 6 weeks treatment with black seed oil, 80.6% had recurrence of their symptoms which was significant (P=0.000) when compared with mild control group. The same pattern reported for moderate group in which, from 79.5% improved at the end of 6 weeks NS oil treatment, 72.7% had recurrence of their symptoms which was significant (P=0.009) as compared to control group. Severe group also showed no significant difference in recurrence rate.

4.14 Side effects

The side effect of systemic NS treatment was diarrhea (10.7%) and nasal dryness (0.9%).

5. Discussion

Allergic rhinitis represents a global health problem. It is a common disease worldwide by which at least 10-25% of the population is affected and its prevalence is increasing. Although allergic rhinitis is not usually a severe disease but it alters the social life of patients and affect school performance and work productivity, and so, the costs incurred by rhinitis are substantial. (2) New knowledge about the mechanisms underlying allergic inflammation of the air ways has resulted to better therapeutic strategies, like immunotherapy with engineered allergen. Even trails of laser surgery for treatment of AR by laser turbinectomy (Tiny biopsy specimens) with local destructive effect of laser energy on the glandular acini and on the surrounding cholinergic nerve fibers which leads to decrease nasal secretions.(21). But still pharmacotherapy is the corner stone in the management of this illness, followed by immunotherapy(22). All these therapeutic strategies have many side effects, some of them may prove dangerous or even lethal, and in addition, there is no curative therapy.

One of the good substitutions is the use of herbal medicine and one of the ancient herbs that was used medically for many diseases was black seed extract(23). This herb has been used for many diseases since no signs of toxicity or serious side effects were known in antiquity (24). The role of herbal medicine in allergic rhinitis as an effective therapy has not been studied extensively (15,16,17,25) and up to our knowledge, the use of topical N.S extract in treating A.R has not been studied yet. Although few studies have been conducted to illustrate the possibility of therapeutic effect of this herb on other allergic diseases like asthma(9,2,10,11,26) and allergic disease of the skin like urticaria(27).

Females were affected more than males. This may be due to the fact that most of our patients came from rural areas where females used to work long hours in the fields. Other studies showed no sex difference or slight male predominance (8) . About 71.7% of the patients were less than 25 years old which means that the onset mainly started during the childhood and adolescence. This goes in line with other studies (28) because allergy is a less common cause of rhinitis in elderly as compared with other forms of rhinitis like atrophic rhinitis (3) . The disease duration has a big correlation with the severity of the disease since the shortest duration was of mild type and the longest duration was of the severe allergic rhinitis group. This may be due to the fact that chronicity of the disease leads to more allergen exposure which, in turn, leads to more non specific hyper reactivity. Non specific nasal hyper reactivity is an important feature of chronic allergic rhinitis and it is defined as: increase nasal response to a normal stimuli resulting in sneezing, nasal congestion and/or secretion[3,8] which lastly leads to more severe and chronic disease.

Perennial type rhinitis were more than seasonal type. This may be due to more exposure since perennial allergens are present every were and at any time. The peak incidence occurred in spring season (from March to May with highest level in the April).This is due to the peak time for tree pollinosis in this area happens during these months which include exacerbation of seasonal type AR as well as perennial type . These results contradicts with the results of some other studies which were done in different geographical areas with different ecological environments [29] .

The highest aggravating factor was allergen exposure simply because of the agricultural nature of the areas with more pollinosis and dampness, then upper respiratory tract infection followed by temperature changes then irritants and lastly hormonal factor. AR has mainly a bad course in the pregnant women since nasal obstruction may be aggravated by the pregnancy itself. [3,5] Allergic disease mainly worsened during pregnancy. This is proved by the following physiological and epidemiological observations[5] :

The major physiologic factors are the direct and indirect effects of pregnancy associated hormones on nasal mucosa, that is estrogen cause nasal mucosal swelling, possibly through stimulation of local Ach production[5].

- Cyclic changes in human female nasal mucus are characterized by the formation of large ferns during ovulation followed by their disappearance premenstrual. [5]
- Recent ultrastructrual and histochemical studies have revealed the increased activity of nasal mucous glands during pregnancy. A change similar to that is found in estrogens and progesterone contraceptive users. [5]
- Pregnancy associated hormones may indirectly affect the nose through their circulatory effect. The increased circulating blood volume during pregnancy combined with nasal vascular smooth muscle relaxation for progesterone may contribute to the nasal mucosal congestion that occurs frequently during pregnancy. Epidemiologic observations showed that allergic rhinitis may occur in up to 20% of the population of women of child bearing age. [5]

It has been noticed that patients with AR have a strong family history of allergic disease. This finding is in accordance with well documented fact in allergic disease. [30-32]the commonest associated illnesses was allergic conjunctivitis which may be as an entity associated with allergic rhinitis due to the same mechanism with the same allergen. Yet, it may be a reflex of histamine granules degranulation and it is considered one of allergic rhinitis co-morbidities.[3] Allergic asthma comes secondly in associated disease's frequency suggesting the concept that say "one air way, one disease". [33] Sinusitis is also one of the associated diseases and contributors to allergic rhinitis.[8,34]

The commonest allergen implicated is house dust mite (HDM) which may be the worldwide commonest cause of allergic rhinitis.[35] One example to the importance of (HDM) in respiratory allergens is that the incidence of the atopy in southern France is 30% but the prevalence of allergic asthma and rhinitis is greater in the low land compared to the ALPS. The reason for this difference in the prevalence of allergies (in the same population type and country) is considered to be the lower HDM population found above 1500 meters, and inhalant allergic patients are cleared an Alpine holiday despite the cold weather and exercise.[36] The severe symptoms patients had higher total serum IgE level then moderate symptomatic patient which in turn had higher level then mild symptomatic one .From this we can conclude that then increased in total serum IgE level correlates with the severity of the diseases.

The mild and moderate active groups patients showed excellent improvement in clinical symptoms at the 3 and 6 week extract treatment which is statistically a highly significant as compared with control groups. The severe group also showed a good improvement in clinical symptoms for active group but was not statistically significant for 3 weeks treatment course. However, the treatment effect was statistically significant after 6 weeks course of therapy with black seed oil. The response to treatment in the severe group was lower than that in mild and moderate groups and this may be due to more associated co-morbidities especially asthma which may need higher doses of N.S. The improvement effect that is seen in different groups may be related to the antihistaminic activity of nigellon through membrane stabilizing action[37] , Anticholinergic activity by competitive property of the pinene[27], Anti inflammatory effect of thymoqunone by effect on cyclo oxyginase & lipo oxyginase pathways) [29,38] , immunomodulatory activity, and antioxidant activity.[23]

The results also showed that the seasonal type has better responses than the perennial type which may be due to less nasal hyper reactivity appears because of less exposure to allergens (seasonal exposure only which don't continue very long) and decrease in the level of pollination may occur through this 6 weeks treatment leads to decrease the triggering factor which result in the decrease of allergic reaction associated with the stabilizing action of N. sativa extract which leads to better response and an improved clinical state.

Males patients show better treatment responses .This may be due to that males had less allergen exposure because of agricultural nature of this area which depends on females and hormonal changes in female through menstrual cycle changes affect the nasal mucosa and enhance disease exacerbations .

IgE level estimation by ELISA showed no switching of any patients from probable allergic group to non allergic group with increased level in some patients even after taking N. sativa extract for 6 weeks. The average of each group patients showed some decline in their level than that of the baseline estimation but this reduction was significant for active and control groups. However, the reduction in serum IgE following 6 weeks of black seed treatment was higher as compared to control group.

Salem [39], reported that administration of nigellone to children and adults during the treatment of asthma, decreased the IgE level and eosinophil count. The reduction in total serum IgE level in control group may be a reflection of reduction in allergen exposure. The patients improved clinically without reduction in total serum IgE level to the level of non allergic individuals was due; firstly, measurement of total serum IgE level is not a measure of a specific IgE Ab which more specific predictor of atopy [28] . Secondly, since mast cell-bound and non circulating IgE Ab are functionally important in initiating atopic reaction upon exposure to allergen. Measurement of the total quantity of IgE fixed to high affinity mast cell and basophile receptors (FC_ER_1) might be more relevant to atopy than serum circulating IgE Ab but since there is no technique for making such measurement currently, there is only an estimation of skin mast cell-bound IgE by thresholds dilution skin testing with heterologous anti-IgE that show the tissue IgE level is much higher in atopic individuals than the normal population. [28]

Improvement in tolerability to the exacerbating factors in active group, as it is compared with the control group after systemic treatment, may be due to the stabilizing effect of N.S on mast cell granules and antihistaminic properties of nigellone thymoquinone and subsequently prevent histamine release from macrophages, intracellular calcium release, protein kinase C activation and oxidative energy metabolism [40]. In a recent study, addition of NS seed to immunotherapy significantly increase the phagocytic and intracellular killing activities of PMNs in patients with AR [16]. Furthermore, NS inhibits the COX and 5-lipoxygenase pathways of arachidonic acid metabolism and decrease the synthesis of thromboxane and leukotrines [23, 41, 42]. Since leukotrines are a potent mediators that play a major role in allergic diseases including allergic rhinitis and histamine plays an important role in immediate hypersensitivity reactions, thus the above findings may explain the mechanism mediating the efficacy of NS in allergic diseases [2,16].

Improvement in associated allergic symptoms of conjunctivitis, asthma, and urticaria in active groups was more than that of control groups revealed clearly the multiple anti allergic actions of N. sativa extract. This may be due to augmentation of PMN function induced by N. sativa seed oil [16, 39], antihistaminic activity [40], antioxidant activity [43], inhibition of prostaglandin production [44] and antiiflamatory activity [45].

Factors associated with poor response to systemic NS treatment include: a) Multiple allergic disorders which may need more dose because the multiple allergic disease especially asthma are more complicated in mechanism than allergic rhinitis and the patients usually have bronchial hyper reactivity. The main antihistaminic action which act on AR occur at the lower doses of N. sativa.[37] While anti-inflammatory action to treat asthma needs higher doses for longer period.[27,38] . b) High IgE level which reflects allergen exposure and correlate with worse atopic state. There are 2-4 fold variations in serum IgE levels with seasonal allergic rhinitis from spring or summer pollens[46] or ragweed pollen [47]. Peak IgE levels are usually reached about 4-6 weeks after the peak pollination period and then decline to a nadir just prior to the subsequent pollination season .Higher IgE level always correlates with a bad clinical features and a more resistance to treatment. c) Gender, Poor response in females may be because of, hormonal changes, more allergen exposure to females (agricultural areas depend mainly on female work). These are leading to many exacerbations which in turn leading to a more chronic symptoms with a more severe condition and a more resistance to treatment. d) Perennial type which is the year round exposure to allergen leads to more nasal hyperreactivity with a more severe cases due to non specific hyperactivity that leads to chronic disease with a more stubborn to treatment. f) High percentage of atopic family history: This makes the patients more vulnerable to allergic disorders at earlier ages than non atopic families patients. Earlier disease, mainly leads to more severe attacks in the future, because more nasal hyper reactivity, high IgE level and multiple allergic disease may happen. g) Older ages: They have more nasal hyper reactivity which is due to more allergen exposures and more attacks, in addition to more chronic disease which leads to non specific stimulation of nasal mucosa which in turn leads to more stubborn to treatment.

Treatment cessation lead to high rate of recurrence rate. However, the rate of recurrence was more in mild group as compared to moderate and severe group. This variation was a reflection of the better response to treatment in mild as compared to other two groups. Thus the response to treatment with black seed oil was severity driven.

The side effects of N. sativa extract used in allergic rhinitis was considered trivial as compared with conventional drugs used for allergic rhinitis like steroids or even antihistamines. One of these side effects of systemic N. sativa use was mild diarrhea which did not affect the administration of the herb. Excessive nasal dryness was much more in topical use; this may be due to more potent anti cholinergic effect in topical use than systemic use.

6. Conclusions

Systemic use of N. Sativa extract is effective in mild and moderate allergic rhinitis symptoms. Factors that may influence the response to systemic N.S treatment in allergic rhinitis include; multiple allergic diseases with high serum IgE level and atopic family diathesis, gender, perennial type, old age group patients. Side effects of N. Sativa extract use are trivial and easily controlled. Nigella sativa extract has proved to have a strong therapeutic effect in allergic rhinitis.

7. Recommendations

N.S extract oil has proved to be very effective in the treatment of AR so it is recommended as adjuvant therapy in patients treated with immunotherapy or conventional treatment. Conduction of long period treatment course clinical trial to elaborate the recurrence rate is warranted. To plan and conduct studies of longer periods and higher doses to clarify the therapeutic effect of this herb.

8. References

[1] Bousquet J, Khaltaev N, Cruz AA, et al. Allergic rhinitis and its impact on asthma (ARIA) 2008 update. Allergy 2008; 63:8-160.

[2] Ulbricht C. Allergic Rhinitis: An Integrative Approach, a National Monograph. Alternative Complementary Therapy 2010; 16:107-111.

[3] Brozek JL, Bousquet J, Baena- Cagnani CE, et al. Allergic Rhinitis and its Impact on Asthma (ARIA) guidelines 2010 revision. J Allergy Clin Immunol 2010;126:466-476.

[4] Bourdin A, Gras D, Vachier I, Chanez P. Upper airway.1: Allergic rhinitis and asthma: united dises through epithelial cells. Thorax 2009;64:999-1004.

[5] Adkinson NF, Holgate ST, Busse WW, Bochner BS, Lemanske RF (eds.). Middleton's Allergy: Principles and Practice, Vol 1 & 2. 8th Ed. 2008.

[6] Yuan CS, Bieber EJ. (eds.) Textbook of Complementary and Alternative Medicine. Boca Raton, Parthenon Publishing, 2003.

[7] Astin JA. Why patients use alternation medicine :Results of a national study. JAMA 1998:279:1548-1553.

[8] Baraniuk JN. Mechanisms of allergic rhinitis. Current Allergy and Asthma Reports.2007;3:207-217.

[9] Mahmood K.S., The role of Nigella sativa Linn seed Extract in treatment of asthma, a thesis, submitted to University of Tikrit ,college of Medicine., 2000.

[10] Ahmad J, Khan RA, Malik MA. A study of Nigella sativa oil in the management of wheeze associated lower respiratory tract illness in children. Afr J Pharm Pharmacol 2010;4:436-439.

[11] Asim MR, Shahzad M, Yang X, et al. Suppressive effects of black seed oil on ovalbumin induced acute lung remodeling in E3 rats. Swiss Med Wkly 2010;140:w13128.

[12] Skoner DP. Allergic rhinitis: definition, epidemiology, pathophysiology, detection, and diagnosis. J Allergy Clin Immunol. 2001; 108(suppl):S2-8.

[13] Fabbri L, Peters SP, Pavord I, et al. Allergic Rhinitis, Asthma, Airway Biology, and Chronic Obstructive Pulmonary Disease in AJRCCM in 2004 Am J Resp Crit Care Med 2005;171:686-698.

[14] Chakrarty H.L. Plant wealth of Iraq A dictionary of Economic plants, Vol. 1, Baghdad 1876: 387-388.

[15] Nikahlagh S, Rahim F, Aryani FH, et al. Herbal treatment of allergic rhinitis: the use of Nigella sativa. Am J Otolaryngol 2010 Oct 12. www.ncbi.nlm.nih.gov/.../20947211. retrived 4/24/2011.

[16] Isik H, Cevikbas A, Gurer US, et al. Potential adjuvant effect of Nigella sativa seeds to improve specific immunotherapy in allergic rhinitis patients. Med Princ Pract 2010;19:206-211.

[17] Ansari MA, Ahmed SP, Ansari NA. Cetirizine and Nigella sativa: comparison of conventional and herbal option for treatment of seasonal allergic rhinitis. Pak J Med Res 2007;46:1-7.

[18] Global strategy for asthma management and prevention (updated 2006): Global Initiative for Asthma (GINA). http://www.ginasthma.org.

[19] Dykeewicz M, Fineman S, Skoner D, et.al. Diagnosis and management of rhinitis. Complete guidelines of the joint task force on practice parameters in allergy, asthma, and immunology. Ann Allergy, Asthma, Immunol 1998; 81:478.

[20] John R.Houck, Rollie E.Rhodes" Immunology" and allergy" in K.J. Lee "Essential otolaryngology, Head and Neck Surgery" 7th edition 1999, ch.12:264-3131.

[21] Elwany-S; Adel-Sallam-S, Laser surgery for allergic rhinitis , the effect on seromucinous glands in Otolaryntologoy. Head and Neck Surg. 1999; 120(5) : 742-4 .

[22] Kalus U, Pruss A, Bystron J, Jurecka M, Smekalova A, Lichius JJ. Effect of Nigella sativa (black seed)on subjective feeling in patients with allergic diseases. Phytother Res. 2003;17: 1209-1214.

[23] Paarakh P. Nigella sativa Linn. – A comprehensive review. Indian J Natu Prod Resources 2010;1:409-429.

[24] Banerjee S, Kaseb AO, Wang Z, et al. Antitumor activity of gemcitabine and oxaliplatin is augmented by thymoquinone in pancreatic cancer. Cancer Res 2009;69:5575-5583.

[25] Ansari MA, Ahmed SP, Haider S, Ansari NA. Nigella sativa: a non conventional herbal option for the management of seasonal allergic rhinitis. Pak J Pharmacol 2006;23:31-35.

[26] Boskabady MH, Javan H, Sajady M, Rakhshandeh H. The possible prophylactic effect of Nigella sativa seed extract in asthmatic patients. Fundam Clin Pharmacol 2007;21:559-566.

[27] Balachandran P, Govindarajan R. Cancer: an ayurvedic perspective. Pharmacological Research 2005;51:19-30.

[28] Yilmaz AAS, Corey JP. Rhinitis in the elderly. Current Allergy Asthma Report 2006;6:125-131.
[29] Fleming D.M. and Crombie D.L. Prevalence of asthma and hay fever in England and Wales. BMJ 1999 294, 279-283.
[30] Erel F, Karaayvaz M, Kaliskaner Z, Ozaguc N. The allergen spectrum in Turkey and the relationships between allergens and age, sex, birth month, birthplace, blood groups and family history of atopy. J Investig Allergol Clin Immunol 2000; 8(4):226-233
[31] Baker JR (ed) Primer an allergic and immunologic diseases. JAMA 1997;278: 1804-2025.
[32] Durham S (ed.) ABC of Allergies. BMJ. 1998.
[33] Grossman J. One air way, one disease., Chest 1997; 111: 11S-16S.
[34] Settipane RA. Complications of allergic rhinitis. Allergy Asthma Proc 1999;20:209-13
[35] Colloff, M.J., Ayres.J., Carswell, F., Howarth.P.H., Merrett.T.G., Mitchell.E.B.et al. The control of dust mites and domestic pets: a position paper. Clinical and Experimental Allergy, 1992;22:1-28.
[36] Cochrance G.M., Rees P.J., A Color Atlas of Asthma, Wolf Medical Publications Ltd, 1989; P 11.
[37] Charkravarty N, Inhibition of histamine release from mast cells by nigelone, Annals of Allergy 1993, 70(3): 237-242.
[38] Houghton, Zarka, Heras and Hoult. Fixed oil N. Sativa and derived thyonoquinone, inhibit eicosanoid generation in leukocytes and membrane lipid peroxidation. Planta Medica 1995, 61:33-36.
[39] Salem ML. Immunomodulatory and immunotherapeutic properties of the Nigella sativa L. seed. Int Immunopharmacol 2005;5:1749-1770.
[40] Broide DH. Immunologic and inflammatory mechanisms that derive asthma progression to remodeling. J Allergy Clin Immunol. 2008;121:560-570.
[41] Gocer P, Gurer SU, Erten N, et al. Comparison of polymorphonuclear leucocyte functions in elderly patients and healthy young volunteers. Med Prin Pract 2005;14:382-385.
[42] Hajhashemi V, Ghannadi A, Jafarabadi H. Black cumin seed essential oil as a potent analgesic and anti-inflammatory drug Phytother Res 2004;18:195-199.
[43] El-Dakhakhny M, Madi NJ, Lembert N, Ammon HP. Nigella sativa oil, nigellone and derived thymoquinone inhibit synthesis of 5-lipoxygenase products in polymorphnuclear lwucocytes from rats. J Ethnopharmacol 2002;81:161-164.
[44] Swamy SMK, Tan BKH. Cytotoxic and immunopotentiating effects of ethanolic extract of Nigella sativa L. seed. J Ethnopharmacol 2000;70:1-7.
[45] El-Mezayen R, El Gazzar M, Nichols MR, et al. Effect of thymoquinone on cyclooxygenase production in mouse model of allergic inflammation. Immunol Lett 2006;106:72-81.
[46] El Gazzar M, El Mezayen R, Marecki JC, et al. Antiinflammatory effects of thymoquinone in a mouse model of allergic lung inflammation. Int Immunopharmacol 2006;6:1135-1142.
[47] Berg, T., and Johansson.S.G.O. IgE concentrations in children with atopic disease .A clinical study, Int. Arch. Allergy Appl.Immunol. 1969, 36:219.
[48] David G. Golding-wood, Mats Holmstran Yvonne DSarby, Glenis K. Scadding, Ralerie T. Lund. The treatment of hyposmia with intranasal steroids, J Laryng. Oto. 1996; 110:93-95.